Ethics and the Kidney

Whilst every effort has been made to ensure that the contents of this book are as complete, accurate and up to date as possible at the date of writing, Oxford University Press is not able to give any guarantee or assurance that such is the case. Readers are urged to take appropriately qualified medical advice in all cases. The information in this book is intended to be useful to the general reader, but should not be used as a means of self-diagnosis or for the prescription of medication.

Analgesic and NSAID-induced kidney disease
Edited by J. H. Stewart

Dialysis amyloid
Edited by Charles van Ypersele and Tilman B. Drüeke

Infections of the kidney and urinary tract
Edited by W. R. Cattell

Polycystic kidney disease
Edited by Michael L. Watson and Vicente E. Torres

Treatment of primary glomerulonephritis
Edited by Claudio Ponticelli and Richard J. Glassock

Inherited disorders of the kidney
Edited by Stephen H. Morgan and Jean-Pierre Grünfeld

Complications of long-term dialysis
Edited by Edwina A. Brown and Patrick S. Parfrey

Lupus nephritis
Edited by E. Lewis, M. Schwartz, and S. Korbet

Nephropathy in type 2 diabetes
Edited by Eberhard Ritz and Ivan Rychlik

Hemodialysis vascular access
Edited by Peter J. Conlon, Michael Nicholson and Steve Schwab

Mechanisms and clinical management of chronic renal failure (Second edition; formerly Prevention of progressive chronic renal failure)
Edited by A. Meguid El Nahas with Kevin Harris and Sharon Anderson

Cardiovascular disease in end-stage renal failure
Edited by Joseph Loscalzo and Gérard M. London

Ethics and the Kidney

Edited by

NORMAN G. LEVINSKY
Boston University School of Medicine
USA

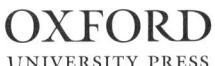

OXFORD
UNIVERSITY PRESS

Great Clarendon Street, Oxford OX2 6DP

Oxford University Press is a department of the University of Oxford.
It furthers the University's aim of excellence in research, scholarship,
and education by publishing worldwide in

Oxford New York

Athens Auckland Bangkok Bogotá Buenos Aires Calcutta
Cape Town Chennai Dar es Salaam Delhi Florence Hong Kong Istanbul
Karachi Kuala Lumpur Madrid Melbourne Mexico City Mumbai
Nairobi Paris São Paulo Singapore Taipei Tokyo Toronto Warsaw

with associated companies in Berlin Ibadan

Oxford is a trade mark of Oxford University Press
in the UK and in certain other countries

Published in the United States
by Oxford University Press Inc., New York

© Oxford University Press, 2001

The moral rights of the author have been asserted
Database right Oxford University Press (maker)

First published 2001

All rights reserved. No part of this publication may be reproduced,
stored in a retrieval system, or transmitted, in any form or by any means,
without the prior permission in writing of Oxford University Press,
or as expressly permitted by law, or under terms agreed with the appropriate
reprographics rights organizations. Enquiries concerning reproduction
outside the scope of the above should be sent to the Rights Department,
Oxford University Press, at the address above

You must not circulate this book in any other binding or cover
and you must impose this same condition on any acquirer

British Library Cataloguing in Publication Data

Data available

Library of Congress Cataloging in Publication Data

1 3 5 7 9 10 8 6 4 2

ISBN 019 263159 4 (Hbk)

Typeset in Ehrhardt MT
by Alliance Phototypesetters, Pondicherry, India
Printed in Great Britain
on acid-free paper by
T. J. International Ltd, Padstow

PREFACE

When I told a colleague that I was editing a book on ethics and the kidney, he replied: 'Why not ethics and the liver?' Superficially it does seem odd but on further thought it is a rational connection. As Richard Rettig points out in the first chapter, historically many critical ethical issues in modern medicine first arose in connection with the treatment of persons with end-stage renal disease (ESRD). Chronic dialysis and kidney transplantation were early examples of a dilemma that has increasingly pervaded all of medicine: how can we provide lifesaving therapy whose costs are beyond the reach of virtually all individuals? Rettig's history of dialysis in the United States illustrates how one nation dealt with scarcity and rationing of lifesaving therapy. The fundamental problem applies in all societies.

In Chapter 2, Ronald Baker Miller, both a nephrologist and a medical ethicist, provides an overview of some key principles and concepts of medical ethics from a general and philosophical viewpoint. He also discusses an illustrative case to show how these principles apply in the care of a patient with renal disease.

As a practical matter, law and ethics are often intertwined. In Chapter 3, Bernard Dickens reviews key legal issues in nephrology. He discusses prenatal issues such as genetic inheritance of kidney diseases, which may raise complex legal and ethical dilemmas such as embryo selection and abortion. Legal considerations about patient autonomy, informed consent and medical futility are involved in initiation and in termination of dialysis. The chapter also reviews laws in the areas of organ retrieval and allocation of kidneys for transplantation. (These controversial issues are discussed from a clinical perspective by Raymond Hoffenberg in Chapter 7 and Robert Sells in Chapter 9.) The very contentious issue of payment to organ donors is discussed from the legal viewpoint in Dickens's chapter, and from an ethical perspective in Hoffenberg's chapter.

Chapter 4 (Eli Friedman) and Chapter 5 (Norman Levinsky) look at allocation of costly dialysis therapy. In general, Friedman takes the 'harder' position that patients may be excluded from dialysis because of advanced age, mental deficiency and extreme non-compliance. I consider the same issue and conclude that the spectrum of patients who should receive chronic dialysis is broader.

Dialysis is a life-preserving treatment; when it is discontinued in patients with ESRD, they inevitably die. Therefore, the issue of discontinuation of dialysis has profound ethical, procedural, and legal aspects. In Chapter 6, Kerry Bowman and Peter Singer provide a broad review of critical issues in this area. Their comprehensive discussion includes consideration of consent, advance directives, and do-not-resuscitate orders, and offers suggestions for resolving conflict in decision making. The chapter is written to emphasize practical answers to the question 'what should the nephrologist do?'

The next three chapters in the book deal with acquisition and allocation of kidneys for transplantation, another area in which there is no lack of contentious issues. In Chapter 7, Hoffenberg reviews measures for increasing the supply of kidneys that have been discouraged or prohibited, such as the sale of kidneys, which is illegal in the United States and many other countries. Hoffenberg provides a salient and thought-provoking argument to favor carefully controlled sale of kidneys. It is interesting to contrast this viewpoint with that by Vivekanand Jha and Kirpal Chugh in Chapter 16. Writing from India, they see very large numbers of desperately poor individuals susceptible to unethical financial pressures. Hoffenberg's chapter also reviews the delicate balance of benefit and risk involved in greater use of living unrelated donors and considers the use of organs from patients in a persistent vegetative state or with anencephaly. Finally, Hoffenberg deals with the use of organs from prisoners or those who have been executed, a topic that is discussed from the Chinese perspective in Chapter 15 by Lei-Shi Li and Xiao-Dan Yao.

Recent advances in biotechnology suggest that experiments with kidney xenotransplantation in humans may be scientifically reasonable within the next few years. In Chapter 8, I consider ethical questions raised by this method for increasing the supply of kidneys for transplantation. Does the potential benefit to individual recipients justify the risk–probably extremely low but definitely not zero–of introducing into the human population potentially lethal new infections?

The supply of kidneys does not meet the needs of potential recipients. In Chapter 9, Sells reviews ethical issues in allocating the inadequate supply of kidneys. He discusses the various medical factors that influence the position of potential recipients on waiting lists. He points out that none of the ingenious systems for organ distribution using medical and non-medical discriminators to achieve fair allocation, priority for the sickest patients, and equity can resolve the fundamental issue: the limited supply of kidneys.

In Chapter 10, Rita Kielstein and Hans-Martin Sass review some of the conceptual, moral and medical issues raised by the 'revolution of Copernican dimension' in genetics. In society at large as well as in the medical profession there is grave concern that genotyping will do more harm than good, because genetic information cannot be kept confidential and will lead to discrimination in employment, medical care, and health insurance based on genetic make-up. The authors very strongly take the opposite viewpoint that appropriate use of burgeoning genetic knowledge will make it possible for individuals to make more educated life choices and reproductive decisions and, through each individual's knowledge of his or her risk factors, enhance the ability of people to receive individualized medication and to undertake preventive measures. Readers will have to make up their own minds, subject to repeated change as the revolution in molecular genetics proceeds.

In Chapter 11, Howard Trachtman and co-authors offer a review of three key issues in the care of children with kidney disease. They present another viewpoint with regard to screening for genetic diseases, explicitly from the point of view of patients who are children. They also discuss informed consent and surrogate decision making in children and issues surrounding kidney donation for transplantation. Children are not just small adults and this chapter brings an appropriately specific perspective to these key ethical issues that affect the care of children.

In the next section of the book, two authors explore some societal and economic issues relevant to the care of patients with kidney disease. In Chapter 12, Daniel Callahan–a medical ethicist widely known for his incisive commentary on medical rationing, among many other issues–reviews the problem of societal allocation of resources. Dialysis is an expensive medical therapy; resources devoted to a small number of ESRD patients could be redeployed to meet other important social needs. Callahan reviews several ways to limit expenditure on the care of patients with ESRD. Whether medical professionals such as nephrologists agree or disagree with Callahan's analysis, they will be stimulated by reading this chapter.

In Chapter 13, William Bennett, a recent president of the American Society of Nephrology, grapples with a different set of economic issues. He reviews the effect of changing mechanisms for health insurance in the United States on the quality of care offered to ESRD patients. He analyzes in detail the impact of the increasing 'industrialization' of nephrology (the majority of dialysis units in the United States are owned by a handful of for-profit companies) on the quality of patient care, on the ethics of physicians, and on academic nephrology programs.

The final section of the book revisits some of the major ethical issues from the perspective of non-Western cultures. Atsushi Asai and co-authors (Chapter 14) provide an excellent review of the health care system, the religions, and ethical precepts in Japan, indicating that these factors markedly impact medical practice in dialysis and organ transplantation. Li and Yao discuss cultural differences and medical ethics as they apply to the care of patients with kidney diseases in China. They provide a fascinating account of the influence of traditional medicine, of the cultural and religious background, and of social and economic status on medical practice. They end with a strong defense of Chinese practices in using organs from executed prisoners for transplantation, an issue considered from a Western perspective by Hoffenberg in Chapter 7. Jha and Chugh review ethical issues in the care of patients with kidney disease in India. They focus on kidney transplantation, since dialysis is very limited because of its high cost. They devote a large part of their chapter to a spirited argument against paid donation by living donors. As noted earlier, this forms a counterpoint to the arguments in favor of paid donation discussed by Hoffenberg in Chapter 7. In the final chapter in the book, Sarala Naicker undertakes no less a task than to review key issues regarding the impact of economics, culture, religion and ethical precepts on the care of patients with renal disease in the entire African continent. She emphasizes the critical impact of poverty on the care of patients in nearly all African countries. Her review provides another view of the impact of scarcity on medical care, in this case from the perspective of very poor nations.

Obviously, this book in the end is–as it must be–non-prescriptive. There is general consensus on many ethical issues in the care of patients with kidney disease but viewpoints continuously evolve, as they should. I hope that the chapters in the book prove as stimulating to other readers as they were to me.

Norman G. Levinsky

November 2001

CONTENTS

List of Contributors — xi

PART I Some general considerations

1 Historical perspective — 3
  Richard A. Rettig

2 Ethical theory and principles — 24
  Ronald Baker Miller

3 Key legal issues — 63
  Bernard M. Dickens

PART II Specific ethical issues in the care of patients with kidney disease

4 Must (Should) all ESRD patients be treated? — 85
  Eli A. Friedman

5 Equity and patient autonomy in dialysis — 99
  Norman G. Levinsky

6 End of life care in dialysis — 110
  Kerry W. Bowman and Peter A. Singer

7 Acquisition of kidneys for transplantation — 130
  Raymond Hoffenberg

8 Xenotransplantation: An ethical dilemma — 144
  Norman G. Levinsky

9 Allocation of kidneys for transplantation — 154
  Robert A. Sells

10 Genetics: Ethical issues in kidney disease — 167
   Rita Kielstein and Hans-Martin Sass

11 Special issues in the care of children — 183
   Howard Trachtman, Mark Grijnsztein, Rachel Frank and Bernard Gauthier

PART III Societal and economic issues

12 Societal allocation of resources for patients with ESRD — 201
   Daniel Callahan

13	Economic issues in nephrology practice: Ethical dilemmas *William M. Bennett*	212

PART IV Ethical issues in non-Western cultures

14	Japan *Atsushi Asai, Yasuhiko Miura, Shizuko Nagata, Shunichi Fukurhara and Kiyoshi Kurokawa*	223
15	China *Lei-Shi Li and Xiao-Dan Yao*	234
16	India *Vivekanand Jha and Kirpal S. Chugh*	241
17	Africa *Sarala Naicker*	255

Index 269

CONTRIBUTORS

Atsushi Asai School of Public Health, Kyoto University Graduate School of Medicine, Yoshida Konoe-cho, Sakyo-ku, Kyoto, Japan 606–8501

William M. Bennett Samaritan Hospital, Solid Organ and Cellular Transplant, Suite 430, 1040 NW 22nd Avenue, Portland, OR 97210, USA

Kerry W. Bowman Mt. Sinai Hospital and University of Toronto Joint Centre for Bioethics, 88 College Street, Toronto, Ontario, M5G 1L4, Canada

Daniel Callahan The Hastings Center, Garrison, NY 10524–5555, SA

Kirpal S. Chugh National Kidney Clinic and Research Centre, 601 Section 18-B, Chandigarh 160 018 India

Bernard M. Dickens Faculty of Law, University of Toronto, 84 Queen's Park, Toronto, Ontario M5S 2C5, Canada

Rachel Frank Schneider Children's Hospital, Division of Nephrology, Room 365, 269–01 76th Avenue, New Hyde Park, NY 11040–1432, USA

Eli A. Friedman Renal Disease Division, SUNY Health Science Center at Brooklyn, Box 52, 450 Clarkson Avenue, Brooklyn, NY 11203, USA

Shunichi Fukurhara Tokai University School of Medicine, Bohseidai, Isehara, Kanagawa, Japan 259–1193

Bernard Gauthier Schneider Children's Hospital, Division of Nephrology, Room 365, 269–01 76th Avenue, New Hyde Park, NY 11040–1432, USA

Mark Grijnsztein Schneider Children's Hospital, 269–01 76th Avenue, New Hyde Park, NY 11040–1432, USA

Raymond Hoffenberg 340/57A Newstead Terrace, Newstead, Brisbane 4006, Australia

Vivekanand Jha National Kidney Clinic and Research Centre, 601 Section 18-B, Chandigarh 160 018 India

Rita Kielstein Medizinische Fakultat, Otto von Guericke Universitat, 39720 Magdeburg, Germany

Kiyoshi Kurokawa Dean's Office Tokai University School of Medicine, Bohseidai, Isehara, Kanagawa, Japan 259–1193

Norman G. Levinsky Boston University School of Medicine, 80 East Concord Street, Boston, MA 02118, USA

Lei-Shi Li Research Institute of Nephrology, Jinling Hospital, 305 East Zhongshan Road, Nanjing, 210002, People's Republic of China

Ronald Baker Miller Program in Medical Ethics, University of California, Irvine, 7001 East Country Club Lane, Anaheim Hills, CA 92807–4414, USA

Yasuhiko Miura Tokai University School of Medicine, Bohseidai, Isehara, Kanagawa, Japan 259–1193

Shizuko Nagata Tokai University School of Medicine, Bohseidai, Isehara, Kanagawa, Japan 259–1193

Sarala Naicker 11 Tunstan Walk, Mobeni Heights, 4092 Durban, Kwa Zulu Natal, South Africa

Richard A. Rettig RAND, 1200 South Hayes Street, Arlington, VA 22202–5050, USA

Hans-Martin Sass Kennedy Institute of Ethics, Georgetown University, Washington, DC 20057, USA

Robert A. Sells Renal Transplant Unit, Link 9C, Royal Liverpool University Hospital, Liverpool, England L7 8XP

Peter A. Singer University of Toronto Joint Centre for Bioethics, 88 College Street, Toronto, Ontario M5G 1L4, Canada

Howard Trachtman Schneider Children's Hospital, Division of Nephrology, Room 365, 269–01 76th Avenue, New Hyde Park, NY 11040–1432, USA

Xiao-Dan Yao Research Institute of Nephrology, Jinling Hospital, 305 East Zhongshan Road, Nanjing, 210002, People's Republic of China

PART I
Some general considerations

1
Historical perspective
Richard A. Rettig

Introduction

This chapter discusses the ethical issues associated with the provision of treatment for end-stage renal disease (ESRD) in their historical context as defined by the public policy issues of the day. The two therapies of dialysis and kidney transplantation raised the dilemma of how clinicians and the broader society should respond to the existence of life-saving treatments whose costs placed them beyond the reach of nearly all individuals. How should one act in a clinically, ethically, socially, and politically defensible way to affirm such fundamental societal values as saving lives when it is technically possible to do so but scarcity imposes limits on what can be done (Calabresi and Bobbitt, 1978)? These issues will be explored principally by a historical analysis of the evolution of ESRD treatment in the United States. While the programs for ESRD treatment differ in detail in various countries, the fundamental dilemma is the same in all nations.

There are two major historical periods for discussing the ethical issues related to dialysis and kidney transplantation in the United States: pre-Medicare and Medicare. The pre-Medicare period dates from the late 1950s and early 1960s, when both therapies first emerged, until the enactment of the Social Security Amendments of 1972, which established the Medicare entitlement for treatment of chronic renal failure. This initial period can be further divided in two. The years from 1960 to (roughly) 1965 are occupied with the emergence and first use of the treatments, the rationing of access, and a vigorous debate within and beyond the medical community. The medical community considered whether these therapies were still experimental or whether their effectiveness had been established. The broader public discussion carried on by the national press and leading clinicians focused on rationing a scarce resource that was assumed to be effective.

The period from 1966 through 1972–73 saw resolution of the experiment versus established therapy argument and was one of an expanding but patchwork commitment to treatment. It was marked by a slowly but steadily increasing patient population, growth in federal and state government programs related to the treatment of chronic renal failure, and a steady stream of legislative proposals being introduced in the US. Congress to deal with the treatment of victims of kidney failure. Toward the end of this period, a substantial literature appeared focused on the legal and ethical issues associated with allocating scarce resources to expensive, life-saving treatment.

The historical link between the pre-Medicare and Medicare periods is the kidney disease treatment provision of the Social Security Amendments of 1972. Public Law 92–603 was signed into law on October 30, 1972, and the kidney failure treatment entitlement became effective on July 1, 1973. Although the Medicare years can be divided historically for some purposes, e.g., discussion of payment policy, there are no neat time periods that serve us well for considering ethical issues. Attention centers, therefore, on Section 299I of PL 92–603, the relief it provided physicians from the hard choices of scarcity-imposed rationing, the ethically ambiguous language of the statute, and the ethical issues created by this new regime. We also consider briefly the continuing manifestations of scarcity in implementation of the entitlement and the effects on ethical and policy issues. We conclude by assaying how the growth of the ESRD program led in time to a clearer understanding of the associated ethical issues, referring to the Institute of Medicine report of 1991 (Rettig and Levinsky, 1991) and to the more recent clinical practice guideline on the initiation of and withdrawal from treatment of the Renal Physicians Association and the American Society of Nephrology (RPA-ASN, 1999). Parenthetically, the ethical issues associated with high reliance on the proprietary provision of dialysis services, an issue having its own unique history within the US, is beyond the scope of this chapter.

The history, to forewarn the reader, is one of disconnects: the clinical community had its issues, journalists and the policy community saw a different picture, and ethical issues were threaded throughout. But none of the professional communities—clinicians, policy makers, ethicists, and journalists—spoke to each other in a systematic way.

An historical baseline

It is worthwhile noting that when hemodialysis and kidney transplantation emerged as treatments for chronic renal failure, virtually none of the institutional and intellectual framework we take for granted today—for assessing the safety and effectiveness, financing, and ethical implications of medical innovations—existed. For example:

- In 1960, the year Belding Scribner placed his first dialysis patient on 'continuous intermittent hemodialysis', the Food and Drug Administration (FDA) regulated only the *safety* of pharmaceuticals. The requirement that new drugs also meet a test of *effectiveness* was not added to the Federal Food Drug and Cosmetic Act until 1962 and then a decade was required to translate the statutory requirement into working regulations and procedures.
- FDA regulation of medical devices, which would have affected the introduction of 'the artificial kidney', was not authorized by Congress until 1976 and again a decade was needed before this new regulatory regime became fully operational.
- Title XVIII (Medicare) and Title XIX (Medicaid) had not been enacted into law. That would come only in 1965 when President Lyndon B. Johnson, working with very substantial Democratic majorities in both the US House and Senate, broke the legislative log-jam that went back to President Truman. Title XVIII established a federal government entitlement for medical and physician services for the elderly (over

65 years of age), and Title XIX created a federal and state-financed and state-administered program of medical services for the poor.
- The protection of human research subjects was in its infancy. The Public Health Service had not yet issued its initial guidelines on this subject (USPHS, 1971), the *Belmont Report* (1979) had not been published, and the Common Rule (45 CFR 46 1991) extending PHS rules to all federal agencies sponsoring research involving human subjects had not been adopted.
- The bioethics community was aborning. The 1960s, which Jonsen (1998) has called 'The Decade of Conferences', preceded the establishment of the Hastings Center (aka the Institute of Society, Ethics and the Life Sciences) in 1969 and the Kennedy Institute of Bioethics at Georgetown University in 1971.

In short, few of the now familiar features of public policy relating to medical financing, regulation of drugs and devices, protection of human subjects, and medical ethics existed when dialysis and kidney transplantation first emerged.

What was in place, of course, was the Public Health Service (PHS) and its crown jewel, then and now, the National Institutes of Health. Although NIH traces its history back to the late nineteenth century and although the National Cancer Institute was established in 1937, it is in the immediate post-World War II period that one sees the creation of the National Heart Institute, the National Institute of Mental Health, and the establishment of the study section, peer-review process for evaluating research proposals. It was also at this time that the political constellation of NIH supporters coalesced around Mary Lasker, Senator Lister Hill, Republican John Fogarty, and NIH Director James Shannon (Strickland, 1972; Rettig, 1977). The Public Health Service, corporate parent of NIH, is much older, going back to the initial decade of the Republic. Nevertheless, it is fair to say that when dialysis and transplantation emerged, NIH was the only federal government game in town.

Pre-Medicare

1960–1965: The introduction of new therapies

The contentious issue of limiting the access of potential patients to life-saving dialysis has existed since the emergence of 'continuous intermittent hemodialysis' in the early 1960s. At that time, the issue was the clinical and ethical bases for accepting patients to treatment for chronic kidney failure.

Belding Scribner and his colleagues at the University of Washington, drawing on the work of Kolff, Teschan, Schreiner, Merrill and others, invented an ingenious device (the AV fistula and shunt apparatus) that enabled repeated connections to be made between a patient and the artificial kidney. Scribner pioneered development and use of hemodialysis and became the foremost advocate in the early 1960s for rapidly financing an expanding treatment capacity across the country and for financing such care.

The dilemma confronting Scribner arose because there were many clinically eligible patients and too few sites of treatment. Scarcity dominated medicine. This led

Scribner and his colleagues to ration access to treatment (Scribner, 1964). Scarcity took many forms. Space and financing constraints and an overriding research commitment led the University of Washington Hospital to refuse to create a dialysis ward. A continuing obligation to care for chronic disease patients could not be justified in the absence of a method for payment for such care. Constraints of machines, beds, space and financing at the newly-established Seattle Artificial Kidney Center (SAKC) in the Swedish Hospital led to the creation of a two-stage patient selection process, which involved rationing access to treatment.

Rationing occurred in this way: beginning in 1962, prospective patients were thoroughly evaluated for treatment in clinical terms, including psychological assessment (Sand *et al.*, 1966). However, clinical evaluation did not reduce the number of potentially eligible patients sufficiently to permit acceptance of all in the limited bed capacity of SAKC. Consequently, a second evaluation occurred, this time for the 'social worth' of the individual. A committee of lay members of the community, whose identities were not known to the prospective patients nor to the public, reviewed potential candidates, accepting some and rejecting others on the basis of the committee's judgment about the relative social worth of the individuals (Murray *et al.*, 1962; Lindholm *et al.*, 1963). The committee had the final word on allocating access to a limited number of beds. Technical innovation provided a partial offset to scarcity. Fully utilized beds at the SAKC led Scribner and his colleagues to develop home dialysis in 1964–1965 as a way to escape its finite capacity (Curtis et al. 1965).*

The anonymous lay committee, sometimes known as the 'God Committee', was prominently featured in a November 1962 cover story in *Life* magazine by Shana Alexander (1962). The Seattle decision process also received national television coverage in November 1965 when NBC did an hour-long documentary narrated by Edwin Newman. (NBC News, 1965). These two national news stories—one print and one television—plus countless local stories in Seattle and elsewhere, generally featured dialysis as a medical breakthrough, while drawing attention to the dilemma created by the financial need to ration access.

Seattle was alone in beginning to provide dialysis treatment. In 1963, the Veterans Administration followed suit, leading the federal government in responding to new treatment capability for chronic renal failure. It announced the initiation of a program to establish dialysis units in 30 VA hospitals across the country over the next decade. The West Los Angeles VAH was the first such unit to be organized (Rettig, 1982). The growth of this VA initiative, coupled with a Public Health Service (PHS) proposal a few years later for a vastly expanded dialysis program, would lead the US Bureau of the Budget (BOB) to create an expert committee to review federal government efforts in this therapeutic area.

However, financial constraints dominated breakthrough medicine. Scribner devoted his 1964 Presidential address to the American Society for Artificial Internal

---

* Home dialysis as an escape from scarcity deserves emphasis. The first home patient was a 15-year-old girl who would not have been admitted to the SAKC on age grounds, the cut-off being 16. The first home dialysis machine was built to save her life. In 1966, I visited the home of Ernie Morelli, a Seattle home dialysis patient, whose Knights of Columbus chapter sponsored an 'Ernie Morelli Night' annually to raise funds for his treatment costs for the coming year.

Organs to a discussion of ethical issues associated with dialysis and kidney transplantation. He estimated that there were 'not more than 50 to 100 patients on transplants plus chronic dialysis' in the entire US in 1964. He decried the fact that 'in the last four years, since these techniques have become available, 10,000 or more ideal candidates have died in this country for lack of the treatment', which he attributed to 'rigid [patient] selection of one sort or another' (Scribner, 1964).

Scribner listed five problems that confronted the medical profession, of which patient selection was the first. The need for such selection, he noted, had driven the profession in Seattle to initiate home hemodialysis training as a way to bring the cost of treatment into a range of affordability. The other items on Scribner's list included: the overt termination of treatment by physicians when multiple organ system failure limited a patient's capacity to benefit from continued dialysis; the overt termination of treatment by the patient; facilitating 'death with dignity' for chronic uremia patients by providing weekly hemodialysis at the end of life 'instead of passively allowing the slow, agonizing death that characterizes terminal uremia'; and donor selection for kidney transplantation (Scribner had already benefited from corneal transplants).

By the end of this initial period, then, it had become dramatically clear that scarcity was driving the rationing of access to life-saving treatment. Although scarcity was widely described as a shortage of machines, its manifestations, however, were space, machines, facilities, trained personnel, and—fundamentally—a sustained stream of resources to pay for treatment. The following questions had been clearly stated: What were the criteria and the processes by which prospective patients were to be selected for life-saving treatment? Who was to make such selection decisions? What obligations did society have through government and community institutions to pay for treatment that was beyond the means of all but a very few potential beneficiaries? How were these obligations affected if the treatments were experimental?

1966–1972

The response to the Seattle experience occurred at two different levels. Much of the medical community was disposed to see dialysis treatment and kidney transplantation as experimental, not proven therapy. Irving Page of the Cleveland Clinic, for example, attacked Scribner and called hemodialysis 'an interesting and important experiment' (Page, 1963). Norman Levinsky, then director of Boston City Hospital's renal service, was quoted saying: 'Chronic dialysis is properly considered a clinical experiment rather than an established mode of treatment at this time' (*Medical World News*, 1964). The Scientific Advisory Board of the National Kidney Foundation (NKF) went through a convoluted debate of this issue in 1964 and emerged the following year with a rather stony-faced turning away from endorsing dialysis as a legitimate treatment of kidney failure. In 1965, however, the NKF declared a policy U-turn and gave its support for dialysis as a treatment for chronic renal failure. The 'intervening variable' in this case was that Senator Henry M. Jackson (Democrat, Washington), a powerful member of the Senate establishment, sponsored legislation that made it imprudent to adhere to this conservative position (Rettig 1976, 206). It was also well known that the founding leadership of the American Society of Nephrology, established in 1966, strongly reflected the research orientation of the East Coast renal physiology establishment and was, to say the least, bearish on dialysis as a treatment. The experimental versus established treatment question was not resolved until 1966–1967.

Kidney transplantation, early favored as an alternative to dialysis by many, also was evaluated in terms of experimental versus established therapy. The National Academy of Sciences, acting through its Committee on Tissue Transplantation, held a conference on kidney transplantation in 1963. The proceedings of that meeting concluded: 'Although the beginnings of clinical success are apparent, strong reservations must be kept in mind regarding the ultimate fate of these patients. Kidney transplantation is still highly experimental and not yet a therapeutic procedure' (*Transplantation Proceedings*, 1964). Opinion had not changed significantly in the follow-up conference held in May 1965 (NAS, 1965).

The other response to Scribner and the Seattle experience was from clinicians around the United States who were beginning to treat patients. As these clinicians sought to provide dialysis therapy, they also confronted the necessity of rationing access to treatment. However, learning from Seattle, they did so generally by burying the need to make invidious distinctions among individuals within the 'medical criteria' for patient acceptance (Nabarro, 1967; Columbia Law Review, 1969: 657–59). Katz and Proctor (1969), reporting the results of a 1967 survey of 93 dialysis centers treating from 1 to 37 patients, wrote:

> The process of selecting patients for hemodialysis included a medical evaluation and frequently social and/or psychiatric evaluations of the patient. A number of non-medical criteria were variously used. A third or more of centers reported 'willingness to cooperate in treatment regimen,' 'intelligence (as related to understanding treatment),' and 'likelihood of vocational rehabilitation' as highly important criteria. However, the variability in applying selection criteria to prospective patients was extensive and was perhaps one of the most impressive aspects noted.

The Gottschalk report

The resolution of the experimental versus established therapy issue occurred in 1967 with the publication of the Gottschalk Committee report. The committee, chaired by Carl Gottschalk of the University of North Carolina, had been convened by the Bureau of the Budget, which was alarmed by the implications of the VA dialysis program and a proposed expansion of the PHS treatment program. The expert committee, which was to operate in secret, was asked to analyze the pertinent policy and budgetary questions and submit its recommendations only to the BoB director.* At that time the number of patients being treated by hemodialysis was about 1000, distributed between VA hospitals and PHS grantees.

The committee report of September 1967 recommended financing treatment for chronic kidney failure through the recently enacted Medicare program, using the disability expansion proposed that year by President Johnson (Report of the

---

* Convening an expert committee for advice was believed to be unique in BoB's history, which typically relied heavily on its own staff and had access to all the expertise of the federal government when needed.

Committee on Chronic Kidney Disease, 1967). Although the 1972 Social Security Amendments closely paralleled this recommendation, there is no evidence that the drafters of that legislation were aware of the Gottschalk Report. However, the impact of the report was significant on clinicians as it indicated that both dialysis and kidney transplantation were effective treatments. Coming from a committee with impeccable nephrology and transplantation credentials, this decisively settled the experiment—treatment issue for the nephrology community.*

Why was the experiment—therapy debate important to the ethical discussion? Simply put, if dialysis and transplantation could be regarded as experimental, one did not then need to confront the ethical issue of what to do with a life-saving technology having an expensive price tag. On the other hand, if these treatments were regarded as clinically effective, then the ethical problems could not be escaped. The issuance of the Gottschalk Report was a watershed. Afterwards, there was no turning back from a search for a way to finance care and resolve the scarcity side of the rationing issue.

Federal government programs

The search for a solution to the dilemma of rationing access to life-saving treatment involved the federal government in various ways. In addition to the VA program, initiated in 1963; an Artificial Kidney/Chronic Uremia contract research program was established at Congressional direction within the National Institute of Arthritis and Metabolic Diseases; a transplant immunology program was created within the National Institute of Allergy and Infectious Diseases; and a Kidney Disease Control Program (KDCP) was created within the Public Health Service.† The KDCP made a very ambitious proposal in 1965 to expand PHS support of dialysis services. (Indeed, this proposal was one stimulus that prompted BoB to convene the Gottschalk committee.) In 1964, KDCP had made a dialysis center demonstration grant award, its first, to the Seattle Artificial Kidney Center. In 1965, it made 10 additional awards to centers across the country, setting in motion the creation of a treatment infrastructure for the non-veteran US population. Over the next several years, the KDCP funded 12 home dialysis demonstration contracts and seven organ procurement contracts, further building the institutional treatment base.

Interestingly enough, the KDCP center and home dialysis grants and contracts were awarded on a declining step-funded basis; i.e., the first year of a 5-year award was the greatest, the fifth year the smallest, and complete phase-out was expected after 5 years. The initial rationale was that awardees would establish community-based funding over the life of the federal grant or contract. However, treatment obligations moved in an opposite direction; i.e., as chronic patients were entered into treatment,

---

* Although BoB did not reprint or distribute the Gottschalk Report, five hundred copies were published by the National Institute of Arthritis and Metabolic Diseases and distributed widely within the nascent nephrology community. The report's influence was far greater among clinicians than policy makers.

† Although this program had several different names over its decade-long existence, we refer to it here by one of its more descriptive names.

a continuing legal and ethical obligation for their care was incurred. Community funding proved very difficult for all but a very few centers and state funding of these initiatives also faced the same resource limitations. The PHS was building treatment capacity but not long-term financing.

In 1969, the KDCP was transferred into the Regional Medical Programs (RMP) and the following year Congress amended the original Heart Disease, Cancer and Stroke legislation by adding 'kidney disease' to the title and legislatively sealing this transfer. The state-based RMP program meshed well with independent state government initiatives in Illinois, California, Washington, and elsewhere. Growth occurred in the number of patients treated (the total reached about 10,000 by 1972), the number of physicians involved, the number of treatment units, and the number of state governments responding to patients at risk. These developments and a steady stream of local and national press (print and television) coverage was instrumental in raising public awareness and understanding of the plight of individuals with kidney failure.

What is the relevance of the above developments to the discussion of ethical issues related to ESRD treatment? First, very ambitious plans for expansion of federal programs were thwarted, essentially for 'opportunity cost' reasons.* Second, the government attacked scarcity by helping to overcome one set of scarce resources—treatment units and clinician capability—but without creating long-term patient care financing.

A blossoming literature

In the late 1960s and early to mid-1970s, a literature on the ethical and legal aspects of life-saving treatment blossomed, often focused on dialysis rationing. Concurrently, the discussion of the ethics of medical experimentation was receiving increasing attention. Paul Freund, a distinguished professor of law at Harvard University, counseled the medical community in the George W. Gay Lecture on medical ethics in 1965 as follows:

> The law on the whole subject of human experimentation will be worked out in close reliance on the moral sensibilities of the community. It therefore behooves the medical profession to take the public into its confidence and to educate public opinion rather than risk the shock and explosion of pent-up revulsion if the lid is pressed down on information and then blown up by some melodramatic case like that of the hospital for chronic diseases. The primary step is to recognize that difficult moral problems—indeed, moral dilemmas—do exist on which help and guidance may be sought from many sources. (Freund, 1965)

He also stated, in a phrase that would reverberate through subsequent legal commentary, that 'The governing standard [for experimentation] is not merit or need or value of the victim but equality of worth as a human being. The governing principle, it might be said, is that man shall not play God with human lives' (Freund, 1965).

Not surprisingly, therefore, in the late 1960s Freund wrote a strong critique of the Seattle practice of rationing access on the basis of social worth.

---

* Charles Zwick, BoB Director in 1967 and 1968, and later a RAND Trustee, said to me after I briefed the RAND board in 1980: 'I remember the Gottschalk Report [and its financing recommendation]. We just parked it. We had a little war going on in Southeast Asia.'

Consider the allocation of the limited and costly renal dialysis machines among sufferers from otherwise untreatable kidney disease . . . In Seattle, a panel of eminent laymen makes the selection on the basis of worth to the community . . . My own submission was that in a matter of choosing for life or death, not involving specific wrongdoing, no one should assume the responsibility of judging comparative worthiness to live on the basis of unfocused criteria of virtue or social usefulness, and that either priority in time, or a lottery, or a mechanical selection on the basis of age should be followed. (Freund, 1969)

Freund was not alone among those distressed by the need for patient selection as a means to ration access to treatment. At the level of the public reaction to rationing, Seattle was subjected to very substantial critical publicity. Others sought to develop various prescriptive approaches to the patient selection problem. Here is a précis of some pertinent papers.

Harry Abram, a psychiatrist, and Walter Wadlington, a lawyer, both at the University of Virginia, focused on 'patient selection of artificial and transplanted organs [where] the patient, if rejected, can find no other treatment even though his situation is terminal.' This area of medicine, along with euthanasia, abortion, and artificial insemination, is characterized by the reluctance of physicians to discuss their practice. The authors raised the questions of who should make patient selection decisions, what criteria should guide those decisions. They suggested the following: that selection should be by a committee, not by an individual physician, composed mainly of physicians but aided by others with backgrounds in 'social work, psychology, and religion.' Each patient should receive a thorough evaluation on 'medical, psychological, and environmental' grounds, rather than on 'such abstractions as social worth' (Abram and Wadlington, 1968).

David Sanders, a physician, and Jesse Dukeminier, Jr, a lawyer, addressed three questions related to the treatment of chronic renal disease by dialysis and transplantation: (1) Who gets the artificial kidney? (2) Who gets the transplanted kidney? (3) How can more cadaver kidneys be secured? (Sanders and Dukeminier, 1968). They listed the following 'subquestions' raised by the first two questions:

Who makes the decision, under what circumstances, applying what criteria? What institutional procedures or restraints are imposed upon the decision makers? What protection do the courts offer against arbitrary or irrational selection procedures? What procedures are arbitrary and irrational? When can the artificial kidney be taken away from a patient who has been using the machine? Are the ethical problems so tough that they should be hidden in a medical judgment? Who bears the cost of treatment? What property arrangements can be devised to shift the cost from the patient to the government? (Sanders and Dukeminier, 1968: 358)

For hemodialysis, the authors reviewed the medical, psychiatric and social worth evaluation of patients and then asked whether the latter should be done at all. Quoting Freund approvingly on the principle of man not playing God with human lives, the application of this principle 'would, in our judgment, proscribe selection for hemodialysis on the basis of ad hoc comparisons of the social worth of the candidates.' They considered then how patients should be selected and, without indicating a preference, listed the following methods: ability to pay; first-come, first-served; lottery or random selection; and 'rules announced in advance that are not unconstitutionally discriminatory.' Although none of these methods was perfect, the authors regarded any of them as 'preferable to selection by an ad hoc comparative judgments of social worth' (Sanders and Dukeminier, 1968: 380).

Regarding the allocation of kidneys for transplantation, they reviewed living donation and sale of organs, displaying a detached ambivalence on both issues. On sale of organs, they did suggest that if a market (or some other means for determining fair market value) for organs was established, organ transplantation 'may raise some knotty tax problems.' Those who received a live kidney donation were, for Sanders and Dukeminier, active finders. Recipients of a cadaver organ, however, were 'presently determined by logistics and medical criteria.' Regarding 'salvaging' cadaver organs, the authors believed that an individual should be granted the right to bequeath her or his organs for medical use prior to death. When conflicts arose between decedent's wishes and those of next-of-kin regarding donation, the authors would deny to next-of-kin the right to override the decedent's expressed wish. 'The first and most important principle of medical ethics,' they write, 'is to save life' (Sanders and Dukeminier, 1968: 410).

In a much shorter piece focused exclusively on 'the artificial kidney,' Dukeminier and Sanders considered the two ways of non-medical patient selection—random selection or selection by social worth (Dukeminier and Sanders, 1971). Regarding social worth evaluations, if selection is to be made on these grounds, the authors warned that selection 'judgments ... should be made explicitly and not be hidden within the verbal formulae of medical requirements.' Indeed, in this medical journal article, they were clearly writing for physicians confronting the selection issue. They reiterated their opposition to playing God, concluding that this proscribed selection on the basis of ad hoc comparisons of social worth of individuals. In this paper, interestingly, they reversed themselves from the prior paper and treat ability to pay not as preferable to social worth but as 'a kind of social worth allocation.'

An unsigned article in the *Harvard Law Review* dealt with patient selection for hemodialysis, noting that a 'narrowing' of selection criteria occurred that basically packed many factors into medical decision making (*Harvard Law Review*, 1969). These factors included age, physical condition, 'cooperativeness' in adhering to the rehabilitation routine, and 'rehabilitation potential.' Whereas equal protection and due process were constitutional principles relevant to patient selection, these concepts had not yet been reduced to administrative routine in allocation of organs. For the benefit of judges and legislatures, therefore, the article set forth the competing interests to be considered in thinking about patient selection: universal treatment; equal opportunity for survival; maximizing use of societal resources; and administration of the selection process. Providing universal treatment for organ failure might appear attractive, but also might fail to maximize total health care. Equal opportunity for survival might be provided by random selection, but choosing beneficiaries on the basis of past service or future promise would result in 'the unwonted normative judgment that one individual's life is more worthy than another's.' Maximizing use of societal resources might provide a utilitarian basis for patient selection, but the net effect would be marginal and offset by the infringement on equality of life. Constitutional principles that might apply included state action, equal protection, and due process. In general, care by hospitals qualified as state action. Regarding equal protection, they argued, a state 'must avoid arbitrary classifications in disbursing funds or benefits.' Thus, ability to pay and social worth criteria (judged by occupation, family, religion and morality) all presented a serious possibility of discriminatory behavior. Due process in selection called for full disclosure of information and procedures used with decisions on the record. 'Anonymous committee decisions, such as those employed by Seattle, are intolerable' (*Harvard Law Review*, 1969: 1336). Addressing legislatures, the paper criticized medical evaluations that used broad, ambiguous criteria such as 'cooperativeness' and 'rehabilitation potential,' and basically argued against social worth evaluations. It concluded by expressing a preference for a first-come, first-served criterion.

An extensive discussion of allocating scarce medical resources appeared in another unsigned law review article in 1969 (*Columbia Law Review*, 1969).* It noted that a number of life-saving medical treatments had developed that were not available to all because of their expense and identified three schools of thought about allocating scarce resources that allowed some to live while denying that opportunity to others: patient acceptance decisions by physicians that take individual social worth into account; acceptance decisions that restrict physicians to medical evaluation and delegate to others the determination of social worth; and acceptance decisions that preclude social worth considerations. The note considered criminal, tort, contract, and fiduciary law as they might apply to the allocation decision and concluded that the law currently had no role in such decisions. Should it? Or 'who should supply the answers?' asked the note. Physicians should have a role but not sole responsibility. The 'black box' of the jury of laymen, guided only by whatever standards they might find useful, should be ruled out as a way to find guiding principles. Lawyers, legislators, and judges had a role in establishing a basis for such allocation decisions.

The empirical analysis suggested to the authors that allocation/acceptance decisions were made in a two-step process: rules of exclusion narrowed the pool of potential applicants; and rules of final selection chose specific individuals. Exclusion rules included: hospital function; age of beneficiary; treatment requirements (psychological stability, intelligence, environment); medical criteria; hospital utilization requirements; ability to pay; and social worth. The authors concluded that exclusion on the basis of medical criteria was generally an acceptable way to narrow the pool from which final selection was made. Final selection may then be approached as a determination of social utility or an arbitrary but egalitarian judgment. Among the medical centers visited, first-come, first-served was the most preferred selection rule; social worth was generally ruled out.

These authors distinguished between micro-allocation (as discussed above) and macro-allocation. The note cites the Gottschalk report's recommendation of a publicly financed program of care, commenting that 'in a great many areas, a macro-allocation decision can reduce—if not altogether eliminate—the problem of scarcity, and alleviate some of the problems of micro-allocation' (*Columbia Law Review*, 1969: 673). Indicative of the relative unimportance of Medicare and the Public Health

* It is a hoary tradition of law reviews that lengthy and often very useful articles by law students are not credited with authorship. Unattributed authorship is especially irritating in this instance, as the note was based on interviews with 78 individuals in 26 cities.

Service in their thinking, the note's authors refer to Medicare only for illustrative purposes. They then engage in a lengthy analysis of the PHS statute and the PHS dialysis program and posit an optimal scheme for making macro-allocation decisions. The note concluded with a recapitulation of the micro-allocation problems, noted that macro-allocation decisions could relieve the burden in many ways, but added—reflective of the time and of the abiding 'opportunity costs'—that 'as long as our cities need rebuilding and Americans suffer from ignorance and malnutrition, the "ultimate" scarce resource—money—will remain unavailable.' Consequently, the allocation dilemma 'is likely to remain as a continuing problem with regard to kidney and other medical treatments' (*Columbia Law Review*, 1969: 691–2).

Several other similar papers appeared over the next few years. They are cited here but not discussed (Childress, 1970; Katz, 1973; Kandoian, 1975). Essentially they elaborated on the above themes. What is noteworthy about this literature? First, many of the authors are lawyers, either professors of law or students writing for law reviews. Second, this literature constitutes a serious body of social commentary, some of which contains a very substantial amount of empirical data about current medical practice in treating kidney failure. Third, it makes a strong case against social worth as a decision criterion in allocation of scarce, lifesaving resources and a corresponding case for a first-come, first-served form of random selection (as distinct from *ex ante* reliance on a lottery). Fourth, this body of thought tends to draw a bright orange line between decisions that are legitimately the province of physicians and those for which physicians lack training and competence and which deserve attention by non-physicians. Fifth, as one might expect of lawyers, the literature has a strong orientation to rules—rules of exclusion and rules of selection. Sixth, it distinguishes between micro-level allocation choices in which a prospective patient encounters a physician and typically other representatives of society and macro—or national—level allocation decisions. Seventh, scarcity is most frequently taken as a given of the current situation. Neither the numerous manifestations of scarcity, nor the social definition of scarcity, nor the manifold ways of responding to it, are dealt with to any extent. The impossibility of escape from scarcity is assumed. For example, although the Gottschalk Report is cited in a number of these papers, no author addressed the Medicare financing recommendation of that report as a way to deal with scarcity. Was this literature relevant to policy makers? This is a question that is taken up in the next section.

The Medicare years

Legislation

Legislative solutions to the problem of scarcity were sought in the US Congress from 1965 onward, which grappled with financing, not with rules for allocating scarce resources at the micro decision-making level. But the Gordian knot of financing was not cut until the inclusion of Sec. 299I in the Social Security Amendments of 1972 (Public Law 92–603). As this legislation was signed on October 30, 1972, and the kidney amendment was offered only on September 30, it qualifies as a genuine eleventh-hour action.

The year 1972 had begun, however, with a search for an appropriate legislative rationale. A number of approaches were under active consideration, of which amending the Public Health Service Act was the most prominent. The PHS Act had provided, after all, the basis for two NIH institutes to engage in related research and development. In addition, it was the sheltering wing under which the Kidney Disease Control Program emerged in 1965, and it was the statutory home to the Regional Medical Program, to which the KDCP was transferred in 1970 (Rettig, 1976; Rettig, 1982). The chief limitation of the PHS Act, however, was the bar against using it as a way to finance patient care. It was the vehicle for funding research, training, facilities, demonstrations but not patient care.

Surprisingly in retrospect, vocational rehabilitation legislation was also actively considered. Why? Dialysis patients were regarded as upstanding, hard-working, tax-paying citizens who needed, among other things, rehabilitative services in order to return to the active labor force. Senator John Tower (Republican, Texas) was the foremost advocate of this approach. Hearings on this approach were held in mid-1972 (US Senate 1972a, b).

In the end, Medicare became the legislative solution to scarcity. When Congress enacted Section 299I of the Social Security Amendments of 1972, it established a near-universal entitlement under Medicare for treatment of chronic kidney disease by dialysis or kidney transplantation. It thus eliminated the need for rationing, which had been explicit in Seattle and implicit elsewhere, whether it involved social worth or only medical criteria.

The original statutory language of Section 299I did include the requirement that there be 'at least . . . a medical review board *to screen the appropriateness of patients for the proposed treatment procedures*' (PL 92–603, 1972 (emphasis added)) No legislative history clarified the meaning of this clinically and ethically ambiguous language.* Nor did the implementing regulations issued by the Social Security Administration or the Public Health Service add clarity. SSA regulations for payment adopted in 1973 were silent (38 FR 1973); PHS regulations proposed in 1975 (40 FR 1975) and adopted in 1976 (41 FR 1976) fell back on process, requiring medical review boards as part of the ESRD 'network' system, but gliding over the screening of the appropriateness of patients. Generally, as medical review boards developed they dealt with other matters. The language was removed in Public Law 95–292 of 1978 and Congress has not seen fit to revisit the thicket implied by the original language.†

---

* In 1990, I was asked to write a paper on the legislative history of Section 299I for a committee of the Institute of Medicine chaired by Dr Carl Gottschalk. In preparation, a group of the principals involved in the 1972 legislation was convened and met for a dinner and a day of structured discussion. Dr James Mongan, who had been staff to the Senate Finance Committee, joined the discussion by telephone at one point. He dimly recalled these words as 'a hook' that Medicare administrators might use to address issues related to problematic patients, but his memory was not as crisp as the reduction of the anecdote to cold print implies.

† In 1995, I testified before the Health Subcommittee of the House Committee on Ways and Means that 'The time has come for Congress to ask the patient and provider communities to address the appropriateness of patients for treatment with respect to developing guidelines for patient acceptance criteria.' Rettig RA. Testimony, pp 38–48, House of Representatives, Committee on Ways and Means, Medicare End-Stage Renal Disease (Kidney Failure) Program, Hearing 104th Congress, 1st Session, April 3, 1995.

Payment policy

Payment for treatment has been the central element of public policy since 1972, including payment for dialysis facilities, physicians, the modalities of home dialysis care, and transplant services. Dialysis payment policy to facilities can be divided into two periods—the interim reimbursement rate, which was uniform across the country and which provided a differential between hospital-based and independent outpatient care (1973–1983); and the composite rate, which introduced a regional wage adjustment (1983 to the present). The reimbursement history has been characterized by the absence of any adjustment for inflation in either period; a substantial one-time rate reduction in 1983 in the shift from the interim to the composite rate; and a $1 per treatment increase in 1990. A 1991 Institute of Medicine (IOM) recommendation that the composite rate be adjusted annually has been ignored. Interestingly enough, a RAND study conducted for the Health Care Financing Administration in the mid-1990s on capitation of dialysis services recommended an upward adjustment in payment as the measured severity of patient increased, a suggestion that moves opposite from a rationing policy. However, in 1999, acting on 1998 and 1999 recommendations of the Medicare Payment Advisory Commission (MedPAC, 1998; 1999), Congress raised the composite rate by 2.4%. No other part of Medicare has been subjected to this severe, even punitive, economic discipline.

The point of the above discussion is simple: there is no escape from scarcity. It will manifest itself in any number of ways of greater or lesser frequency. In the ESRD case, there are two basic aspects of its manifestation: internal to the provision of ESRD care, scarcity defines what services providers can provide, what co-payment burden patients must assume, and how costs are shifted between public and private insurers. Second, the opportunity costs that are borne by bystanders, in this case, non-ESRD Medicare beneficiaries and the general tax-paying public, are diffused across a sufficiently broad base so as to be acceptable or only mildly onerous. The distribution of opportunity costs in this way appears socially, if not morally, preferable to examining the issues directly.

The National Kidney Foundation initiative of the 1970s

The 1972 legislation did not alleviate all ethical anxiety about treating patients by dialysis. Indeed, it gave rise to a new set of concerns. In the 1976, St Francis Hospital, Honolulu, and the National Kidney Foundation co-sponsored a conference on 'emerging medical, moral, and legal concerns' associated with dialysis (Siemsen and Greifer 1976). The initiative, headed by Dr Arnold Siemsen, a nephrologist, originated with a multi-disciplinary committee of the hospital that was seeking to resolve dialysis-related issues, and dovetailed with the creation by NKF of a committee to evaluate the medical, moral, and legal issues related to 'life-sustaining therapeutic procedures.' Seventy-one dialysis centers in 32 states had been surveyed and had identified new technology, increasing chronic illness, and suicide and death by omission as 'common concerns.'

The proceedings contain a number of very thoughtful papers by prominent bioethicists and social scientists dealing mainly with the moral justification for withdrawing treatment from patients with problems resulting from aging, the uremic process, or other comorbid conditions. A review of the extant literature made it clear that 'conclusions and unequivocal guidelines' were not forthcoming. Renee Fox observed that one effect of the 1972 legislation had been to shift the ethical discussion to 'negative selection,' i.e., withholding or withdrawing treatment: 'What seems notable to the sociological observer is that government-supported funding of dialysis has contributed to the slackening, if not elimination, of *biomedical* criteria of judgment and selection, as well as social and psychological ones' (Siemsen and Greifer, 1976: 130).

The Honolulu conference led to panel presentations at the 1977 and 1978 NKF annual meetings of several difficult cases (Siemsen *et al.*, 1977; 1978). The conference and NKF proceedings reflected a very serious and sensitive probing of issues. Regrettably, they were not published in widely circulated documents and the plan to continue the annual presentations failed for lack of financial support (Siemsen, 1992).

Recent efforts to address ethical issues

The Medicare entitlement removed the financial incentive, or need, to ration access to treatment. The nephrology community, moreover, scarred by its experience of the 1960s, was not disposed to dwell on the issue of rationing, occupied as it was with organizing to provide services to an ever-increasing patient population. However, as that growing population became older, as diabetes ceased to be a contraindication for treatment and became the leading diagnosis of kidney failure, as hypertension became the second leading cause of kidney failure, concern was voiced that patients were being accepted whose prognosis was poor and whose quality of life on dialysis was marginal (Cummings, 1993).

The Institute of Medicine (1991)

In response to the above concerns, the 1991 report of the Institute of Medicine, *Kidney Failure and the Federal Government* (Rettig and Levinsky, 1991) included a chapter on ethics.* This chapter addressed the issue of patient acceptance and patient withdrawal from treatment, at least for chronic kidney failure, as well as how to deal with problem patients. The IOM committee articulated the principle that 'patient acceptance criteria should be based on the medical assessment of the benefits and burdens of treatment and on the best interests of individual patients, not on economic objectives of cost containment.' The committee also stated that 'Nephrologists have a professional responsibility to deal with the issues of initiation and termination of treatment' and called for guidelines that would assist patients, families, and physicians 'who must make decisions about the use of any life-sustaining therapy.'

---

* This IOM study had been requested by Congress in the Omnibus Budget Reconciliation Act of 1987. The five questions asked by Congress, however, did not include ethical issues.

The recommendations of the IOM committee are worth citing here, because they stand in some measure as direct antecedents to the current Renal Physicians Association—American Society of Nephrology effort.*

The [IOM] committee recommends that patients, professionals in adult and pediatric nephrology, and bioethicists develop guidelines for evaluation of patients for whom the burdens of renal replacement therapy may substantially outweigh the benefits. These guidelines should be flexible and should encourage the physician to use discretion in the assessment of the individual patient.

Any guidelines for children should be child-specific and should describe the role of the parents in the decision-making process.

Renal professionals should discuss with ESRD patients their wishes for dialysis, cardiopulmonary resuscitation, and other life-sustaining treatments and encourage documented advance directives.

ESRD health care professionals should be encouraged to participate in continuing education in medical ethics and health law.

There is a need for some specialists in the medical ethics of renal disease to educate health care providers, to train members of ethics committees, and to do research on ethical issues in dialysis and transplantation.

Other features of the IOM ethics chapter worth noting in passing are the following. The issues of patient acceptance and withdrawal were proscribed as the domain of patients, families, and caregivers; a role for government was ruled out. Medical assessment in the best interest of the patient was stipulated, ruling out cost containment as a criterion for decision making. Chronological age was deemed unacceptable as a decision criterion for patient acceptance. And the conceptual basis of the discussion was the relation of the benefits and burdens of treatment.

The RPA-ASN guideline (1999)

In November 1999, the Renal Physicians Association and the American Society of Nephrology published Clinical Practice Guideline No. 2 (RPA-ASN, 1999) dealing with the 'appropriate initiation of and withdrawal from dialysis.' The roots of this guideline were, first, the evidence-based clinical practice guidelines movement of the early 1990s and, second, the 1991 IOM recommendation that guidelines for the evaluation of patients be developed. The changing character of the ESRD patient population, including the high proportion of elderly patients voluntarily withdrawing from treatment led the leadership of the two organizations to give the initiation/withdrawal effort highest priority.

The scope embraced acute renal failure and end-stage renal disease, initiation of and withdrawal from treatment, and competent and incompetent patients. The guideline recommended shared decision-making between patient and physician; ensuring informed consent about treatment modality, starting, continuing, and stopping treatment; discussion of a patient's estimated survival; means for resolving conflicts between a patient (or surrogate) and the renal team; the importance of advance

---

* The authors of the chapter were Alvin W. Moss, Christine Cassel, Richard A. Rettig, and Norman G. Levinsky. Moss co-chaired the RPA-ASN effort and Rettig was a member.

directives; guidance for decisions about patients with a non-renal terminal illness; time-limited trials of dialysis; and palliative end-of-life care. With respect to withholding or withdrawing dialysis, the guideline stated:

It is appropriate to withhold or withdraw dialysis for patients with either acute renal failure or ESRD in the following situations:
   Patients with decision-making capacity, who being fully informed and making voluntary choices, refuse dialysis or request dialysis be discontinued.
   Patients who no longer possess decision-making capacity who have previously indicated refusal of dialysis in an oral or written advance directive.
   Patients who no longer possess decision-making capacity and whose properly appointed legal agents refuse dialysis or request that it be discontinued.
   Patients with irreversible, profound neurological impairment such that they lack signs of thought, sensation, purposeful behavior, and awareness of self and environment. (RPA-ASN, 1999: 4)

It is obviously too early to know much about the guideline's reception. But the reviewers of the draft praised it highly, even while making detailed comments for improvement, and both the RPA and ASN endorsed guideline at the respective Fall 1999 meetings.

A comment on the United Kingdom

This chapter has dealt exclusively with the United States, perhaps the only country in the world to provide near-universal care for ESRD and not provide universal care for its entire population for general medical needs. The United Kingdom, on the other hand, has been cited often as a country providing universal care for all of its citizens but which rations access to treatment for renal failure patients.

Aaron and Schwartz (1984) compared the US and the United Kingdom with respect to the impact of medical technology on health care expenditures, focusing especially on ten medical procedures, including dialysis and kidney transplantation. They reported the sharp differences in prevalence of ESRD patients (69 patients per million on dialysis and 56 per million with a functioning kidney in the UK in 1980 compared with 230 per million on dialysis and 57 per million with a functioning kidney in the US) and found that the differences were 'rooted in resource constraints.' In contrast to the US, where the kidney entitlement was a statutorily protected benefit within Medicare, renal services in the UK had to compete with other health services for financing and, within hospitals, for space. Although age appeared to be a criterion for patient acceptance, medical conditions were confounding factors; fewer diabetics were accepted in the UK and the presence of medical problems other than kidney disease often was a reason for not accepting patients. Importantly, the requirement that referral to a specialist (i.e., to a nephrologist) be made by a general practitioner often resulted in screening out candidates at the initial stage of diagnosis in the UK.

Rennie *et al.* (1985) also compared the US and UK, reporting the same striking disparities and citing an instance of physicians rationing access to treatment under explicit orders from a regional health authority official. Among the factors identified as causing the observed disparities were the following: renal services were provided within the NHS overall budget, whereas the 1972 amendment sealed ESRD treatment off from the rest of Medicare; the UK fixed the number of treatment units in the late 1960s and early 1970s, whereas the number of facilities in the US increased as the patient population grew; the number of nephrologists in the UK was constrained by initial appointments and regulated by local decisions of other specialists, where the number in the US was not limited by official policy; and referral to specialists was controlled by GP internists in the UK, where direct access to a nephrologist occurred in the US. By several means, therefore, access to ESRD treatment was limited in the UK. However, the NHS provided universal access to care for general medical needs.

Halper (1989) assayed UK macro-allocation policies toward ESRD. The Ministry of Health, he writes, found dialysis and transplantation 'too valuable to ignore and too costly to embrace.' Consequently, it adopted a policy between these two poles, making a 'cautious beginning with no firm commitments about the future' (p. 35) and followed it by a gradual evolution over time. The controls of the National Health Service (NHS) budget, its downward allocation to regional health authorities, districts, and thence to hospitals and jousting among medical specialties are outlined, as are the disadvantages of financing ESRD care within this system. 'Bureaucratic incrementalism' characterized the UK macro-allocation of resources to ESRD. These societal policies, then, govern the micro-allocation decisions identified by Aaron and Schwartz and Rennie et al.

Halper concludes by asking how to judge UK policy towards ESRD. Scarcity, he argues, is imposed by society, not on society, and ESRD policy can be understood as the UK seeking to live within its means. He reviews the arguments about both an unqualified and qualified 'right to health care,' as well as a libertarian denial of any such right, and finds these of limited value in judging the UK. He asks, then, whether UK policy towards ESRD meets the standards of the NHS's own operating principle of concentrating on providing the health services used by most people most of the time. The policy does 'not at all badly,' in his judgment, by this metric. He also asks whether justice is served by the UK decision-making processes, which hide explicit decisions from full public view and understanding. Halper is reluctant to hold that the 'long utilitarian tradition of balancing interests' is inappropriate.

Conclusions

What conclusions, even lessons, might be drawn from this history of US government policy towards the treatment of permanent kidney failure as that policy has developed over nearly four decades? The following suggest themselves:

- Scarcity in the case of dialysis has been variously defined as machines, beds, clinical experience, trained personnel, and space, but it is basically the absence of money to pay for treatment. Scarcity in the case of kidney transplantation is defined as a physical shortfall between the clinical possibilities for transplantation and the availability of organs.
- In the first instance, that of dialysis, scarcity is a social construct, determined by the choices of public and private decision makers. Payment mechanisms for patient treatment can be designed and implemented.

- Rationing of access to treatment may be required by scarcity in the early stages of a therapy. But as a treatment becomes clinically established, as physicians are trained to provide care, as programs and organizations are created to support treatment, rationing is seen as a temporary expedient that yields to improved treatment effectiveness, increased diagnostic awareness, and a growing population of identifiable patients.
- The criterion of the social worth of individuals has been judged socially unacceptable as a basis for decisions about access to treatment. First-come, first-served emerges as an acceptable criterion for patient selection. Random selection by lottery satisfies fairness *ex ante* but contains the probability of garish unfairness *ex post*.
- Medical decision making carries the responsibility for society in dealing with micro-level manifestations of scarcity. Non-medical personnel may be involved for a time, but such involvement appears transitory.
- The principles, rules, and decision criteria for allocating scarce, life-saving resources that have been designed by lawyers, ethicists, and others are often quite complex and are extremely difficult to implement in public policy.
- Public policy focuses more on resolving scarcity in relatively simple ways and much less on the incorporation of the complex decision rules designed by lawyers and ethicists. How to pay for the treatment of end-stage renal disease was the central policy question of this story.
- The resolution of scarcity in one domain, such as ESRD, imposes opportunity costs on other domains. Resources spent for one purpose are unavailable for other uses.
- In some cases, and life-saving treatment appears to be a signal instance, the opportunity costs imposed by payment decisions appear *ex post* to be worth bearing. The costs of failure to act are much higher for politicians, especially where benefits are clearly identifiable and costs, i.e., opportunity costs, may be widely diffused or hidden.
- Opportunity costs are also imposed within a domain, as no financing scheme is ever adequate for a changing therapeutic capability and a growing patient population. Pay for dialysis treatment but not for the necessary medications that dialysis patients require. Pay for immunosuppressive drugs for transplant recipients, but not forever.
- Averting the eyes from the 'tragic choice' between highly valued social goods, such as saving lives, and scarcity is not without merit. The utility of doing so may be time-limited. (Calabresi and Bobbitt 1978).

Note: This paper was supported in part by grants from the National Library & Medicine, Dialysis Clinic, Inc., and Amgen.

References

Aaron, H. J., and Schwartz, W. B. (1984). *The painful prescription: Rationing hospital care*. Brookings Institution, Washington, DC.

Abram, H. S., and Wadlington, W. (1968). Selection of patients for artificial and transplanted organs. *Annals of Internal Medicine*, 69, 615–20.

Alexander, S. (1962). They decide who lives, who dies. *Life*, November 9, 102–25.

The Belmont Report: Ethical Principles and Guidelines for the Protection of Human Subjects of Research (1979). US Government Printing Office, Washington, DC.

Calabresi, G., and Bobbitt, P. (1978). *Tragic choices*. Norton, New York.
Childress, J. F. (1970). Who shall live when not all can live? *Soundings*, **43**, 339–62.
45 Code of Federal Regulations. Part 46. (June 18, 1991). *Protection of Human Subjects*. Department of Health and Human Services, Washington, DC.
Scarce medical resources. (1969) *Columbia Law Review*, **69** (4), 620–91.
Cummings, N. B. (1993). Ethical considerations in end-stage renal disease. In *Diseases of the kidney, Fifth Edition*, (ed. R. W. Schrier and C. W. Gottschalk), pp. 3097–128. Little Brown, Boston.
Curtis, F. K., Cole, J. J., Fellows, B. J., Tyler, L. L., and Scribner, B. H. (1965). Hemodialysis in the home. *Transactions of the American Society of Artificial Internal Organs*, **11**, 7–10.
Dukeminier, J. Jr. and Sanders, D. (1971). Legal problems in allocation of scarce medical resources. *Archives of Internal Medicine*, **127**, 1133–37.
38 *Federal Register* 17210 (June 29, 1973). Payment for services in connection with kidney transplant and renal dialysis provided to entitled beneficiaries.
40 *Federal Register* 27782 (July 1, 1975). Conditions for coverage of suppliers of end-stage renal disease (ESRD) services. Notice of proposed rulemaking.
41 *Federal Register* 22502 (June 3, 1976). Conditions for coverage of suppliers of end-stage renal disease (ESRD) services. Final rule.
Freund, P. A. (1965). Ethical problems in human experimentation. *New England Journal of Medicine*, **273**, 691–2.
Freund, P. A. (1969). Introduction to 'Ethical Aspects of Experimentation with Human Subjects'. *Daedalus*, Spring 98 (2), xiii.
Halper, T. (1989). *The misfortunes of others: End-stage renal disease in the United Kingdom*. Cambridge University Press, New York.
Patient selection for artificial and transplanted organs. (1969) *Harvard Law Review*, **82**, 1322–42.
Jonsen AR. (1998). *The birth of bioethics*. Oxford University Press, New York.
Kandoian, E. A. (1975). Due process in the allocation of scarce lifesaving resources. *The Yale Law Journal*, **84**, 1734–49.
Katz, A. (1973). Process design for selection of hemodialysis and organ transplant recipients. *Buffalo Law Review*, **22**, 373–418.
Katz, A. H., and Proctor, D. M. (1969). *Social-psychological characteristics of patients receiving hemodialysis treatment for chronic renal failure*. Report prepared for the Kidney Disease Control Program, US Public Health Service. Rockville, Maryland, July, p. 3.
Lindholm, D. D., Burnell, J. M., and Murray, J. S. (1963). Experience in the treatment of chronic uremia in an outpatient community hemodialysis center. *Transactions of the American Society of Artificial Internal Organs*, **9**, 3–10.
Medical World News (1964). Crucial test for hemodialysis, November 6, 97.
Medicare Payment Advisory Commission (MedPAC). (1998). *Report to the Congress: Medicare Payment Policy*. Washington, DC, March.
Medicare Payment Advisory Commission (MedPAC). (1999). *Report to the Congress: Medicare Payment Policy*. Washington, DC, March.
Murray, J. S., Tu, W. H., Albers, J. B., Burnell, J. M., and Scribner, B. H. (1962). A community center for the treatment of chronic uremia. *Transactions of the American Society of Artificial Internal Organs* **8**, 315.
Nabarro, J. D.N. (1967). Selection of patients for haemodialysis. *British Medical Journal*, vol. 1 1, 622.
National Academy of Sciences, Committee on Tissue Transplantation. (1965). Conference on kidney transplants. Transcript of meeting of May 16–17.

National Broadcasting Company, Inc., NBC News. (1965). *Who shall live?*, broadcast November 18, rebroadcast July 1966.
Page, I. (1963). Prolongation of life in an affluent society. *Modern Medicine*, October 14, 89.
Public Law 92–603, Section 299I, Social Security Amendments of 1972, October 31, 1972.
Renal Physicians Association and American Society of Nephrology (November 1999). *Clinical practice guideline on shared decision-making in the appropriate initiation of and withdrawal from dialysis.* Clinical Practice Guideline Number 2. Washington, DC.
Rennie, R., Rettig, R. A., and Wing, A. J. (1985). Limited resources and the treatment of end-stage renal failure in Britain and the United States. Quarterly Journal of Medicine, New Series 56, no. 219, pp. 321–336 (July).
Report of the Committee on Chronic Kidney Disease. (1967) Bureau of the Budget, Washington, DC (aka the Gottschalk Report).
Rettig, R. A. (1976). The policy debate on patient care financing for victims of end-stage renal disease. *Law and Contemporary Problems*, **40** (4), 196–230, but esp. 206.
Rettig, R. A. (1977). *Cancer crusade: The story of the National Cancer Act of 1971.* Princeton University Press, Princeton, NJ.
Rettig, R. A. (1982). The federal government and social planning for end-stage renal disease: past, present, and future. *Seminars in Nephrology*, **2**, 111–33.
Rettig, R. A., and Levinsky, N. G. (eds) (1991). *Kidney failure and the Federal Government.* National Academy Press, Washington, DC.
Sand, P., Livingston, G., and Wright, R. G. (1966) Psychological assessment of candidates for a hemodialysis program. *Annals of Internal Medicine*, **64**, 602–10.
Sanders, D. and Dukeminier, J., Jr. (1968) Medical advance and legal lag: hemodialysis and kidney transplantation. *UCLA Law Review*, **15**, 357–413.
Scribner, B. H. (1964). Ethical problems of using artificial organs to sustain human life. *Transactions of the American Society of Artificial Internal Organs*, **10**, 209–12.
Siemsen, A. W., and Greifer, I. (1976). *Proceedings of the conference on emerging medical, moral and legal concerns.* National Kidney Foundation and Institute of Renal Disease, St. Francis Hospital, Honolulu, Hawaii.
Siemsen, A. W., Beauchamp, T. L., and Robertson, J. A. (1977). Medical, moral and legal aspects of renal replacement therapy. *In Proceedings of the Dialysis and Transplant Forum* (ed. G. E. Schreiner, M. D.), vol. 7, 185–99 printed for the American Society for Artificial Internal Organs.
Siemsen, A. W., Beauchamp, T. L., Hopper, S., and Robertson, J. A. (1978) Medical, moral and legal aspects of renal replacement therapy (Part II). *In Proceedings of the Dialysis and Transplant Forum* (ed. G. E. Schreiner, M. D.), 8, 35–48 printed for the American Society for Artificial Internal Organs.
Siemsen, A. W. (1992). Personal communication, October 9, 1992.
Strickland, S. (1972). *Science, politics, and dread disease.* Harvard University Press, Cambridge, MA.
Human kidney transplant conference. (1964). *Transplantation Proceedings*, **2** (1), 155.
US Public Health Service. (1971). *The institutional guide to DHEW policy on protection of human subjects.* US Government Printing Office, Washington, DC.
US Senate, Committee on Labor and Public Welfare, Subcommittee on the Handicapped. (1972a). *Rehabilitation Act of 1972*, Hearings. 92nd Congress, 2nd Session, May 15, 18, and 23, pp. 305–49.
US Senate, Committee on Labor and Public Welfare. (1972b). *Rehabilitation Act of 1972*, Report. 92nd Congress, 2nd Session, September 20, pp. 3–32.

2
Ethical theory and principles
Ronald Baker Miller

The purpose of this chapter is twofold: (1) to provide an overview of ethical issues of concern to patients with kidney disease and to the physicians and other health care professionals who care for them; and (2) to review both theoretical and practical approaches for the analysis and resolution of clinical ethical problems.

It is only in the 1980s and 1990s that ethics has been taught explicitly in medical schools, internal medicine residencies, and nephrology training programs. This is despite the fact that ethical issues in medicine are as old as medicine itself, for once one asked, 'what is wrong?' and, 'what can be done?' one had also to ask, 'what should be done?' Furthermore, philosophical ethics and its application to medicine in the western world dates to ancient Greece, and major treatises in medical ethics have appeared periodically over the past three centuries.

Contemporary biomedical ethics or clinical ethics is a field of inquiry and knowledge grounded in the ethics subdiscipline of religious studies (theology) and of philosophy. This is an evolving specialty in medicine, nursing, the humanities, and the law which elected—at least with regard to its most practical function, clinical consultation—not to define itself but rather to detail the core competencies, skills, knowledge, and character required for successful consultation by individuals, teams, or committees (Society for Health and Human Values—Society for Bioethics Consultation Task Force on Standards for Bioethics Consultation, 1998). This field is distinguished from professional ethics and etiquette (which deal with the laws, regulations, and professional expectations of physician conduct with patients and with other health care professionals) and from organizational ethics and corporate compliance programs (which deal with the values, mission, and behavior of institutions and their staff). Studies in clinical ethics range from the conceptual terrain of theoretical philosophers and theologians to empirical observations of the behavior of patients and clinicians or surveys of their attitudes and hypothetical behavior.

Can ethics provide answers? James Rachels's answer (in an essay that is also the title of a book of his essays) is, 'Ethics provides answers about what we ought to do, given that we are the kinds of creatures we are, caring about the things we will care about when we are as reasonable as we can be, living in the sort of circumstances in which we live. This is not as much as we might want, but it is a lot. And it is as much as we can hope for in a subject that must incorporate not only our beliefs but our ideals' (Rachels, 1997).

Clinical ethics 'may be defined as the systematic identification, analysis, and resolution of ethical problems associated with the care of particular patients. Its goals include protecting the rights and interests of patients, assisting clinicians in ethical decision making, and encouraging cooperative relationships among patients, those close to patients, clinicians, and health care institutions' (Ahronheim *et al.*, 2000).

History

Western medical ethics is said to begin in the fifth century BC with Hippocrates and the 70 treatises known as the Hippocratic Collection (Jonsen, 1998, 2000). Judeo-Christian tradition (e.g. the sanctity of life) and scholars (Maimonides and St Thomas Aquinas) were important in shaping our tradition. In the eighteenth century, physicians like Samuel Bard of Kings College (now Columbia University) called for integrity and ability and Benjamin Rush (University of Pennsylvania) opposed slavery, the death penalty, and tobacco, and stated, 'a physician should be ever ready to obey the calls of the sick' (Jonsen, 2000). In the nineteenth century Thomas Percival considered medicine a public trust, and the 1847 American Medical Association (AMA) Code of Medical Ethics (Council on Ethical and Judicial affairs, 1998), based on Percival's precepts, endorsed scientific medicine, while Sir William Osler advocated competence and equanimity. In the early twentieth century Richard Cabot (best known for introducing the CPC, the Clinicopathologic Conference) was Professor of Social Ethics as well as Clinical Medicine at Harvard University. He wrote an entire book on honesty, felt that patients should be told their diagnosis, and suggested disputes about appropriate care should be settled by committees. In mid-century, Chauncey Leake at the University of California, San Francisco claimed Percival's ethics was actually etiquette (how doctors should behave toward one another), whereas medical ethics should define how doctors should behave toward patients. He also recommended that medical students have a course beginning with three lectures on 'moral philosophy', followed by a historical survey of ethics in medicine, and thereafter discuss ethical cases with experienced physicians (Jonsen, 1998, 2000). In 1954 the Episcopal theologian, Joseph Fletcher, published the ground-breaking and prescient study, *Morals and Medicine* (Fletcher, 1954; Jonsen and Jameton, 1995).

Near the end of the Second World War Willem Kolff saved the seventeenth patient he hemodialyzed using an artificial kidney whose dialyzing membrane was sausage casing. Following the war the Doctors' Trial at Nuremberg revisited the horrors of the holocaust and of Nazi pseudoscience. The Nuremberg Code for the ethical conduct of human research presaged the development of bioethics.

In 1960 Kouwenhoven and colleagues described closed chest cardiac massage (Kouwenhoven *et al.*, 1960) and soon thereafter the first intensive care unit (ICU) in the United States was opened (Orlowski, 1999). A seminal event in nephrology, the successful identical-twin renal transplant by Joseph Murray and John Merrill at the Peter Bent Brigham Hospital, set the stage for the treatment of end-stage renal failure (Merrill *et al.*, 1956).

These and other scientific and technologic developments (such as the development of antibiotics) allowed unprecedented gains in the capability of medicine to fight disease and extend life, albeit at unprecedented cost. In the United States, the latter was exacerbated by the increasing provision of health care insurance by employers and a cost-plus system of reimbursement. Young physicians increasingly entered subspecialties of medicine and surgery with the consequence that treating physicians were often 'strangers at the bedside' who understood the patient's disease and what could be done for it, but often did not know the 'patient as person' (Ramsey, 1970; Rothman, 1991). There was 'a growing concern about the power exercised by doctors and scientists, which shows itself in concern to assert "patients' rights" and the rights of the community as a whole to be involved in decisions that affect them' (Khuse and Singer, 1998).

As also described in Chapter 1 by Richard Rettig, the stage then was set for spontaneous combustion when a journalist, Shana Alexander (1962), described the consequences of the simple but revolutionary invention of the arteriovenous shunt that enabled ongoing hemodialysis of patients who would otherwise have died of chronic renal failure. She noted that only one in 50 patients with end-stage kidney disease was considered a suitable candidate for this treatment, and that in the first year only five patients were treated. Shana Alexander indicated 'intolerable pressures' for the doctors who were 'receiving agonizing appeals from colleagues to take on more patients than they could possibly care for.' A medical advisory committee of nephrologists (a term not then in existence) and a psychiatrist was appointed by the King County Medical Society to select medically qualified candidates. What caught the national attention was the second committee, also appointed by the County Medical Society, and 'charged with formulating and applying nonmedical criteria to select which medically qualified candidates would receive treatment' (Alexander, 1962; Fox and Swazey, 1978; Darrah 1987). This committee decided to consider factors of age, gender, marital status, number of dependents, emotional stability to accept treatment, education, occupational performance, and potential income and net worth (Alexander, 1962). Alexander (1962) called the committee a 'life or death committee'. It became informally known as the 'Patient Processing Committee' (Fox and Swazey, 1978), but those appalled by the social worth criteria called it a 'God Committee'. In their book Fox and Swazey (1978) stated, 'There is not, and perhaps never can be, any wide accord about what standards and criteria should be used to choose recipients of a scarce medical resource such as chronic hemodialysis, or about who should make this decision . . . Seattle's selection committees are only one imperfect and uneasy attempt to deal with these issues'. In retrospect Swazey (1992) stated, 'The Seattle group was struggling in a much more forthright manner than most medical groups at the time with a number of issues that at once were medical, moral, and social, and would become the major foci of those who . . . became known as bioethicists'.

As David Rothman (1991) said, 'physicians turned to a lay committee because they realized that the traditional medical ethic of each doctor doing everything possible to enhance the well-being of the particular patient could not operate in these circumstances . . . It seemed preferable to empower a lay committee rather than compel doctors to abdicate their responsibilities . . . In making this choice the committee transmitted a message, as Alexander accurately noted: the "acceptance of the principle that all segments of society, not just the medical fraternity, should share the burden of choice as to which patients to treat and which to let die".'

Both preceding and following these events in Seattle, there were other concerns in the academic community: the ethics of clinical investigation, that is of research with human subjects. In 1958 and 1959 Robert Ward, Saul Krugman and colleagues conducted important scientific studies of infectious hepatitis employing a vulnerable population (mentally retarded children). Children were intentionally infected, but it was rationalized that they would have become infected by simply residing in the institution, the Willowbrook School, and that they would receive better medical care by virtue of the study of their hepatitis (Beauchamp and Childress, 1994). In 1963 elderly, debilitated patients in the Jewish Chronic Disease Hospital in Brooklyn, New York were injected with cancer cells without consent (Jonsen, 1998). In 1966 Henry K. Beecher wrote that 'of 100 consecutive human studies published in 1964 in an excellent journal, 12 seemed to be unethical' (Beecher 1966). Concerns over these studies and others such as the Tuskegee study in which African-Americans with syphilis were observed but not offered treatment even after penicillin became available (Pence, 1995) led, in the United States, to congressional legislation and appointment of the National Commission for the Protection of Human Subjects of Biomedical and Behavioral Research in 1974. The commission's Belmont Report, enunciated 'three basic principles: . . . respect for persons, beneficence, and justice' with three derivative requirements for research: informed consent, risk-benefit assessment, and just selection of subjects' (Jonsen, 1998).

If all we have discussed represents its conception and gestation, the birth of bioethics began April 15, 1975 when Karen Ann Quinlan was hospitalized in coma, and ended with the New Jersey Supreme Court decision of March 31, 1976 allowing 'discontinuance of life support . . . even if it meant the prospect of natural death. . . . [The state has no compelling interest in forcing Karen] to endure the unendurable, only to vegetate a few measurable months with no realistic possibility of returning to any semblance of cognitive or sapient life' (In re Quinlan 1976). As Jonsen (1998) wrote 'Karen Ann Quinlan had not died in vain. Because of the sad ending of her short life the American public learned the tragic side of the miracle of intensive care. American law began to move toward views that could accommodate the undesirable consequences of technological medicine. American doctors began to attend more seriously to the ethical dimensions of clinical decisions to forgo life-sustaining treatment'. And perhaps of equal importance, the court recommended an ethics committee to review such cases, based ironically on an article in the *Baylor Law Review* (Teel, 1975) by a pediatrician concerned with having to make, or allowing parents to make, life and death decisions for impaired newborns. Ironic because Dr Teel, the author, was mistaken in her belief that 'many hospitals' had such committees, and doubly ironic because the New Jersey Supreme Court wished the committee to establish the neurologic prognosis of patients like Karen Ann Quinlan rather than to weigh the ethical issues as intended by Teel.

Although it wasn't until the 1990 landmark decision by the United States Supreme Court in the case of Nancy Cruzan, another young woman in a persistent vegetative state, that the constitutional right to refuse medical treatment (even life-sustaining treatment such as artificial nutrition and hydration) was firmly established in the United States, the Quinlan case not only brought societal awareness to the problem but forever changed the practice of medicine in the United States, and established the field of bioethics.

Terminology

For clarity and consistency I will begin with several basic definitions. Ethical and moral are synonymous, interchangeable adjectives (one from Greek, the other from Latin), both meaning: conforming to an accepted code of conduct, i.e., to behavior acceptable to a cultural, ethnic, social, religious, or professional group.

Although the adjectives 'ethical' and 'moral' are interchangeable, the corollary nouns are not. Ethics (or moral philosophy) is the science of morals: the philosophic or religious discipline that systemically examines what is good or bad, right or wrong, just or unjust in human conduct, and the study of cultural, religious, and professional traditions of these values. Morals are cultural, religious, professional and personal standards of ethical behavior. Morality is a cultural, religious, professional or personal tradition of values about what is good, right and just.

There are experts in ethics (the study or discipline) but not in the rightness of moral judgments. That is, no one should be considered an expert in the substance of a moral judgment even though the person may be skilled in how to arrive at a moral judgment; that is, skilled in the process by which moral judgments are made.

An ethical issue is a matter of concern or interest regarding what is good or bad, right or wrong, just or unjust. An ethical problem is an ethical issue that is troublesome or is in dispute. An ethical dilemma is an ethical problem whose resolution is problematic because there is no right, good, or just solution, or because 'there is more than one right thing to do, but to act on one necessarily prohibits you from acting on the other(s)'. Thus, one necessarily does 'something right and also wrong (by not doing the other thing that is also right)' (Purtillo, 1981).

Moral theories and traditions

Moral intuition is generally sufficient to recognize what is ethical and what is not, but if we wish to know why it is (or is not), moral theory (i.e., the discipline of ethics) is helpful. Furthermore, moral philosophy influences the very 'way in which moral problems are described' (Downie, 1996).

The major moral theories, bioethical principles, and several other approaches to the ethical problems in clinical medicine are reviewed in this chapter. Selected concepts in ethics and some of the more popular, though not necessarily defensible, ethical distinctions commonly invoked in discussing ethical issues in medicine are discussed.

An ethical theory provides standards or a basis for judging what is right or wrong, good or bad, just or unjust in human conduct. It should be internally consistent, clear, complete, and preferably simple and practical (Beauchamp and Childress, 1994; Mappes and DeGrazia, 1996). The ultimate test of a moral theory is that it has heuristic value and is helpful when it is needed most—in other words, in the most difficult and complex cases.

Ethical theories can be monistic; that is, have a simple, fundamental principle (e.g., happiness in hedonistic utilitarianism) from which all other principles and all judgments derive, or they can be pluralistic (e.g., W. D. Ross's multiple prima facie duties) (Ross, 1930).

Theories can be categorical, that is, absolute, and admitting of no exceptions (e.g., Kantian deontology) or situational and relative to context (e.g., the situational ethics of Joseph Fletcher) (Kant, 1785; Fletcher, 1954). Alternatively a theory may be intermediate; that is, binding, but not absolutely so, in other words binding unless in conflict with a higher principle or obligation (e.g., the prima facie duties of W. D. Ross) (Ross, 1930).

A final distinction regarding theories is that they may be teleological; that is, consequentialist in which case the rightness of an act is dependent on the consequences of the act or rule (e.g., John Stuart Mill's utilitarianism), or they may be deontologic (or formalist) in which case rightness is independent of consequences and is often based on duty or obligation (e.g., Kantian deontology and his categorical imperative) (Kant, 1785; Mill, 1861a, 1861b). Other examples of deontologic theory are the Decalogue (the Ten Commandments), virtue theory of Plato and Aristotle, natural law theory of Thomas Aquinas, natural rights of John Locke, and the contractarian theories of Thomas Hobbes and John Rawls.

Limitations of space preclude description of the many individual theories but allow brief description of the two major categories (consequentialist and deontologic) and of two theories that are both consequentialist and deontologic.

In a consequentialist theory, right and wrong, just and unjust are empirically discoverable since they are dependent on the consequences of an act or of a rule. In utilitarianism, the best known and most popular consequentialist theory, good is defined as that which promotes happiness (Mill, 1861a and b). Utility, then, can be expressed as a duty ethic: to do that which maximizes happiness or well-being or that which produces the greatest good for the greatest number. It is by necessity a forward-looking theory in that one has to know or predict the consequences in order to know whether an act or a rule is right (Thomas and Waluchow, 1998). What one ought to do (that is a judgment or obligation) is dependent on a judgment of value; that is, of what is good (in turn dependent on what creates happiness) (Thomas and Waluchow, 1998). A contemporary example of a consequentialist approach is cost-benefit analysis of health care interventions or of medical technologies.

'Deontology is, literally, the study of duties persons have toward one another' (Ahronheim *et al.*, 2000). In sharp contrast to consequentialist theories, deontologic theories hold that the rightness or wrongness of actions is independent of the consequences; that is, of whether or not the actions maximize good consequences. Acts are right or wrong due to 'inherent or intrinsic features of acts such as truthfulness or lying' (Childress, 1998). In the most revered deontologic theory, that of Immanuel Kant (Kant, 1785), intention and 'good will' is what matters (Thomas and Waluchow, 1998). In Kantian deontology, the foundational principle is the 'categorical imperative', of which Kant provides at least two formulations: (1) 'so act that the maxim [rule of conduct] of thy act could become, by thy will, a universal law of nature', and (2) 'treat every man as an end in himself, and never as means only' (Kant, 1785). The first formulation, universalizability, is often noted to be equivalent to the 'golden rule' ('whatsoever ye would that men should do to you, do you even so to them ...' Matthew 7:12). The second formulation, to treat persons as ends, not means, embodies the notion of respect for persons or their autonomy (Mappes and DeGrazia, 1996; Thomas and Waluchow, 1998). Thus, in Kantian deontology, a judgment of obligation 'is justified if and only if it meets the categorical imperative test, which ignores consequences altogether' (Thomas and Waluchow, 1998). When it does, the duty is absolute, admitting of no exceptions. However, Flores believes that what makes deontology (rules) acceptable is the consequences (utility) of following the rules (Flores, 2000).

W. D. Ross's (1930) theory of the pluralistic nature of moral obligation is intermediate between, and dependent on, both consequentialist and deontologic notions. 'Promises, contracts, commitments, agreements, loyalty, friendship ... all have moral force, and all can give rise to obligations and responsibilities, independently of good and bad consequences', though consequences are also of importance (Thomas and Waluchow, 1998).

As previously noted, Ross's theory is also intermediate between absolutist and relativistic notions. 'Prima facie' duties are those that are obligatory unless they conflict with other duties, in which case consequences may be determinative in selecting between them. Prima facie duties include: duties of fidelity, reparation, gratitude, justice, beneficence, self-improvement, and non-maleficence. Ross claims these duties are evident through moral intuition, a controversial feature of his theory for philosophers who are often 'suspicious of "self-evident" principles' (Thomas and Waluchow, 1998).

Bernard Gert (1988) distinguishes 'a moral theory, which is an analysis and synthesis of all relevant concepts, and a moral system, derived from that theory, which is what is actually used by people for guiding their behavior and for making judgments'. He defines morality as 'a public system, applying to all rational persons, governing behavior which affects others and which has the minimization of evil as its end, and which includes what are commonly known as the moral rules at its core'. Examples of moral rules are 'Don't kill', 'Don't steal', and 'Don't lie'. Gert aims for simplicity and common sense. An example of the latter is his notion that 'morality is not primarily a system of conduct that a rational person decides to adopt for herself', but rather one that 'rational persons advocate that other people adopt'.

To conclude this section on moral theory, I should quote James Rachels, 'If there is indeed one best overall ethical theory, it is likely to appear as many lines of inquiry converge. The fact that there is still so much disagreement among ethical theorists may be due not to the impossibility of the project but to its complexity ...' (Rachels, 1998). Despite such concerns, we engage in theory, as Aristotle said, because it helps us to deal with practical problems.

Bioethical principles

First order principles

The principles of bioethics articulated in 1979 in the Belmont Report of the National Commission for the Protection of Human Subjects of Biomedical and Behavioral Research (respect for persons, beneficience, and justice) and, in the same year, in the first edition of Beauchamp and Childress's foundational text, *The Principles of Biomedical Ethics* (autonomy, non-maleficence, beneficence, and justice) are so well known that I will describe them only briefly.

Most physicians consider non-maleficence (*primum non nocere*: first, do no harm) the pre-eminent ethical principle as enunciated in the Hippocratic oath. Logicians appreciate non-maleficence as the inverse corollary of beneficence (do or make good), and may prefer the positive rather than a negative statement of the principle. In the United States, which places such a premium on the individual and her freedom, autonomy (self-rule)—or more properly respect for autonomy—is often considered the dominant principle, and neophytes in bioethics not infrequently rely on it to solve almost every ethical problem. Many prefer to emphasize the Kantian notion of respect for persons and think of autonomy as derivative. In turn, derivative from the ethical principle of autonomy are the legal right to self-determination and the legal doctrine of informed consent. Despite its general importance one should consider limiting autonomy when the patient waives it (though this should trigger evaluation of the reason why the patient wishes to waive it and whether it is in the patient's best interest to do so); when the patient would be seriously or irreparably harmed; when identified others (third parties) would be harmed; perhaps when non-identified others (society) would be harmed; when what is requested is unethical; and arguably when what is requested is considered 'futile' (though the goal of the intervention must be defined to assess the probability that it would be ineffective) or is considered outside the limits of the goals of medicine.

The fourth principle in the 'Georgetown Mantra' of Beauchamp and Childress is justice. To treat equals equally and to allocate health care resources fairly are fundamental principles, which implicitly remind us of the importance of the commons, of the greater society, and allow us to balance our emphasis on the individual with communitarian concern.

Some might wish to add utility as a fifth principle either because it also is a 'principle of distribution' or because it is 'an extended version of beneficence' (Downie, 1996). On the other hand Downie (1996) notes that 'defenders of the four principles might also say that the principle of utility ... underlies the other four principles, which are simply expressions of utility in different circumstances.'

Others suggested adding, as a 'fifth principle', 'proportionality: to produce a positive balance of benefits over burdens' (Wicks *et al.*, 1995). However, proportionality may be seen as a corollary of non-maleficence and beneficence and thus not truly a separate principle. On the other hand, as a practical matter it is often clinically very useful to explicitly consider both the benefits and the risks (or harms) for each stakeholder (patient, family, physician, other health care professional, institution, etc.) of each possible solution to an ethical problem.

Second order principles

If non-maleficence, beneficence, autonomy, and justice are considered first-order principles, others may be considered second-order principles or moral rules and action guides. Beauchamp and Childress (1994) further divide these into (1) substantive rules, those for 'truth telling, confidentiality, privacy, fidelity . . ., allocation and rationing . . ., omitting treatment, physician assisted suicide, and informed consent . . .'; (2) authority rules, those regarding decisional authority, surrogacy, professional authority, and distributional authority for scarce resources; and (3) procedural rules, for example those for selecting patients for scarce, expensive, or innovative therapy.

The substantive secondary principles or moral rules and action guides that seem to be most general and regularly applicable to the practice of medicine are confidentiality (secret keeping) and privacy (the right to be left alone), integrity (honesty) and veracity (truth telling), fidelity (promise keeping) and loyalty (devotion), respect for persons and for life (dignity and reverence), and respect for community (solidarity, the golden rule, and compassion).

Approaches to clinical ethical problems

The approach one takes to ethical problems in the care of patients and in interactions with other health care professionals depends on many factors, including one's culture, upbringing, world-view, education and training, mentorship and experience. Knowledge of moral theory, bioethical principles, and the various approaches to be discussed in this section are helpful, particularly in justifying (or rationalizing) one's considered judgments.

The principled approach

The deductivist application of moral theory or of the principles of bioethics to individual cases may be called the principled approach, or, as it is often called by critics of the approach, 'principlism' (Clouser and Gert, 1990). Critics (Clouser and Gert, 1990 and to a lesser extent Jonsen and Toulmin, 1988) notwithstanding, the principled approach remains extremely popular and effectively defended (Childress 1997; 1998; Gillon and Lloyd, 1994), and many believe quite effectively applied.

Clouser and Gert (1990) state the principles are 'merely names for a collection of sometimes superficially related matters for consideration when dealing with a moral problem' and that the principles 'operate primarily as checklists naming issues worth remembering'. They believe 'the "principles" lack any systematic relationship to each other, and that the principles often conflict with each other'. Even if one accepts the Rossian notion of principles as only prima facie correct, Clouser and Gert do not see how to resolve conflicts between principles. Many agree it is not possible to establish a hierarchy of the Georgetown principles, but nevertheless feel comfortable applying them intuitively, i.e., selecting the principle that seems most relevant to the specific case in question. This is not to say there may not be serious conflict: for example, whether to honor a patient's autonomy (when he seems to be making an inappropriate decision) or to be paternalistically benevolent or beneficent. But clearly it bothers the critics who plead for a 'unified moral theory' such as that of Gert (1988) rather than to invoke the principles, which they state 'leads to neglect' of the underlying moral theories, and of the derivative 'rules and ideals that apply to the particular case', and neglect of a 'statement of the particular duties of a profession'.

The casuistic approach

A rather different criticism of the principled approach is the case-based approach or the method of casuistry (Jonsen, 1991; Jonsen and, Toulmin 1988; Kopelman; 1994). In their prologue to 'The Abuse of Casuistry' Jonsen and Toulmin (1988) recount their experience with the National Commission for the Protection of Human Subjects of Biomedical and Behavioral Research. The members of the multidisciplinary commission 'usually agreed in their practical conclusions' but not at all in their reasons for their recommendations, in other words, why they agreed. 'So long as the debate stayed on the level of particular judgments, the eleven commissioners saw things in much the same way. The moment it soared to the level of "principles", they went their separate ways.'

A casuistical approach is analysis of a case by analogy with paradigm cases and maxims (cases and maxims about which one is convinced of the ethical approach) but also with rigorous attention to the particular circumstances of the case and to its context, much as in the narrative approach to ethics. The narrative approach, we might mention, suggests that moral insights are facilitated by rich, full description of the particulars of the case.

Casuistry, then, is ethics 'from the bottom up' in contrast to the deductivist or top-down approach of applying principles. The circumstances and context of particular cases are relevant, often even determinative. Analysis is by comparison with paradigm (archetypical) cases and their associated maxims (folk sayings) and precedents. Judgments are tentative and presumptive, more or less probable, and thus rebuttable and subject to change.

There are four steps in casuistical analysis: (1) discern the grounds (facts) of the case; (2) compare with paradigm cases, noting differences and similarities; (3) consider arguments, maxims and warrants (justifications); (4) make judgments, but realize they have only probable certitude. This case-based approach may be particularly comfortable for physicians and attorneys who seem to learn best from cases. Arras (1998) writes, however, 'this approach, which is essentially backward-looking [because it makes judgments based on prior experience] may have some conservative tendencies', and Kopelman (1994) notes that bias may creep in at each stage of reasoning in casuistry. Arras (1998) also notes that casuistry may work better in cultures with substantial 'agreement on fundamental values' and may 'founder in a highly pluralistic ... culture like our own'. On the other hand he notes this can also be an advantage (as Jonsen and Toulmin had noted), allowing 'parties divided at the level of principle to converge on responses to specific paradigms and cases', which he states is 'a distinct advantage in pluralistic, democratic societies'. But because casuistry is backward-looking it may be less helpful in analyzing the ethical problems posed by new technologies.

Reflective equilibrium

John Rawls (1971) in his extraordinary work on justice introduced the term 'reflective equilibrium' to refer to the equilibrium achieved when 'our principles and judgments coincide'. He suggests that we work from both ends: starting either with our principles or with our considered judgments, we revise either or both so that they do coincide. He adds, however, 'this equilibrium is not necessarily stable. It is liable to be upset by further examination of the conditions which should be imposed on the contractual situation and by particular cases which may lead us to revise our judgments. Yet for the time being we have done what we can to render coherent and to justify our convictions of social justice.' This approach, of course, is not limited to theories and judgments of justice, and accords with a reasoned approach to all of ethics: solutions to problems are suggested by principles, but principles are informed by the circumstances of, and one's judgments about, cases, and may be modified accordingly.

This reflective approach to resolving discrepancies, inconsistencies, imperfect fits or cognitive dissonance should allow either a deductive or inductive approach. Those more comfortable with the application of principles to problems should do so, just as those who prefer to start with a rich understanding of the particulars and the circumstances and context of a case should do so. The conclusion, however, may not be the same, and one should appreciate that reflective attempts to achieve equilibrium are not always effective even when one is motivated to achieve coincidence or at least coherence between one's principles and one's considered judgments. This is even more true when two people have the opposite approach rather than a single individual attempting to view the problem from both sides.

A virtues approach

Yet another approach to moral problems is the virtues approach, which places emphasis on the actor and his or her motives rather than on the act and its consequences. The importance of character was stressed by Plato and Aristotle, who believed virtues could be acquired and character strengthened by training and practice much like language or other skills (Beauchamp and Walters, 1994). We each wish our physician, our nephrologist, to be virtuous: compassionate, conscientious, discerning, fair, honest, humble, prudent, respectful, and trustworthy. The concern with virtues, however, is not suggested in opposition to a principled approach but more often as a supplement to enrich the ethical deliberation. It is, nevertheless, well to acknowledge that the virtues approach is particularly popular with those concerned about the obsession with autonomy in many sectors and the inadequate concern for the commons and the interests of people collectively (society), not just those of individuals (Oakley, 1998).

Prominent advocates of the virtues approach include Foot (1978), MacIntyre (1984), Drane (1988) and Pellegrino and Thomasma (1993).

A relational approach (an ethic of care)

It is intuitively obvious that obligations (and their corollary rights) depend on relationships. The ethical importance of duty or obligation (Kant, 1785), of rights (Dworkin 1977; Locke, 1690), and of the doctor-patient relationship (Brody, 1989; Emanuel and Emanuel, 1992; Veatch, 1991) is patently evident. On the other hand, it was not until Carol Gilligan's (1982) challenge of her Harvard mentor's (Lawrence Kohlberg 1981) thesis of moral development that the feminine perspective and the ethic of care became important contributors to American bioethics. Kohlberg's thesis from studies of boys and men was that people reason morally by applying principles to cases . . . [that] moral progress . . . is cognitive . . . and culminates in principles that are universal and binding on all persons' (Manning, 1998). Gilligan found that girls and women (unlike the abstract, impartial, voice of justice of Kohlberg's men) had a 'voice of care' concerned with social relationships, personal narratives, and sympathetic understanding (Manning, 1998). Indeed, we have come to appreciate the ethic of rights, duties, rules, and justice as masculine, and the ethic of caring, compassion, and the importance of preserving relationships as feminine. Although individuals of both genders in fact have both ethics to varying degrees, these stereotypic gender differences resonate with most of us. But appreciate that the ethic of care is largely a feminine perspective rather than a feminist perspective (Ahronheim *et al.*, 2000), though the latter has impacted bioethics as well, forcing an appreciation of the political importance of power and the subordination of women (card 1991, Holmes and Purdy 1992, Larrabbe 1993, Noddings 1984, Woef 1996).

Yet another variant of the ethic of care and the importance of relationships is the communitarian perspective, as previously noted thought too often lacking in American bioethics. Appreciation of the communitarian view, particularly with regard to the need for fundamental changes in grassroots perspectives and goals if we are to have meaningful change and sustainability in health care, has been repeatedly articulated by Daniel Callahan (1987, 1990, 1993, 1998).

Absolutist versus relativistic approaches

A relativistic, contextual, situational approach to ethical issues is especially in keeping with a pluralistic society, such as the United States. The United States continues to be a melting pot, but one in which diversity is increasingly valued. Acculturation of all who are assimilated is no longer expected, and an ethic of tolerance appears to be developing. It behooves physicians in all countries to learn as much about the cultural values of their patients as possible, though one must be wary of prejudicial assumptions (stereotyping), as there is often more variation within cultures than between them. One factor that may transcend cultural barriers and explain similar values across cultures is socioeconomic class. In any event, as we 'accumulate knowledge about specific ethnic and cultural groups, [we] are challenged to look at both the differences and similarities that exist across cultures' (Purnell and Paulanka, 1998). In an important book, Ruth Macklin (1999) concludes that there are universal ethical principles, but that this does not require ethical absolutism and indeed these universals are compatible with culturally-specific (culturally-relative) interpretations. But, most important, the universally accepted ethical principles are the moral underpinnings of fundamental human rights that transcend cultures.

The pluralistic casuistry of Baruch Brody

The preceding approaches are those many bioethicists have found most helpful with the possible exception of the 'pluralistic casuistry' of Baruch Brody (Brody, 1988). He calls the approach 'casuistry', and perhaps it is case-based in the sense that the particulars of the case determine the principles to be applied to it, but it is otherwise a principled approach as I understand it. In any event, I believe the 'pluralistic' aspect to be the most important, for Brody relies on five different moral appeals: 'the appeal to the consequences of our actions, to rights, to respect for persons, to the virtues, and to cost-effectiveness and justice'. He applies whichever of these appeals or whichever combination of them is most helpful in the given case.

Other approaches

There are still other approaches to ethical problems, some of which are worthy of mention. A *common sense approach* is based on 'intuition', which is, of course, culturally as well as individually determined. The intuitive approach is more 'instinctive' and less cognitive than the *prudential reasoning approach*, which is based on experience and reasoned judgment about what promotes the good of self and of community (an approach that might be attributed to Aristotle and Thomas Aquinas). An *institutional approach* is one in which the values and mission of an institution (for example, a religious hospital) determine its policies. A *professional approach* is one in which professional standards, codes, and oaths guide conduct. The oath of Hippocrates, the prayer of Moses Maimonides, and the periodic iterations of the Code of the American Medical Association (beginning in 1847 and most recently that of 1998–1999 (Council on Ethical and Judicial affairs, 1998)) are the best known to American physicians (Reich, 1995). Virtually all of the health care professions have such codes and standards.

The *economic approach* is one many physicians and patients fear has taken control of the practice of medicine in the guise of concern for maximizing quality care. At one time bioethicists accepted economic concerns as morally relevant in decisions about patient care only when the patient him- or herself was concerned about the cost of health care. For example, in an article written in 1984 Levinsky posited that the doctor can have but one master, the patient, and must advocate only for the patient. Now most physicians take as axiomatic a second responsibility to others whether that be to society in general, to a national health insurance program, to the health maintenance organization or medical group for whom they work or with whom they contract, or to third-party payers. The dominant allegiance remains that to patients, as evident from data concerning physician advocacy for patients that leads them to misrepresent the patients' symptoms or conditions in order to obtain health insurance benefits for those patiente (albeit at times also to ensure payment of the physicians as well) (Bloche, 2000; Freeman et al., 1999; Novack et al., 1989; Ubel, 1999, Webster, 1999; Wynia et al., 2000).

Finally, the *legalistic approach*. If one believes that laws are ethical precepts that are so widely accepted as to be legislated, codified, adjudicated or written as regulatory policy, then this approach can be listed amongst ethical approaches. However, it should be noted that legal or legalistic approaches are minimalist whereas ethical approaches by and large are maximalist or aspirational.

A case example

To illustrate the application of several of these approaches, I will present the case of Jill, who was discovered to have proteinuria at age 18, hypertension at age 20, and mild renal insufficiency at age 22. At age 24 her serum creatinine was 2.5 and she was referred to me for nephrologic evaluation. Her disease progressed to end-stage renal failure.

The patient was thought to have undiagnosable renal disease initially following radiographic, sonographic, and histologic study. Years later, following a second failed renal transplant, subependymal calcifications were discovered in the brain, which were thought diagnostic of tuberous sclerosis (TS). TS may be hereditary, but there is statistically a 40% chance that it may arise *de novo* by gene mutation. If hereditary it might explain renal disease and hypertension discovered in the patient's father and perhaps the red cell casts (without clinical renal disease) in her HLA identical sister, as well as the renal disease of the patient herself. No one in the family had other evidence of TS. If hereditary, since the disease can be an autosomal dominant, the patient's sisters would have a 50–50 chance of the disease and if either was positive, their children would also have a 50–50 chance of the disease. Therefore, we recommended informing the patient's sisters and their pediatricians of the possibility of a hereditary disorder, recognizing the nieces and nephews could be at risk of grand mal seizures and mental retardation as well as of kidney and lung disease if the disease was hereditary. The patient's father felt that this would unnecessarily alarm his children and their families, and adamantly insisted even after repeated discussions that we should not even inform the pediatricians of his five grandchildren. When, after an ethics committee discussion (to which the patient and her father were invited but elected not to attend), I informed the patient and her father that I would inform her sisters, the father threatened a lawsuit.

To simplify discussion we will consider the primary stakeholders as the patient, her nieces and nephews, her father, and the physician. The precise values of the various stakeholders were never clearly elucidated, and some relevant concerns may have been subconscious. The patient hoped that none of her family would develop the problems of health she had suffered, but she may also have feared that her sisters would blame her if they and their children had the same condition. Similarly, her father could not have avoided feeling guilty if it were determined that his genes had caused Jill's renal disease and especially if he were to learn of a similar, albeit latent, condition in his other daughters or grandchildren. With regard to the moral question under deliberation, the primary stakeholders in my opinion were the nieces and nephews, more so than the sisters who were now older than my patient when her renal disease became evident and yet remained clinically healthy. The young children could have severe TS even though there were no obvious manifestations. They might benefit from increased scrutiny and earlier diagnosis if their pediatricians were alerted to the possibility.

I felt an obligation to inform the sisters of the possibility of autosomal dominant inheritance. The options were few: tell, delay telling, don't tell. Surely no one would suggest don't tell if asked. Obviously this is an oversimplification since how one tells may be as important as whether or not one tells.

Now the ethical approaches: Utility holds that the consequences of telling or not telling will determine the good and bad, right or wrong. The consequences for the sisters and the nieces and nephews obviously depend on whether or not they had inherited TS. If they had not, the consequence of telling could be worrying that they had.

Deontology—the ethics of obligation—informs the physician he not only should, but must tell, albeit with full disclosure (that Jill's TS could be a genetic mutation in her, that even if it were hereditary, the sisters have only a 50–50 chance, and their children the same but only if the sisters have TS) and with compassion and care not to unduly frighten the sisters.

The principle-based approach is arguable. Which principles take precedence? For example, non-maleficence or autonomy and if the latter, whose autonomy? Ross's theory suggests the principles are only prima facie applicable, but how does one choose? By initution? I, as a physician, concluded harm to the children (if they had TS but neither they nor their parents nor their pediatricians knew it) was the priority concern. I believe the patient also thought so initially, as for a brief period she agreed with me, but she changed her mind after her father objected, and she never spoke her mind clearly thereafter. And surely the father may have been concerned not only about feeling guilty but quite possibly for fear his relationship with his daughters would be harmed. But the relationships might well be harmed either way (whether he allowed us to tell or refused to allow us to do so).

If we consider autonomy, whose autonomy counts: the patient's, her father's, the nephrologist's? And if we speak of respect for persons (rather than the derivative, autonomy), what about respect for the rights and integrity of the sisters and their children?

Other principles also might be considered: for example, the right to confidentiality of the patient and especially of her father whom I know felt his rights would be violated if I told his daughters or their pediatricians. And what about truth telling? Wasn't that my obligation? I thought also of the golden rule. I knew what I would want if I were one of the sisters, nieces, or nephews, but apparently that was not what the father or even my patient wanted.

Casuistry reminds us to consider the context (family tragedies: my patient's renal failure and its complications and her mother's death from leukemia) and the particulars. The grounds or facts we have already reviewed, but what about paradigm cases? We have already mentioned the utilitarian alternatives, which are obvious, but which is the actual case (inherited disease in the family or mutant gene in my patient only)? What are the applicable maxims? People have the right to know about the possibility of inherited disease, but they also have the right not to know! Or is the relevant maxim, do not stand on principle when someone will sue you for it, or is it, do not give in to unethical threats? In this case I do not find conventional casuistry helpful, nor does it really make me modify my interpretation of the relevant bioethical principles through reflective equilibrium. However, my considered moral judgment in this case made me wish to apply my moral principles with some flexibility or at least with compassion for the different perspectives of different stakeholders, none of whom I disrespected or felt was purposely selfish.

On the other hand the pluralistic casuistry of Baruch Brody is helpful in that it allows analyses of the case from five different moral appeals: consequences (which we have discussed), rights (and rights of the children or of their parents to know imposes an obligation on me, the physician), respect for persons (and I believe respect for the children and their parents outweighs respect for the father), virtues (again I intuitively find honesty outweighs compassion for the father) and cost-effectiveness and justice (which I believe are applicable in a non-economic sense). It could prove very costly (again non-economically) if one of the nieces or nephews had a seizure and died for lack of pediatrician awareness of TS.

One other approach is worth exploring: relational ethics or the ethics of care. From my perspective my primary obligation was to my patient for whom I had cared for 12 years. However, she was not telling me in any detail what she really wanted me to do. I think she was inordinately afraid of hurting her father's feelings if she agreed with me (as she did initially when only she and not her father knew of the problem) and thus she just sat and listened to my debate with him. But this could be rationalization on my part. Furthermore, I had medically evaluated the father and my patient's two sisters, and thus I had a fiduciary, physician-patient responsibility to each of them. How could I show respect to the father and meet my sense of moral responsibility to his daughters and their children?

Finally, we should mention the legalistic approach: I have little doubt that a judge or jury would agree that the nieces and nephews should be protected, and thus that their parents or pediatricians should be told of the possibility that tuberous sclerosis is an inherited disorder in this family. On the other hand if the father were to sue me it would be an inconvenience and take my time that could be better spent in patient care. His threats to sue if I told were not sufficient for me to yield or give up my principles but they did cause me to continue dialogue far beyond what I thought would be effective. At the eleventh hour it suddenly occurred to me to ask, 'What if Jill were to tell her sisters rather than my doing so?' Indeed this was a never-earlier-considered option that solved the dispute. Jill's father said that would be 'okay' with him!

Selected concepts

There are concepts in ethics, familiar to philosophers but often not to physicians, whose understanding is helpful in evaluating relevant circumstances of patients. Several, which are not described elsewhere in this chapter, are defined here.

Affirmative defense

An affirmative defense is a fact or finding that defends against or mitigates the seriousness of a charge. For example, self-defense is usually an effective affirmative defense against a charge of murder. Other affirmative defenses include temporary insanity, coercion, and intoxication (Black, 1991). The affirmative defense is suggested as an alternative to the legalization of euthanasia or physician-assisted suicide (Tulsky *et al.*, 1996). Thus, if certain safeguards are followed (as is true for euthanasia in the Netherlands), Tulsky *et al.* suggest allowing the patient's prolonged and otherwise untreatable suffering to be an affirmative defense for a physician against a charge of assisted suicide.

Death determined by neurologic criteria

This is often called 'brain death' but the more complex term is preferable because so often the term 'brain death' suggests to patients' loved ones that the patient herself is not really dead. In any event, if criteria for death of the brainstem (for example, a compatible neurologic examination and failure of an apnea test), as well as of the cerebral cortex are met, death may be pronounced. Unfortunately, to the non-medical person the concept is counterintuitive since the patient is warm and appears alive albeit in a coma and on a ventilator. In addition, there is a concern that patients might be pronounced dead by neurologic criteria in order to procure organs for transplantation. Hopefully they are never pronounced dead if they are not, but pronouncing death despite continued effective cardiac function (which preserves organs for transplantation) can be misinterpreted. Thus, to avoid such perception, unless family members ask about the possibility of donating organs, transplantation should not be discussed until the patient has been pronounced dead and the rationale of neurologic death thoroughly explained to the patient's family.

Double agency

This is the concept of divided loyalty; that is, of the conflict between one's obligation to a patient and one's obligation to a third party, whether that be to the patient's family, to a provider of the patient's health insurance, to the physician's own employer or contractor, or to the physician's family.

Double effect

The rule or doctrine of double effect is that which permits acts with adverse effects so long as they are only foreseen and not intended. It is often attributed to St Thomas Aquinas but predates him, though he may have clarified the concepts involved. Acts may have bad as well as good effects, and are justified if the good effect is the one intended, if the good effect is not achieved by the bad effect, and if the good effect outweighs the bad effect (and justifies it, should the bad effect supervene). The usual example is pain relief and ventilatory depression due to morphine. One knows that the morphine administration is ethical under the rule of double effect if the rate of administration is no longer increased once the patient's pain is relieved.

Passive euthanasia

Passive euthanasia is 'allowing to die'; that is, withholding or withdrawing life-sustaining therapy to allow a patient to die of the underlying condition. The term has fallen into disfavor because the term euthanasia is increasingly reserved for compassionate, deliberate, active termination of life of a person who is suffering uncontrollably, usually one who has a terminal or severe and irreversible ailment. Terms such as allowing to die, forgoing or withdrawing treatment are more commonly used nowadays.

Paternalism

This is literally acting toward someone, such as a patient, as if one were the individual's father. Parentalism is a gender-neutral term. Although, this is an infringement of the person's rights if he or she is competent, we accept parentalism if: (1) the patient is not an adult (even if competent!); (2) the patient waives the right to self-determination; (3) the patient's condition is truly an emergency; (4) the patient is likely to be seriously and irreparably harmed (for example, loss of limb, sight or life); and (5) the patient's illness (for example, emotional or mental illness) itself precludes rational decision making (though one should then appreciate that the patient is not competent).

Ethicists distinguish 'weak paternalism', in which one infringes the patient's rights during temporary decisional incapacity or pending determination that a patient has capacity, from 'strong paternalism' in which one overrides the patient's voluntary, informed, competent decisions (with benevolent motivation, of course).

Therapeutic privilege or therapeutic exception

This concept, that a physician may withhold information from a patient because the physician believes it would be harmful (for example, to a depressed, anxious or emotionally unstable patient) is rapidly falling out of favor. Whereas it was once widely accepted (as it still as in some countries), a physician in the United States would be hard pressed to defend withholding information, even of a lethal condition, from a competent patient. Similarly the deceptive use of placebos is no longer acceptable except in research studies (where its use is consented to, though the patient and often the investigators are blinded from knowledge whether the patient is getting placebo or active drug).

Ulysses contract

In Homer's *Odyssey* Ulysses commands his men (whose ears he has plugged with wax) to strap him to the mast of his ship so he would not be lured by the irresistible singing of sirens to the lethal whirlpool of the Sicilian sea between Scylla and Charybdis, the redoubtable monsters. Thus, a Ulysses contract is a patient's voluntary commitment to be forceably treated at a future time when she may be mentally ill and would then refuse treatment.

Philosophical distinctions

One of the challenges of ethical practice and assisting patients to make normative decisions is to think clearly. As elegantly described by Ahronheim, Moreno, and Zuckerman (2000), philosophical distinctions need to be logically valid ('capable of sorting actions into two different groups without ambiguity') and morally relevant ('one of the sorts of [i.e., groups of] actions it identifies is morally justifiable while the other is not'). They discuss in detail 'four sets of distinctions that are commonly used in discussions of clinical ethics'. Their analyses are summarized below.

Passive–active distinction

The passive–active or omission–commission distinction is not valid logically because there may be ambiguity in sorting actions into one group or the other. Ahronheim, Moreno, and Zuckerman (2000) give an example: the physician holds a meeting to decide whether or not to forgo life-sustaining treatment. Is this passive or active? Furthermore, the distinction is irrelevant morally because as James Rachels (1975) has pointed out it might be worse (less compassionate) to let the person suffer after omitting life-sustaining treatment than to assist death.

Extraordinary–ordinary distinction

This distinction is also that of non-obligatory–obligatory, optimal–non-optimal, or heroic–non-heroic treatments. It is invalid logically because what is ordinary or customary treatment (that is, the so-called 'standard of care') changes from time to time, sometimes rapidly. Also, the distinction is morally irrelevant because what is ordinarily done may not be what should be done in a given case. Furthermore, I believe this distinction places the emphasis on the treatment, which is relatively unimportant, rather than on the patient who is all-important.

Withholding–withdrawing distinction

This distinction is of uncertain validity logically because it may be difficult to clearly separate acts into the two groups. For example, is it withholding or withdrawing therapy not to give a second course of chemotherapy or not to ventilate a patient manually when there is a power failure which stops a mechanical ventilator? Ahronehim Moreno, and Zuckerman (2000) go on to say the distinction is irrelevant morally if a treatment would not be effective because it is no worse to withdraw an ineffective treatment than to withhold it. On the other hand, it would be relevant morally if an effective treatment were not tried because the patient and physician were not certain it would be effective and would not try it because they believed it wrong to stop a treatment once initiated. Furthermore, the distinction is morally relevant for an Orthodox Jew who is not yet a goses (not yet within 72 hours of death) because the Orthodox believe one can withdraw a treatment or a hindrance to dying only in the final three days of life. Though ethicists and legal scholars generally disagree with the following formulation, if one believes that moral distress is morally relevant and if the patient and physician would be distressed if a treatment was withdrawn (but not if it was withheld) one could say there is a morally relevant preference for withholding treatment. On the other hand, one could say just the reverse, that it is better—more virtuous— to withdraw treatment than to withhold it, because if it is withheld the patient will never know if it would have improved him or her sufficiently that he or she would have wanted it.

Daniel Sulmasy (responding to questions I asked him at a National Kidney Foundation national meeting in the mid-1990s) has suggested other scenarios in which it is morally reprehensible to withdraw therapy. Suppose there is but one bed in the intensive care unit (ICU). If two patients present simultaneously, one with a 30% chance of benefiting from the ICU, the other with a 70% chance, one admits the latter patient. However, if the 30% benefit patient presented first and were admitted to the ICU one would not discharge him from the ICU the next day when the 70% patient presented (even though a physician-director of the ICU might have the moral responsibility to do so).

Letting die-killing distinction

This distinction is usually valid logically. However, the case of assisted suicide is unclear since the physician does not perform the lethal act even though he clearly enables the patient to do so. The distinction is relevant morally (even though in a given case it might be preferable 'for a dying patient to be killed voluntarily rather than to undergo prolonged suffering') because permitting euthanasia by policy lessens respect for life and risks abuse. Note this is a distinction between an act and a rule.

The United States Supreme Court in 1997 allowed states to permit or to ban assisted suicide and held there is no constitutional right to assistance in dying. Nevertheless it held that the distinction between withdrawing life-sustaining treatment and providing assistance with suicide is 'a distinction widely recognized and endorsed in the medical profession and in our legal tradition' (Compassan in Dying v Washington, 1996, and Vacco v Quill, 1997).

Selected ethical issues in clinical practice

In this section, I review several issues that arise frequently in the practice of medicine from an ethical perspective. These are: informed consent and decision making, advance directives, discontinuation of therapy, and futility. Some of these topics are also discussed from a specific nephrological perspective in Chapter 3 by Dickens and Chapter 6 by Bowman and Singer. I do not review the care of 'difficult' patients, which is discussed in Chapter 4 by Friedman and Chapter 5 by Levinsky. I have also reviewed this topic elsewhere (Miller, 1999).

The goals of medicine, for the care of individual patients, are:

(1) promote health and prevent disease (in other words, teach patients about health and illness);
(2) maintain or restore health and prevent or cure illness;
(3) prevent suffering and relieve pain and other symptoms (anticipate and palliate);
(4) reduce impairment and restore function (rehabilitation);
(5) preserve the quality as well as the extent of life;
(6) meet personal, psychological, and spiritual needs;
(7) prepare for death and recognize and ease dying;
(8) provide respect, comfort, care, and hope always.

Key questions of medicine, ethics, and health policy include:

(1) medical questions for physicians:
    (a) What is wrong?
    (b) What can be done?
(2) ethical (value) questions for patients:
    (a) What should be done?
    (b) Who should decide?
    (c) On what basis?
(3) policy (allocation) questions for society:
    (a) What interventions will not be provided?
    (b) What patients or conditions will not be covered by the health care financing and delivery system?
    (c) Are we individually and collectively—for the common good—willing to forego interventions that provide personal but only marginal benefit?
    (d) Should every nation provide universal access to basic health care?

The essential steps to review the ethical problems of a patient and/or the patient care team are:

1. Review the medical facts: diagnosis or condition, prognosis, degree of certainty of diagnosis and prognosis, treatment options (and their risks, benefits, and expected outcomes), and the patient's capacity for decision making. If the patient lacks decisional capacity, determine the appropriate surrogate and ascertain whether or not the patient has completed an advance directive (or has made explicit statements) regarding preferences for proxies and/or for treatment.
2. Elicit the values, beliefs, preferences, and concerns of the patient, family (including significant others), physician, other health care professionals and the institution—but first and foremost those of the patient.
3. Identify the conflict(s) of values or of principles; that is, identify the ethical problems or dilemma(s). Also, discern relevant social, legal, and economic issues.
4. Consider the benefits and burdens of all ethically acceptable solutions: rank and communicate them for consideration by the attending physician, the patient, and concerned others.

Decision making

Decisional capacity in common parlance is competence. However, technically competence can be determined only by a court whereas decisional capacity is a determination that any physician is entitled to make.

The three components for truly informed and valid consent are: (1) the threshold component, decision-making capacity; (2) information components, disclosure of information and understanding of information; and (3) consent components, voluntariness of choice and voluntary, uncoerced authorization or refusal of treatment. Competent, voluntary, valid informed decision making requires:

- freedom from duress or from coercion;
- recognition of one's values and goals;
- receipt of adequate medical information (it is wise to ask the patient what he or she heard);
- ability to understand it (also ask what he or she understood);
- ability to reason about options and their consequences;
- ability and willingness to communicate and explain the decision (this is desirable, but not required);
- in addition the decision should be stable over time and authentic (that is consistent with the patient's values and goals).

Ethical disclosure for informed consent or refusal, in other words the medical information required for informed decisions, includes:

- the nature of the patient's condition (that is, of the ailment, illness, or injury);
- expected consequences of the illness (that is, the prognosis and its degree of certainty);
- the consequences of forgoing therapy;
- the nature of the proposed treatment (or intervention) and its purpose;
- the probability of success of the treatment, and the risks and benefits of the intervention;
- alternative treatments (or interventions) and likely outcomes, risks, and benefits;
- the risk of unfortunate results (from the proposed and alternative treatments);
- the chance of unforeseen conditions within the body;
- any conflict of interest of the physician, hospital, or health maintenance organization;
- the patient's right to ask questions or to seek second opinions without prejudice to her care.

Informed consent is much easier said than done. There are many constraints on patient comprehension in informed consent. These include: inadequate information; excessive information (information overload); unexplained information; irrelevant information; distorted information; the use of technical jargon; irrationality or immaturity of the patient; fear or other controlling influences; and coercion or manipulation by the health care professional or others.

Furthermore, there are circumstances under which intentional non-disclosure may be appropriate, for example when:

- there is an emergency circumstance and delay to obtain informed consent might occasion loss of life, limb, or sight;
- the patient prefers to waive the right of informed consent. (Should a physician ever force information on a patient?);
- the patient requests coercive treatment in advance of its need because the patient fears he or she will change his or her mind inappropriately (the Ulysses Contract);
- to disclose would be harmful to the patient psychologically (such withholding of information is allegedly justified as 'therapeutic privilege'); and
- a placebo is used. Placebo therapy is purposeful deception of the patient in using an agent that is believed by the physician not to be effective (other than by way of belief on the part of the patient that it would be effective) but believed by the patient to be effective. In the past the use of placebo medication or placebo statements was thought acceptable: as Socrates stated, physicians need to be aware of the 'healing effects of fair words'; and as Plato said 'Physicians employ lies for good and noble purposes'; Hippocrates stated a patient would think a physician the worst doctor in the world 'if he does not promise to cure what is curable and to cure what is incurable'. Today, however, we believe one should have the patient's consent, in advance, if placebo medication is to be used therapeutically just as we require informed consent for a placebo-controlled clinical trial.

Capacity to make health care decisions and incapacity

Decision-making capacity is an ethical or common sense concept regarding a patient's ability to make decisions regarding his or her health care. It can be assessed by medical personnel and does not require a court hearing. It is defined in the State of California Probate Code (Section 4609) as 'a patient's ability to understand the nature and consequences of proposed health care (including its significant benefits, risks, and alternatives) and to make and communicate a health care decision.'

Thus decision-making capacity is the ability to: understand one's medical condition; appreciate the benefits and burdens of treatment options or of forgoing treatment; reason and deliberate about these options; make decisions consistent with one's values, preferences, and goals; and communicate one's decisions.

In contrast to 'decisional capacity', 'competence' is a legal term, and technically a patient is competent until a court determines otherwise. Indeed, the California Probate Code (Section 810) states 'there shall exist a rebuttable presumption affecting the burden of proof that all persons have the capacity to make decisions . . . A judicial determination that a person . . . lacks capacity . . . should be based on evidence of a deficit . . . rather than on a diagnosis of a person's mental or physical disorder.'

Decisional incapacity may be: complete (global) or partial (that is, task-specific); temporary or fluctuating or permanent; certain or probable or possible or unlikely. It is customarily determined by the patient's attending physician, although it may be wise to consult a neurologist or psychiatrist if dementia or depression are not easily excluded. Whenever he or she is uncertain about a patient's decisional capacity, it is also wise for the responsible physician to ask other members of the health care team and members of the patient's family or friends if the patient is his or her usual self and is capable of making decisions. Asking the patient open-ended questions often is revealing.

Criteria for lack of decisional capacity are:

- inability to understand disclosed information;
- inability to understand one's situation and relevantly similar situations;
- inability to analyze risks and benefits;
- inability to state a preference or to make a choice or decision;
- inability to give a reason for the preference or choice; and
- inability to make a reasonable decision; that is, a decision most reasonable persons would make under the same or similar circumstances.

To be sure, there are a number of pitfalls in assessing decisional capacity. These include: belief that a patient is incompetent just because he or she disagrees with the physician's recommendation; belief that failure on a mental status exam is evidence of global incompetence; and belief that a psychiatric diagnosis is evidence of incompetence. Furthermore, critical illness and/or medication may impair decisional capacity, as can simply being informed of a serious or especially a lethal diagnosis.

In the assessment of decisional capacity, it is often wise specifically and explicitly to consider whether the patient might have depression or dementia (cognitive impairment). Further discussion of such assessment is beyond the scope of this chapter but in the new clinical practice guideline of the Renal Physicians Association and the American Society of Nephrology on Shared Decision-making in the Appropriate Initiation of and Withdrawal from Dialysis (RPA and ASN Working Group 2000) there is a 'toolkit for assessing or documenting decision-making capacity, depression, mental status, advance directives, prognosis and quality of life'.

Preparing for the care of patients who might lose decisional capacity

It is better to prevent a problem than to treat it. Our concern is to avoid the circumstance in which we don't know what the patient who has become decisionally incapacitated would want under the present circumstances because we never took the time to discuss such hypotheticals. A good preventive technique is to know the patient well: to know the patient's goals, values, beliefs, and concerns, which often allows one to predict what the patient would want. This is called 'substituted judgment': judging what the patient would want in a given circumstance without having discussed the specific circumstance with the patient. One can have an even higher level of confidence in making decisions for a decisionally incapacitated person if one has reviewed the precise or very similar circumstances in a hypothetical scenario to which the patient made an explicit statement.

The values history

I wish to recommend including values questions in every medical history. Collectively such questions comprise a 'values history', a term first used by Joan McIver Gibson, PhD of the University of New Mexico when studying the training necessary for public guardians of patients who have no surrogates (Gibson, 1990). Many of the questions that follow were suggested by Dr Gibson.

What are your thoughts about: life in general? independence and control? health and illness? doctors and hospitals? disability and nursing home care, home care, hospice? death and dying? resuscitation? an afterlife?

If you were to develop a serious illness, what would you want to know? Your diagnosis? Your prognosis? Your treatment options? What would you want us to tell your family? Your referring physician? Anyone else? Under several circumstances that you might imagine could befall you, what would be your wishes regarding: hospitalization? nursing home care? home care? hospice? artificial ventilation (use of a breathing maching)? cardiopulmonary resuscitation (CPR)? enteral (tube feeding) or parenteral (intravenous) nutrition and hydration? transfusion? dialysis (use of an artificial kidney)? organ transplantation? surgery of various sorts (for example, amputation)? organ or tissue donation after your death? autopsy? funeral? euology? obituary?

What conditions are so unacceptable to you that, if you developed a life-threatening condition you would prefer not to be treated?

Whom would you want to make decisions for you should you ever be unable to make decisions for yourself? If different members of your family have different recommendations for your treatment, whose decisions should guide us in your care? Do you have: an advance directive? a living will? a durable power of attorney for health care (DPAHC)?. If you have a proxy directive or DPAHC: may we meet with your surrogate or health care agent to discuss your preferences? What is your surrogate's name, phone, address? An alternate's? If your surrogate and your physician believed that what you had indicated in an advance directive was not in your best interest, should they override it?

Where would you wish to be cared for if you were terminally ill? What does your medical insurance cover? And not cover? Do you have medical financial concerns?

Questions suggested by Lo, Quill, and Tulsky (1999) include: What are your expectations? What are your fears? What are your hopes? What is the best and worst that might happen? What matters the most to you? What do you want to accomplish before you die? How do you want your children and grandchildren to remember you? These authors also advised: 'Physicians naturally want to reassure patients. However, reassurance may deter patients from disclosing their concerns and emotions . . . In addition, offering reassurance prematurely before fully understanding patients' concerns, may paradoxically increase their worry . . .'

All of the above questions are recommended to be asked in every routine, thorough medical history where one will become the patient's primary physician in order to better know the patient and his or her values and concerns in order to help guide shared decision making *with* the competent patient or *for* an incompetent patient should he or she have lost decisional capacity. Realistically, these questions will need to be spread over a number of visits but they should be asked early to avoid the possibility of never having the opportunity because of unexpected loss of decision-making capacity.

Advance directives

The routine values history by the primary care physician (which of course is the nephrologist for many patients and most particularly for all those with end-stage renal disease) is strongly advised but not often accomplished, at least to the extent that would be truly helpful should the patient develop a life-threatening condition at a time when he or she no longer had decisional capacity.

Even when a values history has been obtained, and certainly if it has not been, it is wise to recommend to all patients that they have an advance directive. This is absolutely crucial for patients who do not have a surrogate or proxy, of particular importance for patients with end-stage renal disease, but truly wise for every patient as encouraged but not required in the United States by the Patient Self-Determination Act of 1990 (PSDA, 1990; Wolf *et al.*, 1991).

Advance care planning is the process of a patient's effective communication (in advance of possible loss of decision-making capacity) with the physician, chosen surrogate, and family regarding his or her preferences for a surrogate and for future medical care. This may include a formal written advance directive and—whether formal or informal—the process should be flexible and repeated periodically (Emanuel, 1991; Sehgal *et al.*, 1992).

In advance planning, the physician should:

- anticipate incapacity and recommend detailed discussion between the physician, patient, and surrogate;
- get to know the patient as person and his or her values; ask whom he or she would wish as a proxy (surrogate decision maker);
- establish trust and obtain the confidence of the surrogate as well as of the patient;
- discuss the goals the patient would want for treatment;
- review current treatment in view of the goals for treatment;
- when uncertain, consider a time-limited trial of treatment; and
- when treatment should be limited, avoid inducing guilt: make a firm recommendation to limit treatment (rather than asking if it should be limited).

An advance directive may be: durable such as a living will or a durable power of attorney for health care, or non-durable such as a Do-Not-Attempt-Resuscitation (DNAR) order written in the hospital. Many jurisdictions now permit a durable prehospital DNAR, which may cover patients at home or in a long-term care facility as well as in transit to a hospital.

Durable advance directives are of two types: one is an instructional directive, which is a statement (such as a living will) made in advance to guide the nature, extent, and intensity of care in the event decisional incapacity develops. Often the intent is to limit care but this need not be the case: one can also request care in an advance directive. The second is a proxy directive (such as a DPAHC), which is a statement made in advance to indicate who should make medical decisions in the event that incapacity develops.

Decision making for decisionally incapacitated patients

The three ethical and legal bases for decisions for decisionally incapacitated patients are, in descending order of preference:

1 Explicit statements (of the now-incapacitated individual) made previously when he or she had capacity.
2 Substituted judgment: judgment based on knowledge of the patient's values and beliefs. Substituted judgment is sometimes called the 'subjective test' for determining appropriate care of the patient.
3 Best interests: judgments as to what would be best for the patient in the absence of knowledge of the patient's preferences or relevant values. The best interests judgment is sometimes called the 'objective test' for determining the patient's care.

Children

Ahronheim, Moreno, and Zuckerman (2000) in their text, *Ethics in Clinical Practice*, state 'until about age 9, most children are unable to conceptualize disease ... Many early adolescents, up to around age 15, are unable to identify a preference that is not unduly influenced by some authority figure. Thus, while the cognitive ability to comprehend the "information" necessary for informed consent may be present, the emotional capacity for voluntary choice is ordinarily not available until later.'

Thus, parents are the presumed surrogate decision makers for children and non-emancipated adolescents. They have extensive but not absolute moral and legal authority. They can be disqualified if their decisions are not in the best interests of the child. Sometimes, understandably, parents consider the interests of other children and of themselves. Although the impact of decisions on parents and siblings is not irrelevant (since it may affect the welfare of the patient), the best interest of the child (even if foster home placement were to be necessary) limits parental discretion.

The surrogate hierarchy

In some jurisdictions a surrogate hierarchy is established by legislation. In others the surrogate hierarchy is dependent on case law and common law tradition. In most cases, precedence is given to an agent named in an advance directive or to a legally appointed conservator or guardian *ad litem*. A general durable power of attorney may or may not allow an agent to make health care decisions, though the DPAHC always does. Next in line is the spouse (and in some states, a domestic partner) followed by adult children, parents, siblings. Some states then allow persons who are not relatives but have had significant involvement with the person (for example, caretakers, those with caring relationships, etc.) to participate in health care decisions. Morally valid surrogates are those who have had significant involvement with the patient, have knowledge of the patient's values, are willing to express the patients' values or wishes, and have no emotional or other conflict of interest.

In bygone days when physicians were generally trusted implicitly, physicians customarily made decisions for incapacitated patients (particularly indigent patients) without surrogates. In the past several decades, except in emergency circumstances, physicians in the United States have no longer been allowed to make unilateral decisions, and surrogate decision makers have been thought mandatory for patients without surrogates. In most jurisdictions this requires legal intervention, and decisions by judges are sometimes made after no more than a telephone discussion. Although courts often expedite decision making (usually by appointing a guardian or conservator, sometimes however without authority to refuse treatment as well as to consent to it), the process is cumbersome and, many believe, flawed.

In New York State in two institutions for mentally handicapped children, committees of hospital professionals were allowed by temporary statute to make health care decisions. The experiment was judged a success, and the legislation was renewed. In some other jurisdictions, as in California nursing homes but not acute care hospitals, professional committees are similarly empowered. This remains a highly controversial approach.

Forgoing or limiting treatment

This is a constitutional right in the United States. The 1990 Cruzan decision of the US Supreme Court held that: the right does not require a terminal condition; the right survives the development of incompetence; the right may be exercised by a surrogate; artificial nutrition and hydration may be refused like any other treatment; but the State may require clear and convincing evidence of the individual's intentions (Crusan v Director, 1990).

Except in an emergency or when it would endanger another individual, a competent adult may refuse any treatment, at any time, at any place, for any reason (or for no reason). The individual need not be informed, be rational, or tell the reason and rationale. There are irrational reasons for treatment refusal (fear, delusion, depression) but if they invalidate refusal they do so by virtue of the impairment of decisional capacity (competence).

Conversely the 'Four P's' define the traditional interests of the State in: preservation of life, prevention of suicide, protection of innocent third parties, and preservation of the integrity of the medical profession. Even this latter tradition was upheld by the US Supreme Court in 1997 (Washington versus Glucksberg and Vacco versus Quill) when it held there is no constitutional right to physician-assisted suicide, though it also held that states may permit as well as prohibit assisted suicide.

Thus, a physician may forgo treatment if: it is refused by the patient, it is illegal, it is harmful (burdens substantially greater than benefits), or it is ineffective, non-beneficial, or 'futile' (a topic to be discussed separately), and—arguably—if it is too costly (at least if society or one's health insurance has decided not to pay and the patient is unable to pay).

The Los Angeles County Medical and County Bar in 1993 stated: 'The best interests of the patient do not require that life support be continued in all circumstances such as when the patient is terminally ill and suffering, or where there is no hope of recovery of cognitive function. Even a treatment which is only minimally painful or intrusive may be disproportionate to the potential benefits if the prognosis is virtually hopeless for any significant improvement in the patient's condition.'

Robert D. Orr, MD, Clinical Ethicist at Loma Linda University (personal communication, 1990) states that forgoing treatment falls into the following categories (see Table 2.1).

Table 2.1 The emotional consequences of forgoing treatment

Consequences are:	Less difficult	More difficult
If the treatment is:	complex expensive risky of marginal benefit or there is alternative treatment	simple available safe effective the only treatment
If the patient is:	elderly demented	young alert
Or if the disease is:	irreversible spontaneous	reversible iatrogenic

Withdrawing versus withholding treatment

Emotionally it is much more difficult for patients, families, physicians, and other health care professionals to withdraw than to withhold therapy, though both are less traumatic if the patient is suffering or is permanently unconscious. However, withholding and withdrawing are usually ethically and legally equivalent.

Withholding and withdrawing may not be equivalent when the patient does not know about the treatment and would wish the treatment. In that case, he or she cannot object to its being withheld. On the other hand, if the patient is told of the treatment or if it is tried and withdrawn, he or she can object. This view can be oversimplified by stating that it is more ethical to withdraw than to withhold treatment. However, there are some patients (and even some physicians) who believe once a treatment has been instituted it is unethical to withdraw it. It would be more appropriate to dissuade the individual from this belief than to withhold treatment without a trial when the benefit/burden calculus is marginal or uncertain. (Miller, 1992).

Even legally there may be differences: A physician might be guilty of abandonment if he or she withdraws from the care of a patient without adequate notice and arrangement for transfer, whereas she is free to choose which patients she accepts (if other care is reasonably available and the patient does not have an emergency).

Limiting as opposed to forgoing treatment

Clearly if patients have the right to refuse treatment, they have a right to limit it. However, the physician must be cautious if the patient's goals are not clear or if the patient's understanding of what various treatment options can or cannot achieve is not correct. In general the patient decides on the goals after receiving information and recommendations from the physician, but how best to achieve the goals is properly the physician's responsibility (albeit subject to acquiescence or approval or to a request for a second opinion by the patient). Limiting treatment is appropriate if that which is limited is unduly burdensome or if the treatment cannot achieve goals acceptable to the patient. Unfortunately patients often do not receive the limitation of treatment they desire (SUPPORT Principal Investigators, 1995).

The consensus of most people in the United States, of most religions, of bioethicists, and of the US Supreme Court is that competent adults have the right to refuse any treatment including life-sustaining treatment unless:

1 third parties, for example a fetus (or perhaps young children of a single parent), would be harmed;
2 the patient is mentally ill or emotionally distraught from an accident or because he or she was just informed of a serious prognosis (which would challenge the competence of the patient);
3 there is an emergency threat to life, limb or sight (for example, a ruptured aortic aneurysm) that precludes the informed consent process.

Medical futility

'Futile' therapy is therapy unlikely to achieve the goal of the physician ('most often') or the goal of the patient (preferably, unless the goal is unrealistic or improper). Some say the term, 'futile therapy' is an oxymoron: if futile, not therapeutic; if therapeutic, not futile. Others find the term pejorative or conclusory. Although Lantos and colleagues introduced the concept in an article about CPR in neonates (1988) and defined medical futility (1989) clearly, it was Schneiderman, Jecker, and Jonsen (1990) who brought such attention to the issue that it has been on the bioethical agenda ever since. Lantos *et al.* (1989) said, 'Decisions to withhold therapy that is deemed futile, like all treatment choices, must follow (1) judgement about the chance of success of a therapy, and (2) consideration of the patient's goals for therapy.' Schneiderman, Jecker, and Jonsen (1990) defined futility as therapy that fails to improve the person as a whole, therapy that was useless in the last 100 cases, or therapy that merely prolongs the life of a permanently unconscious person. Furthermore, they suggest treatment is futile if the patient can survive only in an intensive care unit. They are very careful to point out, however, that 'our' notion of futility does not come from considerations of scarce resources. Arguments for limiting treatments on grounds of resource allocation should proceed by an entirely different route and with great caution in our open system of medical care.'

From a pragmatic standpoint, there are three senses of 'futile':

1. useless—for example, an antibacterial drug for a viral illness,
2. unlikely to succeed—for example, CPR for a person with multiorgan system failure,
3. not worth it—either because it is expensive despite little chance of benefit or because the non-economic burdens outweigh the benefits.

The topic of futility is discussed at length in an anthology of Zucker and Zucker (1997).

The concept of futility has had great appeal among physicians because it wrests back some of the decisional authority and power (or physician autonomy) lost in the worship of patient autonomy brought about by the bioethics movement. There are three practical implications of a judgment or determination that a treatment is 'futile': the physician is not obligated to offer it; the physician may withhold or withdraw it; the physician is not obligated to discuss it unless the patient asks. Some even hold that the physician is obligated to withhold or withdraw therapy that is judged to be futile even if the patient does not ask. But beware: a determination of futility may hide paternalism, social prejudice and discrimination, or a resource allocation decision.

Nevertheless, as Schneiderman has argued, the concept of futility does have heuristic value:

- It encourages clarity of thought: that is, it requires defining the goal of therapy (from the patient's point of view and perhaps from the physician's perspective as well) and the probability of achieving the goal (a judgment to be made by the physician, perhaps confirmed by a consultant).
- It distinguishes gatekeeping (omitting treatment of no or only marginal benefit) from rationing (omitting a beneficial treatment that society has decided not to provide or not to reimburse).
- It encourages publication of scientific studies showing negative as well as positive therapeutic outcomes.
- It allows futile treatment to be offered only as an experiment, with Institutional Review Board (IRB) approval, and with the subject's consent.
- It recognizes that patients do not have entitlement or a right to unproven therapy on the grounds that their illness is serious, and that the requested therapy has not been proven ineffective or dangerous, and that no therapy of proven benefit is available.

Compassion is an acceptable response to some requests for 'futile' interventions. The classical example is to temporarily continue mechanical ventilation of a dying patient pending the arrival of a relative from out of town. Ahronheim, Moreno, and Zuckerman (2000) go further, stating, 'Beneficence often requires a more flexible view of the physician's response to [a request for a futile intervention] particularly when patients are gravely ill. It is entirely appropriate to provide interventions that will not affect the underlying condition but will provide comfort, even if . . . only the patient's loved ones are those comforted.' Kate Christensen (1998, in a discussion of Developing Standards of Practice at a conference held by Lawrence Schneiderman at the University of California, San Diego, February 20, 1998) notes that hospital futility policies may increase, not decrease, conflict. She and I both believe that occasional irresolvable cases may be the price we must pay to respect the diversity of our society's values and to maintain the public trust.

Resources for assistance with ethical problems

There are many resources to assist the ethically uncertain or conflicted clinician, some of which are available to patients and their families as well. One may begin with a literature search and reference to journals and books (Council on Ethical and Judicial Affairs 1998; Dunn *et al*; 1994; Siegler *et al.*, 1988), and increasingly the Internet (Ahronheim *et al.*, 2000; National Reference Center for Bioethics Literature, 2000). One may discuss problems informally or obtain formal consultation with colleagues, social workers, chaplains, or with the patient's relatives or friends. A patient care conference with all the professionals caring for the patient can be extremely useful. Often one should include the patient and/or family for at least part of the meeting. Such a conference is less intimidating than an ethics committee meeting for health care professionals as well as for patients and often achieves the same goals. It may be helpful to include an ethicist or an ethics-experienced health care professional for facilitation of the discussion.

Clinical practice guidelines, clinical pathways, and disease management are contemporary approaches that parallel case management, managed care, and policies of health maintenance organizations (HMO) but are much more acceptable to most physicians (Bodenheimer, 1999; Committee to Advise the Public Health Service on Clinical Practice Guidelines, 1990; Culpepper and Gilbert, 1999; Eknoyan and Levin, 1999; Miller 1992 and 1999; Moss *et al.*, 1993; National Institutes of Health Consensus Development Conference, 1993; National Kidney Foundation Dialysis Outcomes Quality Initiative, 1997; National Kidney Foundation K/DOQI Nutrition Working Group, 2000; Paris and Moss, 1995; Patient Services Committee, National Kidney Foundation, 1996; Price 1992; RPA-ASN Working Group 2000).

Clinical practice guidelines ideally are evidence-based and summarize the literature in order to provide a useful framework for the care of patients. When data are insufficient, expert opinion is sought, preferably from a multidisciplinary group, and preferably with documentation of the rationale for recommendations. Guidelines are intended to provide evidence to allow informed decision making, to improve clinical outcomes, and to reduce practice variation, all in order to protect patients from inappropriate interventions, physicians from malpractice claims, and society from excessive costs. Criticisms of guidelines include the fact that they tend to oversimplify the complexities of medicine (and suggest cookbook approaches to complex problems) and that they cannot take into account the uniqueness of each patient and his or her illness (Fauci *et al.*, 1998). Stross (1999) reviews the barriers to effective dissemination and implementation of guidelines.

A major concern is the development of guidelines by almost every department in every hospital. Such efforts are naïve, failing to take into account the enormous effort in sophisticated and critical analysis of the literature along with expert, multidisciplinary experience and judgment required to develop a reliable, valid, clear, and relevant guideline. Furthermore, institutional guidelines that do not have such attributes are dangerous not only medically but medicolegally. Far more appropriate than developing guidelines in small hospitals would be the adoption of nationally developed guidelines, such as those of the US Agency for Health Care Policy and Research, and the US National Institutes of Health consensus process, or those of specialty societies.

Disease management is a population-based approach to identify persons at risk of a disease, to intervene with specific programs, and to measure clinical and other (for example, cost) outcomes (Epstein and Sherwood, 1996; Gunter, 1999). Like practice guidelines, disease management has become an important initiative in nephrology particularly with regard to the management of renal insufficiency as early in its course as possible with interventions aimed at slowing, if not preventing, progression.

For review of ethical problems of individual patients (or of the health care professionals who attend them) ethics consultation by an individual ethics consultant or by several members of an ethics committee, or case discussion by a multidisciplinary ethics committee can be extremely helpful. By consultation I mean first-hand evaluation of the patient and of all relevant material and persons, whereas by case discussion I imply an unbiased, reflective discussion by a committee that receives information about the patient and problem second-hand from a presentation by a member of the patient's care team. Although such discussion is vulnerable to the misinformation or biased information of an inexperienced presenter, such discussion can also be powerfully creative in thinking of options that might otherwise never even be conceived. The advantages and disadvantages of consultants, teams, and committees have been reviewed by Swenson and Miller (1992), and committees have been well discussed by Cranford and Doudera (1984), Ross et al. (1986), and Ross et al. (1993).

Ethical problems that are not resolved at the level of an institution (for example, when a patient believes the hospital ethics committee may be biased or may have a conflict of interest) may require external review, for example, by a regional network of hospital ethics committees if there is one and if it is willing to hear such a case. I have recommended that county medical societies might also provide such a service but this is not yet a reality (Miller, 2000). I believe there is a need for extramural ethics committees in the renal community especially as many dialysis facilities are free-standing and not affiliated with a hospital. The only such committee I am aware of in the United States is in Kansas City where the National Kidney Foundation affiliate and the Midwest Bioethics Center have a joint committee, which is described by Grochowski and Blacksher (in press 2000) and is said to have effectively met their community's needs. The 17 regional ESRD networks, which are under federal contract, like the National Kidney Foundation, have patient as well as physician participants and thus might also develop ethics committees to hear ethical concerns of patients, professionals, or facilities. For clinical investigation and research, human subjects review by an institutional review board (IRB) regarding the scientific validity and safety of the protocol and regarding the adequacy of the informed consent process and form is mandatory.

The Joint Commission on Accreditation of Healthcare Organizations (JCAHO) mandates policies in United States hospitals for organizational ethics and patients' rights. Ethical issues include those related to access to care, payment for care, quality of care, and the like. Institutional mission and values are ethical matters of the greatest moment, but virtually all hospital policies and procedures have ethical ramifications. Some hospitals emphasize corporate compliance whereas others espouse more aspirational institutional or organizational ethics. Virtually all hospitals have risk managers and legal counsel, and where legal considerations are relevant these resources, rather than or in addition to, ethics consultants and committees, may wisely be consulted. Where conflict arises one may wisely seek the advice of risk management or legal counsel, but the advice of an ombudsman or a mediator may be particularly helpful (Miller, 1997). Indeed if both parties in good faith hope to resolve a dispute, mediation is more likely to achieve a mutually satisfactory and lasting compromise than is negotiation, arbitration or adjudication.

Internet resources

Finally, below is a list of several Internet resources and addresses, as provided in an appendix by Ahronheim, Moreno, and Zuckerman (2000), which contains a number of others as well.

American Society of Bioethics and Humanities
  http://www.asbh.org
American Society of Law, Medicine, and Ethics
  http://www.aslme.org
National Bioethics Advisory Commission
  http://www.bioethics.gov
National Reference Center for Bioethics Literature
  http://www.georgetown.edu/research/nrcbl/
National Library of Medicine
  http://www.nlm.nih.gov/databases/freemedl.html
  (free Medline using Internet Grateful Med or Pub Med)
National Guideline Clearinghouse
  http://www.guideline.gov

References

Ahronheim, J. C., Moreno, J. D., and Zuckerman, C. (2000). *Ethics in clinical practice* (2nd edn). Aspen Publishers, Gaithersburg, MD.

Alexander, S. (1962). Medical miracle and a moral burden of a small committee: They decide who lives, who dies. *Life Magazine*, **53**, 102–25.

Arras, J. D. (1998). A case approach. In *A companion to bioethics* (ed. H. Kuhse and P. Singer), pp. 106–14. Blackwell Publishers, Oxford.

Beauchamp, T., and Childress, J. F. (1979 and 1994). Principles of biomedical ethics (1st edn 1979, 4th edn 1994). Oxford University Press, New York.

Beauchamp, T. L., and Walters, L. R. (1994). *Contemporary issues in bioethics* (4th edn). Wadsworth Publishing Co., Belmont, CA.

Beecher, H. K. (1966). Ethics and clinical research. *New England Journal of Medicine*, **274**, 1354–60.

Black, H. C. (1991). *Black's law dictionary* (6th edn). West Publishing Co., St. Paul, MN.

Bloche, M. G. (2000). Fidelity and deceit at the bedside. *Journal of the American Medical Association*, **283**, 1881–4.

Bodenheimer, T. (1999). Disease management–promises and pitfalls. *New England Journal of Medicine*, **340**, 1202–5.

Brody, B. (1988). *Life and death decision making*. Oxford University Press, New York.
Brody, H. (1989). The physician-patient relationship. In *Medical ethics* (2nd edn), (ed. R. M. Veatch). Jones and Bartlett Publishers, Sudbury, MA.
Callahan, D. (1987). *Setting limits: medical goals in an aging society*. Georgetown University Press, Washington, DC.
Callahan, D. (1990). *What kind of life: The limits of medical progress*. Simon and Schuster, New York.
Callahan, D. (1993). *The troubled dream of life: Living with mortality*. Simon and Schuster, New York.
Callahan, D. (1998). *False hopes: Why America's quest for perfect health is a recipe for failure*. Simon and Schuster, New York.
Card, C. (1991). *Feminist ethics*. University Press of Kansas, Lawrence, KS.
Childress, J. F. (1997). *Practical reasoning in bioethics*. Indiana University Press, Bloomington, IN.
Childress, J. F. (1998). A principle-based approach. In *A companion to bioethics* (eds H. Khuse and P. Singer), pp. 61–71. Blackwell Publishers, Oxford.
Clouser, K. D., and Gert, B. (1990). A critique of principlism. *Journal of Medicine and Philosophy*, **15**, 219–36.
Committee to Advise the Public Health Service on Clinical Practice Guidelines, Institute of Medicine (1990). *Clinical practice guidelines: Directions for a new program*. National Academy Press, Washington, DC.
Compassion in Dying v Washington, 79 F. 3d 790 (97th cir. 1996), (en banc), rev'd subnom. Washington v Glucksberg, 117 S. Ct. 2258 (1997).
Council on Ethical and Judicial Affairs (1998). *Code of medical ethics*: Current opinions with annotations, 1998–1999 edn. American Medical Association, Chicago, IL.
Cranford, R. E., and Doudera, A. E. (1984). *Institutional ethics committees and healthcare decision making*. Health Administration Press, Ann Arbor, MI.
Cruzan v Director, Missouri Department of Health, Supreme Court of the United States, 1990. 497 U.S. 261:110S.Ct. 2841, 111L. Ed. 2d 224.
Culpepper, L., and Gilbert, T. T. (1999). Evidence and ethics. *Lancet*, **343**, 829–31.
Darrah, J. B. (1987). The committee. *Transactions of the American Society of Artificial Internal Organs*, **33**, 791–3.
Downie, R. S. (1996). *Medical ethics*. Dartmouth Publishing, Aldershot.
Drane, J. F. (1988). *Becoming a good doctor: the place of virtue and character in medical ethics*. Sheed and Ward, Kansas City.
Dunn, P. M., Gallagher, T. H., Hodges, M. D., *et al.* (1994). Medical ethics: An annotated bibliography. *Annals of Internal Medicine*, **121**, 627–32.
Dworkin, R. (1977). *Taking rights seriously*. Harvard University Press, Cambridge, MA.
Eknoyan, G., and Levin, N. W. (1999). An overview of the National Kidney Foundation–Dialysis outcomes quality initiative implementation. *Advances in Renal Replacement Therapy*, **6**(1), 3–6.
Emanuel, L. L. (1991). The health care directive: learning how to draft advance care documents. *Journal of the American Geriatrics Society*, **39**, 1221–8.
Emanuel, E. J., and Emanuel, L. L. (1992). Four models of the physician-patient relationships. *Journal of the American Medical Association*, **267**, 2221–6.
Epstein, R. S., and Sherwood, L. M. (1996). From outcomes research to disease management: a guide for the perplexed. *Annals of Internal Medicine*, **124**, 832–7.
Fauci, A. S., Braunwald, E., Isselbacker, K. J., *et al.* (1998). *Harrison's principles of internal medicine* (14th edn). McGraw-Hill, New York.

Fletcher, J. F. (1954). *Morals and medicine: The moral problems of the patient's right to know the truth, contraception, artificial insemination, sterilization, euthanasia*. Princeton University Press, Princeton, NJ.

Flores, A. (2000). Talk addressed to the Medical Ethics Committee, University of California, Irvine, 16 May.

Foot, P. (1978). *Virtues and vices*. University of California Press, Berkeley, CA.

Fox, R. C., and Swazey, J. P. (1978). *The courage to fail: A social view of organ transplants and dialysis* (2nd edn, revised). University of Chicago Press, Chicago, IL.

Freeman, V. G., Rathore, S. S., Weinfurt, K. P., Schulman, K. A., and Sulmasy, D. P. (1999). Lying for patients: physician deception of third-party payers. *Archives of Internal Medicine*, **159**, 2263–70.

Gert, B. (1988). *Morality: A new justification of the moral rules*. Oxford University Press, New York.

Gibson, J. M. (1990). National values history project. *Generations*, **14**, 51–64 (Suppl.).

Gilligan, C. (1982). *In a different voice*. Harvard University Press, Cambridge, MA.

Gillon, R., and Lloyd, A. (1994). *Principles of health care ethics*. John Wiley and Sons, Chichester.

Grochowski, E. C., and Blacksher, E. (2000). Collaborative ethics: a standing renal dialysis ethics committee. *Advances in Renal Replacement Therapy*, 7(4): 355–7.

Gunter, M. J. (1999). A practical guideline to disease outcomes. Lecture at DCA Research Foundation Conference, Integrating Informatics and Telemedicine to Improve Clinical Outcomes, Las Vegas, February 4–5, 1999.

Holmes, H. G., and Purdy, L. M. (1992). *Feminist perspectives in medical ethics*. Indiana University Press, Bloomington, IN.

In re Quinlan, Supreme Court of New Jersey, 1976. 70 N. J.10, 355 A. 2d 647, certiori denied 429 U.S. 922, 97 S.Ct. 319, 50 L. Ed. 2d 289.

Jonsen, A. R. (1991). Casuistry as methodology in clinical ethics. *Theoretical Medicine*, **12**, 295–307.

Jonsen, A. R. (1998). *The birth of bioethics*. Oxford University Press, New York.

Jonsen, A. R. (2000). *A short history of medical ethics*. Oxford University Press, New York.

Jonsen, A. R., and Jameton, A. (1995). History of medical ethics: The United States in the twentieth century. In *Encyclopedia of Bioethics* (revised edn) (ed. W. T. Reich). Simon and Schuster-MacMillan, New York.

Jonsen, A. R., and Toulmin, S. (1988). *The abuse of casuistry*. University of California Press, Berkeley, CA.

Kant, I. (1785). *Groundwork of the metaphysics of morals*, translated and analyzed by H. J. Paton (3rd edn 1956). Harper and Row, New York.

Khuse, H., and Singer, P. (1998). What is bioethics? A historical introduction. In *A companion to bioethics* (eds H. Kuhse and P. Singer), pp. 3–11. Blackwell Publishers, Oxford.

Kohlberg, L. (1981). *The philosophy of moral development*. Harper and Row, New York.

Kopelman, L. M. (1994). Case method and casuistry: The problem of bias. *Theoretical Medicine*, **15**, 21–37.

Krugman, S., Ward, R., Giles, J. P., Bodansky, O., and Jacobs, A. M. (1959). Infectious hepatitis: Detection of virus during the incubation period and in clinically inapparent infection. *New England Journal of Medicine*, **261**, 729–34.

Kouwenhoven, W. B., Jude, J. R., and Knickerbocker, G. G. (1960). Closed chest cardiac massage. *Journal of the American Medical Association*, **973**, 1064–7.

Lantos, J. D., Miles, S. H., Silverstein, M., and Stocking, C. L. (1988). Outcome after cardiopulmonary resuscitation in babies of very low birthweight: Is CPR futile therapy? *New England Journal of Medicine*, **318**, 91–5.

Lantos, J. D., Singer, R. A., Walker, R. M., *et al.* (1989). Illusion of futility in clinical practice. *American Journal of Medicine*, **87**, 81–4.

Larrabbe, M. J. (1993). *An ethic of care: feminist and interdisciplinary perspectives*. Routledge, New York.

Levinsky, N. G. (1984). The doctor's master. *New England Journal of Medicine*, **311**, 1573–5.

Lo, B., Quill, T., and Tulsky, J. (1999). Discussing palliative care with patients: ACP-ASIM End-of-life care consensus panel. *Annals of Internal Medicine*, **130**, 744–9.

Locke, J. (1690). Natural rights in *Two Treatises of Government* in a critical 1960 edition by Peter Laslett, Cambridge, England.

MacIntyre, A. (1984). *After virtue* (2nd edn). University of Notre Dame Press, Notre Dame, IN.

Macklin, R. (1999). *Against relativisim: Cultural diversity and the search for ethical universals in medicine*. Oxford University Press, New York.

Manning, R. C. (1998). A care approach. In *A companion to bioethics* (eds H. Khuse and P. Singer), pp. 98–105. Blackwell, Oxford.

Mappes, T. A., and DeGrazia, D. (1996). *Biomedical ethics* (4th edn). McGraw-Hill, New York.

Merrill, J. P., Murray, J. E., Harrison, J. H., and Guild, W. R. (1956). Successful homotransplantation of the human kidney between identical twins. *Journal of the American Medical Association*, **160**, 277–82.

Mill, J. S. (1861a). *Utilitarianism* (1979 edn) (ed. G. Sher). Hackett Publishing Co., Indianapolis, IN.

Mill, J. S. (1861b). *Utilitarianism and other writings* together with selected writings of Jeremy Bentham and John Austen (ed. 1962 with an introduction by Mary Warnock). New American Library, New York.

Miller, R. B. (1992). Selection of patients for chronic dialysis: Let society decide whether rationing is needed. *Nephrology News and Issues*, **6**(2), 36,40,41,43.

Miller, R. B. (1997). Mediation for challenging patients–A promising approach. *Advances in Renal Replacement Therapy*, **4**, 372–6

Miller, R. B. (1999). Ethical issues in the care of patients with ESRD treated by dialysis. In *Dialysis and transplantation: A companion to Brenner and Rector's The Kidney* (Eds W. F. Owen, B. J. G. Pereira, and M. H. Sayegh). W. B. Saunders and Co., Philadelphia, PA.

Miller, R. B. (2000). A call for regional ethics committees for ESRD patient problems. A web only editorial. www.arrtjournal.org. *Advances in Renal Replacement Therapy*, **7**(4): E5.

Moss, A. H., Rettig, R. A., and Cassel, C. K. (1993). A proposal for guidelines for patient acceptance to and withdrawal from dialysis: A follow-up to the IOM Report. *American Nephrology Nurses Association Journal*, **20**, 557–61, 617.

National Commission for the Protection of Human Subjects of Biomedical and Behavioral Research (1979). *The Belmont Report: Ethical principles and guidelines for the protection of human subjects of research. Federal Register*, **44**, 23192–7, 18 April.

National Institutes of Health Consensus Development Conference on Morbidity and Mortality of Dialysis (1993). *NIH Consensus Statement: Morbidity and Mortality of Dialysis*, **11**(2), 1–33.

National Kidney Foundation Dialysis Outcomes Quality Initiative (1997). *Clinical practice guidelines*. National Kidney Foundation, New York.

National Kidney Foundation K/DOQI Nutrition Work Group (2000). K/DOQI clinical practice guidelines for nutrition in chronic renal failure. *American Journal of Kidney Diseases*, **35**(6), Suppl. 2, S1–140.

National Reference Center for Bioethics Literature (2000). Basic resources in bioethics: 1996–1999. Scope note 37 in *Kennedy Institute of Ethics Journal*, **10**(1), 81–102.

Noddings, N. (1984). *Caring: A feminine approach to ethics and moral education*. University of California Press, Berkeley, CA.

Novack, D. H., Detering, B. J., Arnold, R., Forrow, L., Ladinsky, M., and Pezzullo, J. C. (1989). Physicians' attitudes toward using deception to resolve difficult ethical problems. *Journal of the American Medical Association*, **261**, 2980–5.

Oakley, J. (1998). A virtue ethics approach. In *A companion to bioethics* (eds H. Khuse and P. Singer), pp. 86–97. Blackwell, Oxford.

Orlowski, J. P. (1999). *Ethics in critical care medicine*. University Publishing Group, Hagerstown, MD.

Paris, J. J. and Moss, A. H. (1995). Control of services in managed care: guidelines for use in renal disease. *Trends in Health Care Law and Ethics*, **10**, 101–4.

Patient Self-Determination Act (1990). Sections 4206, 4751 of the Omnibus Reconciliation Act of 1990, Public Law No. 101–508, Nov. 5, 1990.

Patient Services Committee, National Kidney Foundation (1996). *Initiation or withdrawal of dialysis in ESRD: Guidelines for the health care team*. National Kidney Foundation, New York.

Pellegrino, E. D., and Thomasma, D. C. (1993). *The virtues in medical practice*. Oxford University Press, New York.

Pence, G. E. (1995). *Classic cases in medical ethics: Accounts of cases that have shaped medical ethics, with philosophical, legal, and historical backgrounds* (2nd edn). McGraw-Hill, New York.

Price, C. A. (1992). Is it time again for patient selection criteria? *Nephrology News and Issues*, **6**(2), 18–20.

Purnell, L. D., and Paulanka, B. J. (1998). *Transcultural health care: a culturally competent approach*. F. A. Davis Co., Philadelphia, PA.

Purtilo, R. (1981). *Ethical dimensions in the health professions* (2nd edn). W. B. Saunders Co., Philadelphia, PA.

Rachels, J. (1975). Active and passive euthanasia. *New England Journal of Medicine*, **292**, 78–80.

Rachels, J. (1997). *Can ethics provide answers? And other essays in moral philosophy*. Rowman and Littlefield Publishers, Lanham, MD.

Rachels, J. (1998). Ethical theory and bioethics. In *A companion to bioethics* (eds H. Kuhse and P. Singer), pp. 15–23. Blackwell Publishers, Oxford.

Ramsey, P. (1970). *Patient as person: Explorations in medical ethics*. Yale University Press, New Haven, CT.

Rawls, J. (1971). *A theory of justice*. Harvard University Press, Cambridge, MA.

Reich, W. T. (1995). *Encyclopedia of bioethics* (2nd edn). Simon and Schuster-MacMillan, New York.

Renal Physicians Association and American Society of Nephrology Working Group (2000). *Clinical practice guideline: Shared decision-making in the appropriate initiation of and withdrawal from dialysis*. Renal Physicians Association, Rockville, MD.

Ross, J. W., Bayley, C., Michel, V., and Pugh, D. (1986). *Handbook for hospital ethics committees*. American Hospital Publishing, Chicago, IL.

Ross, J. W., Glaser, J. W., Rasinski-Gregory, D., Gibson, J. McI., and Bayley, C. (1993). *Healthcare ethics committees: The next generation*. American Hospital Publishing, Chicago, IL.

Ross, W. D. (1930). *The right and the good*. Clarendon Press, Oxford.

Rothman, D. J. (1991). *Strangers at the bedside: A history of how law and bioethics transformed medical decision making*. Basic Books, New York.

Schneiderman, L. J., Jecker, N. S., and Jonsen, A. R. (1990). Medical futility: Its meaning and ethical implications. *Annals of Internal Medicine*, **112**, 949–54.

Sehgal, A., Galbraith, A., Chesney, M., *et al.* (1992). How strictly do dialysis patients want their advance directives followed? *Journal of the American Medical Association*, **267**, 59–63.

Siegler, M., Singer, P. A., and Schiedermayer, D. L. (1988). *Medical ethics: An annotated bibliography*. American College of Physicians, Philadelphia, PA.

Society for Health and Human Values–Society for Bioethics Consultation Task Force on Standards for Bioethics Consultations (1998). *Core competencies for health care ethics consultations*. American Society for Bioethics and Humanities, Glenview, IL.

State of California. Probate Code, Section 4609.

Stross, J. K. (1999). Guidelines have their limits (editorial). *Annals of Internal Medicine*, **131**, 304–6.

SUPPORT Principal Investigators (1995). A controlled trial to improve care for seriously ill hospitalized patients: The *S*tudy to *U*nderstand *P*rognoses and *P*references for *O*utcomes and *R*isks of *T*reatment. (SUPPORT). *Journal of the American Medical Association*, **274**, 1591–8.

Swazey, J. (1992). Discovering the ethical dilemma. Paper read at the Birth of Bioethics Conference, Seattle, Washington, September 23–24, 1992. (And quoted in Jonsen (1998).)

Swenson, M. D., and Miller, R. B. (1992). Ethics case review in health care institutions: Committees, consultants, or teams? *Archives of Internal Medicine*, **152**, 694–7.

Teel, K. (1975). The physician's dilemma: a doctor's view: what the law should be. *Baylor Law Review*, **27**, 6–10.

Thomas, J. E., and Waluchow, W. J. (1998). *Well and good: A case study approach to biomedical ethics* (3rd edn). Broadview Press, Peterborough, Ontario.

Tulsky, J. A., Alpers, A., and Lo, B. (1996). A middle ground on physician-assisted suicide. *Cambridge Quarterly of Healthcare Ethics*, **5**(1), 33–43.

Ubel, P. A. (1999). Physicians' duties in an era of cost containment: advocacy or betrayal? *Journal of the American Medical Association*, **292**, 1675.

Vacco v. Quill, 117 S.Ct., 2293 (1997), rev'g 80 F. 3d 716 (2nd cir. 1996).

Veatch, R. M. (1991). *The patient-physician relation: The patient as a partner*, Part 2. Indiana University Press, Bloomington, IN.

Ward, R., Krugman, S., Giles, J. P., Jacobs, A. M., and Bodansky, O. (1958). Infectious hepatitis: Studies of its natural history and prevention. *New England Journal of Medicine*, **258**, 407–16.

Webster, G. (1999). Serving two masters: medical practice vs administrative ethics. *Journal of the American Medical Association*, **282**, 1678–9.

Wicks, A. C., Spielman, B. J., and Fletcher, J. C. (1995). Survey of ethical orientations and theories. In *Introduction to Clinical Ethics* (1st edn) (eds J. C. Fletcher, C. A. Hite, P. A. Lombardo, and M. F. Marshall). University Publishing Group, Frederick, MD.

Wolf, S. M. (1996). *Feminism and bioethics: Beyond reproduction*. Oxford, New York.

Wolf, S. M., Boyle, P., Callahan, D., *et al.* (1991). Sources of concern about the Patient Self-Determination Act. *New England Journal of Medicine*, **325**, 1666–71.

Wynia, M. K., Cummins, D. S., VanGeest, J. B., and Wilson, I. B. (2000). Physician manipulation of reimbursement rules for patients: between a rock and a hard place. *Journal of the American Medical Association*, **284**, 1858–65.

Zucker, M. B., and Zucker, H. (1997). *Medical futility and the evaluation of life-sustaining interventions*. Cambridge University Press, Cambridge.

3
Key legal issues
Bernard M. Dickens

Introduction

Kidneys are paired in the human body, like lungs, to serve highly particularized and distinctive functions, but legal issues related to kidney function and replacement affect the entire body of legal regulation of human life. Legal issues extend beyond cradle to grave or 'womb to tomb' concerns, since they arise before individuals are conceived, and extend to posthumous use of their remains. Parents' legal claims have been recognized when they were denied proper counselling regarding the risk of their unconceived children inheriting polycystic kidney disease (*Park* v *Chessin* 1976), and claims by affected children themselves following birth are at the centre of complex legal 'wrongful life' controversies (Kennedy and Grubb, 1998: 679 *et seq.*). Legal systems approach recovery (or 'harvesting') of transplantable kidneys following death by different techniques, some depending on consent by individuals in anticipation of their deaths or by their family members thereafter, others creating an automatic right of recovery unless individuals while living record their refusal of posthumous recovery (WHO, 1994).

The allocation of posthumously recovered kidneys among potential recipients raises scientific concerns of tissue compatibility, but also human rights concerns regarding legally prohibited grounds of adverse selection. Discrimination on grounds such as race, religion, sex, age, marital status, physical or mental disability and lifestyle is barred under many national laws, and under international legal conventions that many countries have ratified consistently with the 1948 Universal Declaration of Human Rights. Further, to resist objectionable commerce through which persons vulnerable to exploitation might be induced to provide kidneys from their living bodies in exchange for payment, laws may prohibit live donation except to close blood relatives or spouses. The defence of human dignity to which such prohibitions are directed may be questioned, however, on both ethical (Radcliffe-Richards *et al.*, 1998) and legal human rights grounds. A related concern is the legal status and control of a kidney from a live donor while in transit to a designated recipient (Dickens 1991).

Access to dialysis raises comparable legal concerns regarding discrimination on grounds, for instance, of age or disability, but patients' refusals or requests for discontinuation of dialysis may create concerns, perhaps from patients' relatives, of medically assisted suicide. Physicians' refusal or discontinuation of dialysis raises additional legal concerns, including of criteria of futility and euthanasia (Otlowski,

1997). Accordingly, legal issues in nephrology include many of the most sensitive, complex and vital topics in contemporary medical law and legal accommodation of ethical options.

Many practical problems in nephrology raise profound issues of professional and social ethics. Relationships between law and ethics are therefore of concern (Dickens, 1994a), even in countries where the 'pervasive, unwelcome crushing embrace of medicine by law' (Rosenberg and Calabresi, 1986) is not as oppressive as it is sometimes seen to be in the United States. Law is often described as a minimal ethic, meaning that medical practitioners are required at least to observe legal requirements in their care of patients and discharge of administrative functions. Laws considered excessively oppressive of ethical options may be legally challenged, and law itself recognizes grounds of legitimate dissent on grounds of conscience. Where an option is considered intolerable it will be legally prohibited, for instance by legal definitions of murder, but law often tries to accommodate ethical options, such as offering or not offering a patient treatment that an attending physician considers futile. Some laws, such as those against murder and criminal negligence, require obedience, but most are designed not to supersede but rather to accommodate ethical judgment. The law aims to set a general, usually permissive, framework within which ethical judgment is to be exercised. However, politically-inspired legislation may depart from the generally tolerant approach of law to professionally skilled, disinterested judgment, such as that in the US that prohibits physicians giving treatment in federally funded family planning clinics from raising the lawful option of elective abortion (*Rust* v *Sullivan* 1991).

Prenatal issues

Legal concerns about genetic inheritance of kidney diseases are likely to become more significant with advances in genetic understanding, particularly as studies of the human genome generate improved awareness of genetic transmission. Nephrologists may be anticipated to be at the front edge of advances in interpretation of genetic data relevant to kidney diseases that may affect future children. However, in time, which with rapid growth of genetic comprehension may be relatively short, general medical practitioners may be expected to recognize warning signs of conditions that are genetically transmissible as part of the legal standard of care of patients which they are required to maintain. Professionalism includes awareness of limits of one's knowledge, and of the need to advise referral to appropriate specialists. That is, general practitioners uncertain of which conditions of kidney or other disease in patients may be inherited by their children should advise patients of which types of specialists may help them.

Developments in human reproductive biology and embryology, allied with the new reproductive technologies, have opened pathways to preconception and preimplantation diagnosis of the genetic characteristics that born children would inherit, and of harmful conditions that embryo selection can avoid. Wastage of embryos created *in vitro* because they show dysgenic characteristics, such as inherited kidney diseases, will be unacceptable to some patients, who may accordingly be expected to decline recourse to preimplantation genetic diagnosis. Similarly, practitioners concerned about their complicity in deliberate embryo wastage may decline to undertake diagnosis of *in vitro* embryos, although they may remain obliged to inform patients of alternative diagnostic services (Tasca and McClure, 1998). In many medical professional ethical codes, practitioners who have conscientious objections to particular procedures are required so to inform patients, and offer them timely referral to other practitioners (Kennedy and Grubb, 1998: 636–40).

Many ethical and legally enforceable codes of research conduct prohibit creation of human embryos for purposes only of experimentation. Research with embryos intended to be implanted *in utero* for gestation to birth is for infertile patients' therapy rather than for experimentation. Where the purpose of embryo creation *in vitro* is to avoid dysgenic traits that patients might transmit, the activity may also be classified as therapy rather than research, and not be bound by research guidelines even when innovative.

Legal concerns may be deeper where prenatal genetic diagnosis involves an embryo or fetus *in utero*, because identification of a dysgenic trait legally requires disclosure to the patient, and may raise the option of abortion. This option will not be pursued when a pregnant patient finds it unacceptable, but raises the concerns addressed above when the patient would want to consider the option but a health care practitioner is conscientiously opposed to abortion. Concerns are amplified where hospital or associated clinics reject the option of abortion on religious grounds, whatever a particular practitioner's disposition. In several of the United States, state legislation renders hospitals with a Roman Catholic affiliation and their staff members legally immune from liability not only for not offering abortion services, but also for not counselling patients about the option and not referring them elsewhere. Patients unaware of their liability to transmit polycystic kidney disease or a like trait to the children they conceive, and unaware of the religious affiliation of the clinic on which they depend for genetic services, may thus be left without legal recourse on delivery of an affected child. Where no legislated immunity exists, practitioners and facilities face legal liability for denying patients informed choice on continuation of pregnancy.

Initiation of dialysis and transplantation

Initiation of any medical procedure directed to a particular patient legally requires consent. For a patient capable of exercise of reason and judgment, this means the patient's own consent. Capacity to consent is dependent on maturity and comprehension rather than chronological age. Even where legislation establishes a minimum age for medical consent, law often recognizes that mature minors below that age may be legally capable of making autonomous medical decisions. They may therefore legally authorize interventions their parents would deny them. Laws differ on whether, as for instance in Canada, mature minors' refusals override parents' consent (*Van Mol* (*Guardian ad Litem of*) v *Ashmore* 1999), or, as in England, parents in principle may legally authorize treatments their mature minor children refuse (Re R. [1991]: 185–6).

Capacity to consent to medical treatment is a pervasive issue, without regard to age, where individuals decline to consent to treatment, such as dialysis, that in clinical judgment appears necessary for their survival and ability to maintain functions of everyday living. Legal capacity is decreasingly considered global, in the sense that those who possess intellectual ability to understand the implications of medical information have capacity for all medical decisions, and those who lack this ability are comprehensively incapacitated and amenable to others' medical choices for their care (Dickens, 1997). Capacity is now increasingly considered specific to particular functions, so that, for instance, patients incapable of exercising choice over some matters may be legally competent to make decisions regarding others. Recognition of so-called asymmetrical medical competence or capacity is particularly significant, since the law sets a low threshold of capacity to consent to medically indicated treatment. That is, patients willing to accept treatments recommended by their clinicians may be considered legally competent. Those who decline such care but insist on remaining untreated or on recourse to unproven or contraindicated interventions raise concerns about their legal capacity.

It may at first appear cynical and self-serving that physicians whose recommendations are accepted consider their patients mentally competent, but question their patients' intellectual capacity when their advice is rejected. When dialysis appears indicated in clinicians' skilled and disinterested medical judgment, however, the question is legally appropriate, and necessary to ask. Patients may more clearly decline experimental treatments, and more invasive, even though established, interventions such as kidney transplantation from a cadaveric or living related donor. However, refusal of available and indicated institutional or home dialysis triggers questions of patients' mental capacity and emotional status, and whether, for instance, depression or denial of their pathology is distorting their judgment. Patients' refusals may be found legally competent, since for their own reasons, patients may reject even life-prolonging interventions, such as indicated blood transfusions (*Malette* v *Shulman* 1990). Patients may be apprehensive, for instance, about financial costs and health insurance coverage. Refusals of indicated dialysis should not be passively accepted, however, but should cause medical care-givers to question their basis and patients' legal competence as autonomous decision makers. If refusal is based, for instance, on patients' fear of inadequate health insurance, care-givers may have legal duties to represent patients' health service needs to insurers (*Wickline* v *State* 1986).

In cases of medical emergency, it may not be possible to obtain consent by or on behalf of patients when withholding or postponement of dialysis appears to leave them in peril of death or in serious danger to health. Legal doctrines of medical necessity may then excuse any assault that initiation of dialysis is alleged to constitute (Giesen, 1988: 361–69). Further, in many circumstances, initiation of dialysis may be justifiable under principles of implied consent, based on the legal proposition that peril invites rescue. However, implied consent is unavailable if a person when competent executed an advance medical directive clearly refusing this intervention if it was indicated when the person could not express a choice, or perhaps if the person's peril is a consequence of attempted suicide (Giesen, 1988: 358–61). In these types of cases, only the excuse of necessity is legally available. A legal limit of this excuse is that, even when courts of law are prepared to excuse the wrong the intervention constitutes, professional licensing authorities may not find the wrong excusable. Legal counsel cannot advise behaviour they know to be legally wrongful, and can only inform clients of the wrong, and possible judicial and professional responses.

Information for decision making by or on behalf of patients has different theoretical orientations. Increasingly, disclosures for informed choice or decision making, that is for so-called 'informed consent', are to be based on information that would be material to a reasonable or prudent person in the particular patient's circumstances. This orientation of disclosure originated in California (*Cobbs* v *Grant* 1972) but became widespread throughout the US (*Canterbury* v *Spence* 1972) and was adopted in Canada (*Reibl* v *Hughes* 1980) and, for instance, Australia (*Rogers* v *Whitaker* 1992). The highest court in England maintains principles of disclosure based on information that would be given by a professional peer of the practitioner in question (*Sidaway* v *Board of Governors of the Bethlem Royal Hospital* [1985]). The court rejected patients' rights to give, or refuse, 'informed consent', incorrectly supposing informed consent to be a 'transatlantic doctrine' responsible for a flood of malpractice litigation in the US. In fact, the principle is widely applied in France, Germany, Switzerland and elsewhere in Europe (Giesen, 1988: 289–97).

Information material to the decision on initiation of dialysis includes: the patient's prognosis if it is not initiated; the prognosis with the alternative of kidney transplantation and the patient's likelihood to receive a transplant and chances of its success; health effects of continuing dialysis and its effects on lifestyle; and implications of the alternative, where it exists, of hospital-based or home-based dialysis. Similarly, when transplantation is available, patients should be informed of dialysis alternatives and their implications. Differences between transplantation from a cadaver and from a living donor may not have to be addressed unless a living person, such as a relative of the patient's, offers donation, or the patient asks questions about differences.

Patients' refusal and termination of dialysis

Unless medically indicated dialysis is terminated because a patient has received a transplanted kidney, termination of dialysis leads in time to a patient's sickness and death. Accordingly, the legal issues arise of suicide, medically-assisted death, euthanasia and murder, and the contrast between each of them and natural death. Some philosophers, ethicists and theologians have denied that any morally significant difference distinguishes murder from termination or omission of life-sustaining treatment when it is known and intended that the consequence will be a dependent patient's death. In law, however, the distinction between killing and letting die is critical.

Because courts of law have come to give decisive significance to competent individuals' autonomy, they empower competent persons to decline medical care and not become patients, and to refuse the only medical interventions, such as kidney dialysis, that will save or prolong their lives. When mentally competent, adequately informed patients whose lives have been sustained by dialysis, ventilators, drug treatments or other artificial means, including artificially supplied nutrition and hydration, refuse its continuation in order to die, the courts will find them to experience natural death (*Nancy B.* v *Hôtel-Dieu de Québec* 1992). The same applies to withdrawing care from patients in persistent vegetative state when care is found futile (*Airedale NHS Trust* v *Bland* [1993]). Patients are found to have died not from the refusal or discontinuation of treatment, but from the condition that treatment was only optional to relieve. However, grieving relatives may deny that the deceased patient, when competent, had declined life-sustaining care, and the US Supreme Court requires that there be 'clear and convincing' evidence of the patient's refusal (*Cruzan* v *Director, Missouri Department of Health* 1990).

It has been seen that patients' refusal of life-prolonging medical interventions raises the issue of their mental capacity. Historically, religions have considered suicide a mortal sin, and attempted suicide was a crime. This remains a crime in some legislation, although England, Canada, many of the United States and many other jurisdictions have decriminalized attempted suicide. The purpose of decriminalization has not been to create a legal right to commit suicide, however (*Rodriguez* v *British Columbia (Attorney-General)* 1993), but rather to allow attempted suicide to be approached as a mental health concern, and as a cry for help not to die, but to live better. It was considered that treating the attempt as criminal was dysfunctional because it led to suppression of evidence of a person's suicidal disposition, and so obstructed the introduction of preventive assistance and counselling. Coroners' inquests still tend to record verdicts of 'suicide while the balance of the mind was disturbed,' sometimes in order to preserve deceased persons' eligibility for burial in consecrated ground. Recognition of rational suicide has been advanced by the advocacy of those anticipating non-demented AIDS-related deaths, and various organizations that support Death with Dignity goals. Legislation in Oregon and the Northern Territory of Australia and more visibly in the Netherlands has approved medically-assisted suicide (Otlowski 1997). However, Supreme Courts for instance in the US (*Washington* v *Glucksberg* 1997; *Vacco* v *Quill* 1997) and Canada (*Rodriguez* v *British Columbia (Attorney-General)* 1993) have denied that there is a constitutionally-protected right to suicide or to medically-assisted death.

However, patients' informed refusal of initiation or continuation of dialysis or other life-prolonging intervention is not legally considered suicide. Accordingly, healthcare providers who provide comfort measures only and who, on patients' request, withdraw them from dialysis, face no legal liability, for instance in criminal law or the civil law of negligence, for consequent death. Their legal responsibilities particular to their patients' deaths are discharged once they are satisfied of their patients' mental capacity and that patients are not, for instance, clinically depressed or cognitively impaired, and ensure patients' comfort. Care must be taken in assessing patients' mental health status, for instance by reference to their recent life-experiences, because patients are entitled to conventional medical confidentiality. Family members may be asked if, for instance, patients have experienced bereavement or grief, but no disclosure may be made of intentions to die from natural causes unless the patients have consented to such disclosure.

Denial and involuntary termination of dialysis

Termination of dialysis, and its denial on diagnosis of patients' impending kidney failure, are somewhat more problematic when patients are not competent to approve and have given no clear advance medical directive. Concerns are aggravated when patients' family members insist on initiation or continuation of dialysis to preserve loved ones' lives, but the attending physicians consider the intervention to be futile or contrary to the patients' best interests, such as when dialysis would prolong the process of death and make it more painful or distressing for the patient.

Relevant to the legal approach to a patient's treatment, but not necessarily decisive, is the attending physician's clinical assessment of the patient's best interests. Competent patients are entitled, as a key aspect of their autonomy, to be treated in accordance with their wishes, even when these contradict their best interests as assessed by attending or other physicians, family members and judges. The doctrine that wishes prevail over interests has been shaped, however, and limited, by patients' rights to refuse medically indicated or advised resuscitation and surgical, pharmacological or other interventions. This doctrine applies when patients competently refuse offered care at the time of offer or by an advance medical directive. There is no comparable autonomy, however, for patients or their family members to demand care that is neither medically indicated nor clinically recommended, for instance because attending physicians consider it futile or to violate their historic ethical duty, to do no harm (Newdick, 1996).

There is no comprehensive legal definition of medical futility, but courts consider a patient's prognosis as determined by the clinician in charge in accordance with a body of professional opinion. In a leading case in the highest court in England, Lord Goff said that:

I cannot see that medical treatment is appropriate or requisite simply to prolong a patient's life when such treatment has no therapeutic purpose of any kind, as where it is futile because . . . there is no prospect of any improvement in his condition. It is reasonable also that account should be taken of the invasiveness of the treatment and the indignity to which . . . a person has to be subjected . . . (*Airedale NHS Trust* v *Bland* 1993)

Physicians have no legal duty to undertake treatment they consider will not help their patients, and may have a duty not to impose invasive, undignified treatments that are of no established therapeutic potential. Accordingly, if attending physicians consider dialysis to be futile, they can decline to order it for both competent and incompetent patients, without need of consent by or on behalf of their patients. To initiate or continue dialysis without consent legally constitutes a criminal assault or in civil law (that is, non-criminal law) a battery. However, physicians need no consent if in their clinical judgment they propose not to initiate or to continue dialysis. Incompetent patients may, when earlier competent, have appointed another, by independent power of attorney or by an advance medical directive, to make personal care decisions for them. Even when such legal instruments clearly express patients' wishes, however, or authorize others to attribute or impute wishes to the patients and to express them on patients' behalf, they do not oblige physicians to initiate or continue contraindicated or futile care. Legal instruments allow consent to be given to offered care, but create no power to compel care that is not offered. Patients have no rights to futile or contraindicated care, and third parties cannot be empowered to claim such care when attending physicians consider it clinically inappropriate.

When incompetent patients' wishes are unknown and no others claim to make medical care decisions for them, physicians must give treatment according to their clinical, disinterested judgment of their patients' best interests. This includes power to not initiate or to discontinue dialysis. As against this, if physicians consider dialysis to serve patients' best interests, they may initiate or continue treatment even over the protests of incompetent patients' family members. Legal doctrines of patients' implied consent to receive care that their attending physicians consider to be in their best interests will protect health care providers. Grounds to not initiate or to discontinue dialysis may arise, however, when incompetent patients show resistance to procedures by struggling against them, and, more materialistically, when patients lack financial means, insurance coverage or, for instance, charitable support to meet the costs. This is relevant not only in the private health insurance system of the US, but also to patients ineligible for coverage under public health insurance arrangements, such as new immigrants, refugees and visitors.

Treating dependent people in ways intended to result in their deaths appears in principle to constitute criminal homicide, but courts have given prior approval of medical management of both competent (*Nancy B.* v *Hôtel-Dieu de Québec* 1992) and incompetent (*Airedale NHS Trust* v *Bland* 1993) patients for this purpose. In the sad *Airedale* case concerning a brain-damaged young man named Anthony Bland, who could breathe without support but had been in a persistent vegetative state for three years and whose family members had urged the hospital to let him die, the highest court in England approved withdrawal of artificial feeding and hydration. The court was concerned with moral factors, but concluded that since the patient would not regain consciousness and felt no pain, feeding served no interest of his, and could accordingly be lawfully withdrawn, resulting in his natural death. Physicians terminating feeding would control the time of death, but were not its legal cause. The same would have applied had the patient's death been postponed by dialysis. The court favored a prior judicial hearing before such steps to end life were taken, because of the novelty of the issue, but this may become less necessary when courts have decided enough cases to indicate the principles they will apply.

Recovery of transplantable cadaveric kidneys

Historically, law regarded bodies of deceased persons as a matter of religious or ecclesiastical concern rather than as objects of utility. In the Anglo-Saxon customary or common law tradition, dead bodies are still not generally regarded as governed by the law of property, because property interests protect value, which arises principally from utility and scarcity (Dickens, 1977). Dead bodies, however cherished and revered on spiritual grounds, had no utility and so no commercial value that property law addressed. On grounds of decency and public order, a crime has been recognized of causing indignity to a corpse (Kennedy and Grubb, 1998: 888), and public health law requires those administering deceased persons' assets to dispose of their bodies in sanitary ways, usually by burial or cremation, by paying associated costs. It is only in recent times that recoverable organs from dead bodies have become useful, and highly valuable. However, for fear of an unsavoury market in human organs, efforts have been made to prevent commodification and commercialization of organs, by legal prohibition of sales, purchases and advertising of and for human organs.

Many countries have enacted specific legislation to provide for posthumous recovery of kidneys and other transplantable organs, and to prevent commercial trafficking. Laws follow one of the two major patterns, described as the express consent or 'opting in' and the implied consent or 'opting out' patterns respectively, with minor variants within each pattern. English-speaking jurisdictions, including those of the UK, the US, Canada and Australia tend to have 'opting in' legislation, while 'opting out' laws are common in Western Europe and a growing number of countries beyond (WHO, 1994).

Opting in laws empower people, in anticipation of their own death, to state their approval of posthumous recovery of their organs for transplantation. Legislation often couples donation for transplantation with other uses for therapy, scientific research and medical education. If at death the deceased person is found not to have opted into donation, but not to have stated or indicated any personal opposition to posthumous organ recovery for transplantation or associated uses, a family member may approve organ recovery. Legislation often differs on the priority of family members authorized to consent, such as a spouse, child, parent, sibling or sibling's child, and on whether a single consent at the highest available level of priority is legally adequate, or whether one person at that level, such as a child of the deceased person, may veto consent given by another of the same rank. Laws often provide that consent given by the now deceased person is complete legal authority for organ removal, but in practice physicians are often unwilling to recover, or 'harvest' organs, when aware of family members' opposition.

The basis of opposition to opting in may be, for instance, personal aversion or a distrust of medicine, but it often reflects the religious setting in which treatment of dead bodies has historically been situated. Several major religions include beliefs in resurrection, but have not clarified whether the raising of the dead is to be a purely spiritual or an actual biological phenomenon. The physiology of resurrection is unclear, and those who envision the event in physiological terms require that their bodies be buried intact. They may be willing to receive transplanted organs to prolong duration of their mortal lives, but oppose posthumous donation in order to protect their afterlife and hope of resurrection. Accordingly, individuals' religious faith may cause them expressly to refuse posthumous organ removal, and, in the absence of their express refusal, will prevent family members aware of such faith from consenting to organ removal from the person's dead body.

Some opting in laws include so-called 'required request' provisions, which require physicians and perhaps others to request attending family members' consent to recovery of organs when the deceased had neither opted in nor opposed posthumous recovery. Legislation is usually not specific, however, regarding whether consent is given to a specific physician, clinic, hospital, university or other person or institution.

Consent is usually given at large, enabling the hospital or other agent managing organ recovery to determine its use, unless legislation also provides an organ allocation system. Similarly, legislation may leave organ recovery co-ordinators or organizations to facilitate recording options to donate in a systematic way. Private completion of an organ donation card may be known only to a person's family members and personal physician. A practical concern may be payment of organ removal surgeons. Those engaged on salary have less concern than those paid on a fee-for-service basis, for instance by national or public health service agencies or from private insurance plans. Fees may be difficult to claim, since dead patients are not eligible to receive funded services, and transplant recipients may be unknown and may be covered under different health insurance plans.

Legislation that gives effect to implied consent or 'opting out' provisions can be more systematic, because it is based on the premise that recoverable cadaveric organs are a public resource or asset, amenable to public regulation. Such laws create a legal presumption that those who did not opt out of organ donation in an appropriate form consented to posthumous organ recovery. As with opting in laws, legislation may cover transplantation and other therapeutic use of organs, scientific research and medical education. Because organ implantation is undertaken only in specialized medical facilities, the presumption is that the donation is to a centre capable of transplantation, although organ recovery may be undertaken elsewhere. Legislation usually includes arrangements by which persons who do not consent to posthumous removal of any or particular organs record their refusal. Electronic data recording systems now allow facilities capable of organ recovery to learn quickly whether a deceased person had refused organ removal.

Legal and human rights issues are raised when the system recording refusal of posthumous donation is publicly maintained and easily accessible, because individuals may consider their personal preferences, based perhaps on their religious convictions, to be a private matter. This is particularly so when religious or racial minorities fear oppression or discrimination, and do not want to risk public identification as individuals or members of a group or community who refuse to contribute to public resources or assets. They may also fear that their known refusal to contribute organs will compromise their eligibility to receive them when indicated.

Implied consent laws do not necessarily eliminate the need for family members of deceased persons to be counselled regarding the benefits of organ recovery for transplantation and other uses. Some laws may allow family members' objections, particularly on the ground that the deceased persons opposed perceived mutilation or desecration of their bodies. Even without legal provisions, staff of facilities capable of organ recovery may defer to family members' opposition to organ removal. Accordingly, it remains a matter of evidence whether legal transition from an opting in to an opting out system significantly increases the supply of transplantable cadaveric kidneys and other organs, and a matter of policy whether any increase justifies the social, psychological, human rights and political costs of legal change. A helpful variant of the opting out legislation exists, where laws permit family members to opt out of recovery of a deceased relative's organs, but not if the person when alive specifically opted for posthumous recovery of his or her organs.

Organ allocation

Whether the imposition of legally directive recovery of cadaveric organs is justifiable is related in part to the justice of their allocation among patients eligible to receive them. If everyone is expected to allow posthumous organ recovery but allocation will primarily benefit a socially, financially or otherwise privileged elite or socio-economic class, injustice may be apparent. Similarly, opting in may not be attractive to members of a group, such as a racial or socio-economic group, unconvinced that they will be treated justly in allocation policies or practices. In the US, for instance, Afro-Americans are under-represented among posthumous organ donors, although, due perhaps to genetically-linked high blood pressure, they are over-represented on waiting lists for transplantation. Their reluctance to donate may be because they perceive that they are disadvantaged in the national organization of health care. They were also sensitized to racial inequity in organ transplantation in observing highly-publicized pioneering initiatives in South Africa under the regime of apartheid.

International, regional, national and state or provincial human rights laws or codes uniformly condemn discrimination on grounds such as race, ethnic origin, sex and religion, reflecting the conditioning influence of the 1948 Universal Declaration of Human Rights. Also condemned is discrimination on grounds of age and physical and mental disability. The legal concern this raises in equitable kidney transplantation policies and practices is that factors of age and disability may affect patients' comparative prognoses with and without transplantation, their capacity to cope with dialysis, and, for instance, their compliance with medical care in the aftermath of transplantation that would affect its success and their survival. Tissue compatibility between donors and prospective recipients continues to be a factor where access to or tolerance of immunosuppressive drugs is uncertain (Claas, 1997).

Legitimate organ allocation policies include those that favour patients closer to death without transplantation over those whose prospects of untransplanted survival appear better. More utilitarian policies may also be applied, however, that favour patients with longer survival prospects over those whose more serious impairments such as multiple organ failure reduce their likelihood to survive even if kidneys are successfully transplanted. It seems to contradict utility in employment of a scarce resource to postpone transplantations for relatively healthy patients with superior survival prospects until their health and survival prospects have deteriorated and they are closer to death. Where prospective length of survival is influential, however, younger patients are liable to be favoured over more elderly patients, violating legal principles prohibiting discrimination on grounds of age. Nevertheless, a leading American ethicist has advanced the concept of intergenerational justice, claiming that ethics require, and law should allow, that the young be favoured in allocation of scarce health-care resources, in order to enhance their prospects to survive to the advanced age of patients competing against them for life-prolonging resources (Callahan, 1987).

Further concerns of an ethical nature, including regional inequities within countries in donation and recovery of organs, transplantation of intellectually impaired patients and, for instance, of those in persistent vegetative states, are addressed in other chapters of this book. Regional differences in transplantation rates and waiting times became a particular concern in the United States, where in April 1998 the federal Department of Health and Human Services (DHHS) issued regulations on organ allocation. These provoked considerable controversy in requiring comparable rates and waiting times among quite different regions, and discounting organ deterioration in transit over distances. Consequently, the US Institute of Medicine was asked to study and report on relevant policies and options (Institute of Medicine, 1999). Following the report and its recommendations, the DHHS issued amended regulations in a Final Rule (Rules and Regulations, 1999).

Of legal concern is whether alleged inequities are open to legal challenge and remedy. It is notable that, even in the litigation-prone US, court challenges against organ allocation policies and practices have been very rare. This may be due in part to the evidentiary difficulty of proving in law that a policy adverse to the interests of a particular patient, such as an aged patient suffering multiple organic disabilities, is based on an intention to deny a class of persons a benefit generally available to others, or that the policy even inadvertently has that effect, and that the policy is not based on *bona fide* medical, diagnostic and prognostic considerations. Courts will be likely to condemn, however, as violations of human rights to non-discrimination, allocation policies that state, and systemic practices that show, disfavour of classes of patients on grounds such as mental disability or race unrelated to medical or health-related factors.

Another reason for allocation policies and practices remaining almost unchallenged may be legal analysis that deters lawyers from advising challenge. In developed countries where legal challenge tends to be more feasible and likely, the ordinary medical response to kidney dysfunction is dialysis. Patients may successfully challenge a decision to deny them ordinarily indicated dialysis. Even where transplantation is the treatment of choice according to a patient's diagnosis and prognosis, however, transplantation depends on access to an appropriate waiting list, equitable progress on the list, availability in time of a compatible and otherwise suitable organ, and availability of facilities and personnel to undertake the procedure. The high and perhaps rising proportion of patients who die while on waiting lists for organ transplantation shows, on a balance of probability, that obtaining an organ is extraordinary.

Patients have legally enforceable rights to ordinary care, which dialysis might now be found to be, but not to extraordinary care, such as organ transplantation or sophisticated biotechnological devices. In the well-known case of Karen Quinlan, the Chief Justice of the New Jersey Supreme Court observed that 'the use of the same respirator or like support could be considered "ordinary" in the context of the possibly curable patient, but "extraordinary" in the context of the forced sustaining . . . of an irreversibly doomed patient' (Quinlan 1976: 667–68). In many developed countries, where dialysis is now considered routine, ordinary care may also include placement on a waiting list for transplantation, but progress to the offer of an available, adequately compatible organ depends on issues so particular to individual patients and to other, competing candidates, including patients whose earlier transplants have failed and who have become closer to death, that rules of legally enforceable practice and of legal generalizability become inapplicable. An allocation manager who acts negligently or in conflict of interest may be sued, but this concerns an alleged personal failure, not failure of the allocation system itself. A particular patient in a conscientiously managed transplantation programme who is disfavoured to another may find it impossible to show on a balance of probabilities any individual or systemic denial of a legal entitlement to care.

So peculiar to particular patients and circumstances are organ allocation decisions that courts may decline to review them. For instance in the English Court of Appeal hearing a challenge to a denial of an operation, a judge observed that:

> It is not for this court, or indeed any court, to substitute its own judgment for the judgment of those who are responsible for the allocation of resources. This court could only intervene where it was satisfied that there was a *prima facie* case, not only of failing to allocate resources in the way in which others would think that resources should be allocated, but of a failure to allocate resources to an extent which was . . . [so] unreasonable [that no reasonable person addressing the issue could have come to such a decision] (Walker 1992: 35).

Live donation

Allocation concerns rarely arise when people offer to donate one of their kidneys while they are living, because donations are made to specifically designated recipients, usually donors' close family members. Legal issues regarding live donors include but go beyond conventional concerns with free and informed consent. Legislation in some jurisdictions prohibits parents or other legal guardians from authorizing donations by legal minors and mentally disabled persons, and prohibits such persons from consenting to donate on their own behalf, although mature minors may be entitled to consent for themselves to receive transplanted organs (*Gillick* v *West Norfolk and Wisbech Area Health Authority* 1985). However, from the origin of organ transplantation, some courts in the US approved minors as organ donors to close family members when satisfied that the risks of donation were heavily outweighed by emotional and other benefits to the minors themselves of survival of the recipients, who were their siblings or parents (*Strunk* v *Strunk* 1969). Courts applied the test of whether donation was in the best interests of the minor donors, requiring clear evidence that the balance of benefit to risk was heavily in the minors' favour.

Information for competent prospective donors' decisions includes risks to them of the preparation for donation, surgical removal of one of their kidneys, recuperation from surgery and of living thereafter with a single kidney. The prognosis if the intended recipient does not receive a kidney from the prospective donor must be placed in the context of alternative sources of donations, and also of the possibility of the prospective donor's kidney being rejected following implantation. Information for a possible donor's decision may affect freedom of consent, since informing a prospective donor that no other family member is suitable to donate and an alternative source is unlikely to arise may create pressure in favour of consent. Care must therefore be taken to reduce a potential donor's motivation to consent primarily for avoidance of guilt, or of blame from other family members, if donation is refused and the potential recipient, a close family member, should die.

The requirement that patients' consent to medical procedures should be freely given is designed to preclude physicians and other health care providers from bringing pressure to bear in order to serve some interest of their own, such as a financial interest in earning fees or in serving their promotion of, or research into, a particular product or procedure. It is a legitimate motivation that a patient consents out of a feeling of commitment to a particular personal, altruistic or other cause not influenced by the physician, including a feeling of obligation to another person. A prospective donor's genuine concern for the welfare of a close relative does not vitiate the legal validity of consent to organ donation. However, when family members create pressure on one of them to agree to donation, that one may be moved by fear of family recrimination and alienation rather than by independent dedication to the intended recipient. Consent induced by this pressure is legally questionable. A physician apprehending that consent is so conditioned may seek an independent assessment of the prospective donor's suitability, and may find psychological unsuitability, due for instance to ambivalent motivation, as a ground for not proceeding.

Alternatively, a prospective donor may be genuinely and fully willing to consent to organ removal, because of the promise or prospect of receiving payment or other material reward for donation. Legislation prohibits all forms of commerce and exchange for reward concerning human organs from both living and cadaveric sources. Although plausible and principled arguments have been presented against the paternalism and moral panic such legislation reflects (Radcliffe-Richards *et al.*, 1998), particularly as market forces are more strongly supported in health service delivery (Dickens, 1994b), national governments and intergovernmental agencies remain strongly opposed to any apparent commodification of human organs. Indeed, the suspicion of commercial exchange raised by a person intending living donation to an unrelated recipient has caused the UK to establish the Unrelated Live Transplant Regulatory Authority (ULTRA), without whose approval following examination, particularly of the intended donor's motivation, participation in such donation is a criminal and professional disciplinary offence. (Kennedy and Grubb 1998, p. 830).

The belief that any gift or reciprocity in exchange for organ donation is necessarily commercial in character reflects capitalist values that predominate in Westernized cultures. There is accordingly heavy scepticism and rejection of the claim that, in cultures where strangers interact on a basis of personal reciprocity, so-called 'rewarded gifting' is *hors de commerce* and does not violate laws against trading in human organs (Daar *et al.*, 1997). This negative approach may impair the development of living organ exchanges that, for instance, Israel has legalized (Frenkel, 1998; Menikoff, 1999). Exchange arises when, for instance, Mr A requires a kidney that Mrs A is willing but incompatible to donate to Mr A. Mrs A is a compatible donor to Mr B, whose wife is compatible to donate to Mr A, whether or not she is also a suitable donor to Mr B. Mrs A agrees to donate to Mr B, provided that Mrs B will donate her kidney to Mr A. Mrs A is conscientiously motivated by her concern for Mr A, and, if Mrs B could donate to Mr B, her willingness to donate to Mr A instead appears altruistic rather than commercial. Nevertheless in the UK, ULTRA has stated that the Authority would prohibit an exchange of this nature as offending the prohibition in the Human Tissue Act 1961 against exchanges 'for money or money's worth' (Sells, 1997).

More legally problematic even where organ exchange is considered non-commercial is a variant by which Mrs A will donate her kidney to an anonymous recipient on a transplantation waiting list, provided that Mr A will be given priority to receive the next compatible cadaveric kidney that becomes available. The advantage of earlier transplantation for the recipient of Mrs A's kidney is offset by the disadvantage to the potential recipient who is displaced on the list by the priority given to Mr A. From a macroethical perspective, society benefits by Mrs A's addition to the number of kidneys available for transplantation. However, those on the list whose receipt of an organ would be postponed if priority was given to Mr A might legally claim that they would suffer unlawful prejudice from such management of the waiting list.

Legal control of kidneys outside the body

It has been seen that, historically, remains of deceased people were not considered in law to be property (Dickens, 1977). Similarly, since abolition of slavery, living people are not considered to be property. This has recently raised the question of the legal status and control of cadaveric organs, and organs in transit between a living donor and a recipient. Opposition to considering such organs to be property arises from the supposition that a person holding a property interest would be free to sell the organ, and others would be free to buy it. Those conditioned by capitalism find it difficult to accept that items of demonstrable value can be exchanged between strangers *hors de commerce*, and argue for legal non-marketability or 'market inalienability' of organs (Radin, 1987). Laws can prohibit commerce in tangible items, such as drugs, and it is increasingly difficult to contend that in law organs would not be treated as property.

The key issue, however, may not be the legal status of extracorporeal organs *per se*, but their legal control (Dickens, 1991). Cadaveric organs for transplantation are under the control of the agencies that legislation directly or indirectly appoints or permits to possess them pending implantation, or wastage and disposal when they are unsuitable to transplant. Control over them may be unchallengeable by private persons, since even patients with legal power to challenge management of their waiting lists cannot claim a legal interest in any particular cadaveric kidney. In the leading case on the legal status of a living person's cells outside his body (Moore 1990), the Supreme Court of California denied his claims that they were to be treated as his property. The court's judgment was based, however, on the therapeutic and other beneficial uses to which they might be put, and the restraining effect his property rights would have. The court deliberately left open the possibility of finding a property interest in them, saying that: 'We do not purport to hold that excised cells can never be property for any purpose whatsoever' (*Moore v Regents of the University of California* 1990: 493). If the court had addressed kidney transplantation, it would probably have found the procedure beneficial, and might well have recognized a property interest where this would have protected or advanced that goal (Dickens, 1992).

The court did find that the physicians and others in the case were bound by a fiduciary duty to deal with the patient and his cells in good conscience. The Supreme Court of Canada has similarly found physicians under fiduciary duties to deal conscionably and equitably with information in patients' medical records that physicians possess, but that the patients own (*McInerney v MacDonald* 1992). Courts may treat the relationship between a person who has factual possession of property and another who has a beneficial interest in it as comparable to a trust. The possessor is trustee of another's interest, and must in conscience serve and protect that other's interest. That is, while the possessor holds the property, it is under the legal control of the beneficiary, whose directions the possessor must heed. A court is likely to find that, when a living person gives a kidney for transplantation into a designated recipient, it is not property while in the prospective donor, nor when implanted into the intended recipient, but is within the donor's beneficial interest while possessed by physicians and others in transit from donor to recipient. Physicians and other relevant personnel are not legally free to deal with the kidney as they wish, but are legally empowered only to serve the donor's intentions, which cannot lawfully be commercial. Whether designated recipients can claim beneficial interests is less clear, but it seems from the limited cases that have been decided that living donors of organs for transplantation would have legal control of them while physicians and hospital or other authorities possess and manage them.

Conclusion: Health and human rights

There are, already, new issues in kidney transplantation, which the law has not begun deliberately to address. Xenotransplantation, for instance, falls uncomfortably between legislation on animal welfare, patients' clinical care and public health protection against diseases that may cross the species barrier into humans (Daar, 1999). Cloning kidneys for implantation into patients who face kidney failure and lack an alternative to kidneys cloned from their own cells may in time be accommodated by law. This may be when the rush to legislate prohibitions of human cloning, founded on the panic-based over-reaction against the prospect of cloning entire persons, has abated, and religiously-based objections to creating human embryos other than for birth have been moderated by the spiritual and pragmatic values of prolonging and improving human survival.

Legislation restricting these and other technological innovations will be reviewed by courts, even when enacted by democratically constituted legislatures, according to human rights principles. The European Convention on Human Rights has long been applied to require national legislatures to take account of its provisions, and for instance in the UK, the Human Rights Act 1998, in force from October 2000, will increasingly require and empower domestic courts directly to enforce its provisions. Canada has quickly ratified all of the leading international human rights treaties, and has given the force of domestic law to the International Covenant on Civil and Political Rights through the Canadian Charter of Rights and Freedoms, which since 1982 has been an influential element of Canada's constitution. Under provisions of the Charter, for instance, the Supreme Court of Canada held inoperative Criminal Code prohibitions of abortion, with punishment of up to life imprisonment, because they violated women's rights to security of the person (*Morgentaler, Smoling and Scott* v *The Queen* 1988). The same right may be found to support patients' pursuit of kidney transplantation.

For constitutional reasons concerning relations between federal and state authority, the US has not ratified many of the leading international human rights conventions, although the United Nations' 1948 Universal Declaration of Human Rights was strongly influenced by Eleanor Roosevelt's sense of liberties founded on the US Bill of Rights. Nevertheless, human rights, often described as civil rights, have in recent decades been firmly defended by the US Supreme Court, even under a conservative influence. Liberal judgments of the Supreme Court of Canada, for instance on the human right to abortion, have been influenced by judgments of the US Supreme Court. The post-1945 human rights movement, based on the 1948 Universal Declaration, was a reaction against Nazi totalitarianism and abuse of state legal power to oppress its own citizens and pave a legal path to the Holocaust.

Legislation based on religious, political or other fundamentalism that impairs patients' preservation of their lives by access to replacement kidneys without material loss or harm to others may be invalidated for violation of patients' human rights (Mann et al., 1999). The International Covenant on Economic, Social and Cultural Rights recognizes everyone's right to the highest attainable standard of health, and the International Covenant on Civil and Political Rights protects every person's right to life. These rights may be found to protect patients' rights to non-oppressive access to replacement kidneys, through techniques such as xenotransplantation and cloning that may offend particular religious and philosophical sensitivities. These sensitivities are conscientious and warrant protection but, as in the case of abortion, courts may not let them prevail by obliging individuals involuntarily to forfeit their health and lives for their defence.

References

Airedale NHS Trust v *Bland* [1993] Appeal Cases 789 (House of Lords).
Callahan, D. (1987). *Setting limits: medical goals in an aging society*. Simon and Schuster, New York.
Canterbury v *Spence* (1972). 464 Federal Reporter 2d 772 (U.S. Court of Appeals, District of Columbia Circuit).
Claas, F. H. J. (1997). Kidney allocation in highly sensitized patients. In *Procurement, preservation and allocation of vascularized organs* (eds G. M. Collins, J. M. Dubernard. W. Land and G. G. Persijn), pp. 217–22. Kluwer, Dordrecht.
Cobbs v *Grant* (1972). 502 Pacific Reporter 2d 1 (California Sup. Ct.).
Cruzan v *Director, Missouri Department of Health* (1990). 110 Supreme Court Reporter 2841 (U.S. Sup. Ct.).
Daar, A. S. (1999). Animal-to-human organ transplants–a solution or a new problem? *The International Journal of Public Health*, 77, 54–61.
Daar, A. S., Gutmann, T., and Land, W. (1997). Reimbursement, 'rewarded gifting', financial incentives and commercialism in living organ donation. In *Procurement, preservation and allocation of vascularized organs* (eds G. M. Collins, J. M. Dubernard, W. Land, and G. G. Persijn), pp. 301–316. Kluwer, Dordrecht.
Dickens, B. M. (1977). The control of living body materials. *University of Toronto Law Journal*, 27, 142–98.
Dickens, B. M. (1991). Who legally owns and controls human organs after procurement? In *Procurement, preservation and allocation of vascularized organs* (eds G. M. Collins, J. M. Dubernard, W. Land and G. G. Persijn), pp. 385–92. Kluwer, Dordrecht.

Dickens, B. M. (1992). Living tissue and organ donors and property law: More on *Moore*. *Journal of Contemporary Health Law and Policy*, **8**, 73–93.

Dickens, B. M. (1994a). Legal approaches to health care ethics and the four principles. In *Principles of health care ethics* (ed. R. Gillon), pp. 305–17. John Wiley, Chichester.

Dickens, B. M. (1994b). Morals and legal markets in transplantable organs. *Health Law Journal*, **2**, 121–34.

Dickens, B. M. (1997). Legal aspects of the dementias. *Lancet*, **349**, 948–50.

Frenkel, D. A. (1998). Organ transplantation from live donors in Israel. *Annals of Transplantation*, **3**, 42–44.

Giesen, D. (1988). *International medical malpractice law*. Mohr (Paul Siebeck), Tübingen; Martinus Nijhoff, Dordrecht.

Gillick v West Norfolk and Wisbech Area Health Authority (1985). [1986] Appeal Cases 112 (House of Lords).

Institute of Medicine (1999). *Organ procurement and transplantation*. Institute of Medicine, Washington, DC.

Kennedy, I. and Grubb, A. (eds) (1998). *Principles of medical law*. Oxford University Press, Oxford.

Malette v Shulman (1990). 67 Dominion Law Reports (4th) 321 (Ontario Court of Appeal).

Mann, J. M., Gruskin, S. Grodin, M. A., and Annas, G. J. (eds) (1999). *Health and human rights*. Routledge, New York.

McInerney v MacDonald [1992] Supreme Court Reports 138 (Sup. Ct. Canada).

Menikoff, J. (1999). Organ swapping. *Hastings Center Report*, **29**(6), 28–33.

Moore v Regents of the University of California (1990). 739 Pacific Reporter 2d 479 (California Sup. Ct.).

Morgentaler, Smoling and Scott v The Queen (1988). 44 Dominion Law Reports (4th) 385 (Sup. Ct. Canada).

Nancy B. v Hôtel-Dieu de Québec (1992). 86 Dominion Law Reports (4th) 385 (Quebec Superior Ct.).

Newdick, C. (1996). *Who should we treat? Law, patients and resources in the N. H. S.* Clarendon Press, Oxford.

Otlowski, M. F. A. (1997). *Voluntary euthanasia and the Common law*. Clarendon Press, Oxford.

Park v Chessin (1976). 387 New York Supplement 2d 204 (New York Sup. Ct.).

Quinlan (In the matter of Karen Quinlan) (1976). 355 Atlantic Reporter 2d 647 (New Jersey Sup. Ct.).

Radcliffe-Richards, J., Daar, A. S., Guttmann, R. D., *et al.* (1998). The case for allowing kidney sales. *Lancet*, **351**, 1950–52.

Radin, M. (1987). Market-inalienability. *Harvard Law Review*, **100**, 1849–936.

Re R. [1991] 4 All England Reports 177 (English Court of Appeal).

Reibl v Hughes (1980). 114 Dominion Law Reports (3d) 1 (Sup. Ct. Canada).

Rodriguez v British Columbia (Attorney-General) (1993). 107 Dominion Law Reports (4th) 342 (Sup. Ct. Canada).

Rogers v Whitaker (1992). 175 Commonwealth Law Reports 479; 109 Australian Law Reports (High Court of Australia).

Rosenberg, L. E., and Calabresi, G. (1986). *Law and medicine in confrontation: a deans' dialogue*, Yale Law School Program in Civil Liability, Working Paper No. 45. Yale Law School.

Rules and Regulations [Organ Procurement and Transplantation Network]. 64 Federal Register [U.S.] (October 20, 1999) 56649–56661.

Rust v Sullivan (1991). 500 United States Reporter 173 (U.S. Sup. Ct.).

Sells, R. A. (1997). Paired kidney-exchange programs (letter). *New England Journal of Medicine*, **337**, 1392.
Sidaway v *Board of Governors of the Bethlem Royal Hospital* [1985] 1 All England Reports 643 (House of Lords).
Strunk v *Strunk* (1969). 445 South Western Reporter 2d, 145 (Kentucky Court of Appeals).
Tasca, R. J., and McClure, M. E. (1998). The emerging technology and application of pre-implantation genetic diagnosis. *Journal of Law, Medicine and Ethics*, **26**, 7–16.
Vacco v *Quill* (1997). 117 Supreme Court Reporter 2293 (U.S. Sup. Ct.).
Van Mol (Guardian ad Litem of) v *Ashmore* (1999), 168 Dominion Law Reports (4th) 637 (British Columbia Court of Appeal).
Walker—R. v *Secretary of State for Social Services*, ex p. *Walker* (decided 1987) reported in (1992). 3 British Medical Law Reports 32 (English Court of Appeal).
Washington v *Glucksberg* (1997). 117 Supreme Court Reporter 2258, 2302 (U.S. Sup. Ct.).
Wickline v *State* (1986). 239 California Reporter 810 (California Court of Appeals).
World Health Organization (WHO) (1994). *Legislative responses to organ transplantation*. Martinus Nijhoff, Dordrecht.

PART II

Specific ethical issues in the care of patients with kidney disease

4
Must (should) all ESRD patients be treated?
Eli A. Friedman

Introduction

Allocation, defined as 'the action of apportioning or assigning to a special person or purpose' (*Oxford English Dictionary*, 1971) has as synonyms: appropriation, ration, allotment, distribution, quota, and share. In terms of treatment for end-stage renal disease (ESRD) it is evident that throughout the world rationing (allotment, quotas) of ESRD treatment are realities forced by financial limitation. As shown in Fig. 4.1, there are sharp national differences in the rate of treatment for ESRD depending on the income of individual countries (United States Renal Data System, 1999).

This pragmatic conclusion is no surprise and is consistent with the existence of rich and poor economies. Annual income of $23,240 in the USA is 123 times greater than that in Tanzania ($180) where ESRD therapy is non-existent. Starting in the 1980s, the European Dialysis and Transplant Association (EDTA) demonstrated a direct

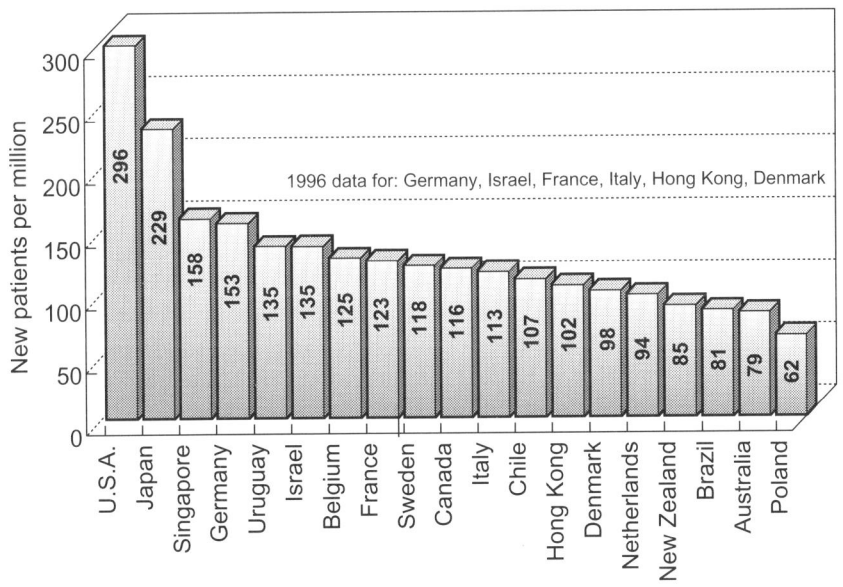

Source: USRDS, 1999

Fig. 4.1 Newly treated ESRD patients by country.

relationship between a country's per capita income and the number of patients enrolled in ESRD therapy (Jacobs et al., 1981). In its eleventh combined report on dialysis and kidney transplantation in Europe, the EDTA registry deduced that: 'It is difficult for countries with a gross national product (GNP) lower than 2,700 US dollars to put many patients on treatment. Three-quarters of the world's population live in countries where the per capita GNP is below 2,700 US dollars.' From EDTA data, it was obvious (Friedman and Delano, 1981) that for the foreseeable future, the world will be unable to afford uremia therapy, a conclusion unaltered by collapse of the Soviet Union and the end of the cold war (Friedman, 1995).

How can nations too poor to afford physicians, safe water or supervised pregnancies consider establishing renal failure programs matching America's cost that exceeds $60,000 per patient per year (Bruns et al., 1998)? They can't (Friedman, 1996). Consider that of every five women giving birth in Senegal, four receive no professional medical care, leading to a first year infant mortality rate of 68 per 1000 compared with 5.2 per 1000 in Sweden. Lacking both funds and skilled professionals, developing nations like Cambodia, Chad, Ethiopia, and Tanzania must bypass the ethical stresses of allocating uremia therapy, at least until more basic survival concerns are resolved.

Appreciating the distinction between have not and have nations, I will therefore focus on industrialized developed nations. A hopeful note is provided by experience indicating that a changed political system and/or improving economy, may permit nations with minimal ESRD facilities to expand remarkably rapidly as evidenced by a tripling in acceptance for dialysis in the former East Germany within three years of the fall of the Berlin Wall (Friedman, 1994). The point of the foregoing comments is that any discussion of an ethical approach to treatment of kidney failure must begin with the stark verity that the majority of the world's population who develop ESRD—including nearly everyone with ESRD in Africa, China, India, Indonesia, Mexico, Pakistan, and Vietnam—will die with no possibility of dialysis or a kidney transplant.

Rationing in industrialized nations

The broad variation in incident treatment of ESRD in industrialized nations (Fig. 4.1) can be explained in one of three ways: (1) *There are extraordinary differences in ESRD 'attack rates' by country*. Australia, for example, has only 21% as many cases of renal failure as does the United States. (2) *Overtreatment of inappropriate patients is practiced in the United States*. By this interpretation, the United States enrolls into dialysis programs agonal, moribund, and senile individuals who ought best be allowed to die undisturbed. (3) Undertreatment of rehabilitatable patients in some countries sentences salvageable patients to death. Evidence supporting this contention can be gleaned from multiple sources. For example, once French dialysis programs began accepting diabetic patients in large numbers, their formerly exemplary annual survival rate (Laurent et al., 1983) decreased to levels reported (and criticized) typical of the United States (Friedman, 1999). Illustrating this point is the report by Chantrel et al. lamenting their program's high mortality in type 2 diabetic hemodialysis patients treated in Strasbourg (Chantrel *et al.*, 1999): Of 84 type 2 diabetic patients begun on dialysis, 27(32%) died in a mean follow-up of 211 days. Thus, although diabetes accounted for 40% of newly dialyzed patients in the Strasbourg program, a pervasive bias against accepting diabetic patients for uremia therapy is present in France, their nationwide acceptance rate for dialysis is only 15.7% (Maghlaoua *et al.*, 1997).

Perhaps the most analyzed exclusion of uremic patients from therapy took place in the United Kingdom between 1965 and 1990 following the introduction of maintenance hemodialysis. From introspective studies in the United Kingdom (Berlyne, 1982; Mallick, 1997), it is clear that the treatment acceptance rate for renal failure patients is governed both by governmental policies and economic pressures (Schena, 1997). Canada, although adjacent to the United States, practices dialysis restriction through non-referral of uremic patients by generalists and nephrologists to dialysis facilities (Mendelssohn *et al.*, 1995; McKenzie *et al.*, 1998). Kjellstrand added substance to the inquiry into government and physician restriction to patient referral for dialysis warning that: 'Not-so-subtle economic pressure by managed care, government, administrators, and politicians, is already in force' (Kjellstrand, 1996). Entering this turbulent sea, nephrologists desiring placement for their uremic patients face resistance and obstruction that is likely to grow as the budget for ESRD therapy grows ever larger.

Should every uremic patient be treated?

Given the actuality that everyone manifesting kidney failure cannot be treated by dialysis or a kidney transplant because of economic limitation (Ozminkowski *et al.*, 1998) and a shortage of cadaver organs, rationing is inevitable (Hauptman and O'Connor, 1997). Although many schemes have been proposed to allocate medical resources that are scarce, all distill down to restriction by age, diagnosis, economic and/or political status (citizenship). A personal exclusion (rationing) preference list is given in Table 4.1. Observing what happens when government alone, or undisciplined managed care companies determine who gets what in medical care, I urge that physicians participate in every aspect of medical resource allocation. Appreciating that as a group, physicians elected medicine as a profession with the highest motivation of serving others, it is difficult to imagine non-physicians making the crucial decision of 'who shall live'.

Table 4.1 Exclusion from government-funded ESRD therapy: author's bias

	Hemodialysis	Peritoneal dialysis	Cadaver kidney transplantation
Age restriction	>80 years	>80 years	>60 years
Futile prognosis	All	All	All
Overt psychosis	Non-comprehending	Non-comprehending	Non-comprehending
Mental deficiency	Non-comprehending	Non-comprehending	Non-comprehending
Non-citizen	Case by case	Case by case	All
Infants	Unless transplant	Unless transplant	Evaluate individually
Non-compliance	Case by case	Case by case	All
HIV+	None	None	All

Despite admitted sometimes egregious behavior by a small minority of doctors who place the business of medicine above the calling of medicine, I believe the patient's interests are best served when physicians decide their fate.

Variables used to limit dialysis include age of the patient (Chandna et al., 1999), extensive disability (Gladman and Sackley, 1998), persistent vegetative state (Payne and Taylor, 1997), adverse psychiatric evaluation (Corley et al., 1998; Klapheke, 1999), and citizenship (Maxwell, 1995).

Age

Ethicists split hairs when contending with the issue of age as a legitimate criterion for limiting resource allocation. Consider the following: 'Rationing according to social worth, ability to pay, or age is not ethically justifiable, but it is justified to ration according to medical benefit' (Glover and Moss, 1998). What does that mean? Is it not self-evident that any medical benefit derived from a kidney transplant will be greater for a 40-year-old than a 90-year-old, all other factors being equivalent? Similarly, (Nilstun and Ohlsson, 1995) expound:

Health care rationing by age is inconsistent with the principles of equality and liberty. But in some situations such rationing has support from the principles of solidarity and efficiency. The compromise suggested is that, as a rule, rationing by age should not be permitted, except in situations with intrinsic scarcity (as is the case with transplantation) and in situations with temporary extrinsic scarcity (as was the case with dialysis for a period of time).

Again, interpretation provides sufficient substrate to occupy a Talmudic scholar for weeks.

Opposing age, *per se*, as reason to exclude individuals from dialytic therapy for uremia, Chandna and co-workers conducted a hospital-based cohort study of 292 patients of mean age 61.3 years (18–92 years) starting dialysis over a 4-year recruitment period (follow-up 15–63 months). They concluded 'Severity of comorbid conditions and functional capacity are more important than age in predicting survival and morbidity of patients on dialysis' (Chandna et al., 1999). Also supporting dialysis without age restriction, Neves et al. conclude from an experience in treating 50 hemodialysis patients aged over 80 years at the beginning of dialysis that 'haemodialysis is the best available choice for treating very old chronic renal failure patients.' Actuarial survival in their patients was 48% at 36 months (Neves et al., 1994).

Although kidney transplants are performed in recipients in their eighth decade, consensus thinking recognizes that a high mortality and aggravated morbidity accompany the stress of surgery and immunosuppression in those older than 60 years (Morris et al., 1991; Hestin et al., 1994). Cadaveric renal transplantation in the elderly is advised only if undertaken after careful selection; excluding serious cardiovascular disease; and giving truthful counseling as to the greater risk of death (approximately one-third of recipients are likely to die within three years). There are no reports of kidney transplantation in a series of patients in the eighth or ninth decade.

Transplant surgeons have long accepted imposition of the stricture on successful outcome imposed by advancing age. Evidence that this is so is afforded by perusal of the chapter on 'World transplant records' in *Clinical Transplants 1998* (Cecka and Terasaki, 1999). No living double-lung recipient was older than age 60 at the time of transplantation. No recipient of a small bowel transplant older than age 57 was alive. Of the registry's solid organ allografts, the oldest given a pancreas (age 62), liver (age 76), or heart (age 74) were all younger than age 80. Furthermore, while four renal allograft recipients were older than age 80, only 23 of approximately 50,000 kidney recipients since 1995 were given to recipients older than 75 years when transplanted. From the foregoing, it is reasoned that even though the adverse impact of age may be objectionable when allocating organ transplants, the reality of predictable failure has defined age as a key criterion for selecting potential recipients.

As noted in Table 4.1, kidney transplantation using the common pool of cadaver kidneys should not be applied in recipients older than 60 years. Setting an upper age limit for initiating dialytic therapy is less supportable by outcome-based trials though as a generalization, few individuals older than 80 will achieve even marginal rehabilitation.

James A. Michener, author of the Pulitzer Prize-winning *Tales of the South Pacific* and more than 40 other books with combined sales of more than 75 million, said: 'A person on dialysis undergoes very heavy and irritating treatment and in time it seems more than you can bear. There's always an easy out, just don't go to the hospital. Then after two weeks, you're dead.' At the age of 90, after three years of hemodialysis, Michener concluded: 'For the first time I could understand how a person could say "the hell with it".' Michener died, days after ordering his doctors in Austin, Texas to stop dialysis (Channel 4000, 1997). As illustrated by the sad outcome of initiating dialytic therapy in a renowned public figure, biological aging cannot not be ignored as factor in determining ESRD therapy.

Few individuals, in my experience, attain satisfactory rehabilitation when dialysis is started after the age of 75 years. Just as surgeons decline to operate when the chances for success are minimal, so should nephrologists withhold *imposition* of dialytic therapy on the very old. All of society understands the need for age limits at both extremes of life: those younger than age 18 will not be granted a license to drive in New York State, while individuals older than age 55 must yield their license as commercial pilots. Recognizing the need and practicality of setting limits to a stressful regimen, I believe that restricting dialysis to ESRD patients younger than 75 is a rational policy.

Psychosis, mental deficiency

Few reports examine the application of ESRD therapy in patients who are unable to comprehend what is happening to them. Reports of satisfactory treatment of ESRD in Down's syndrome by kidney transplantation (Edvardsson *et al.*, 1995), or peritoneal dialysis (Kupferman *et al.*, 1994) attest to the perseverance and dedication of responsible pediatric nephrologists. Nevertheless, individuals who are unaware of the rationale for their uremia therapy should not undergo long-term dialysis. I have observed and lamented treatment of combative, screaming, adult psychotic patients, made irreversibly uremic by lithium, whose dialysis regimen was conducted using restraints and powerful sedation. Similarly, I watched premature infants with multiple congenital anomalies—including renal agenesis—begin dialysis realizing that there was a negligible probability of their reaching adulthood. There are no easy answers to the ethical questions provoked by the challenge of managing uremia in the unaware. At morning report discussions, renal fellows and elective residents are about equally aligned favoring or opposing such therapy. I believe it unwise, a waste of resources, and even unkind to subject those without comprehension to the rigors of a dialytic regimen or immunosuppression for a renal allograft.

Medical futility

Futile (from the Latin *futilis*) means incapable of producing any result, serving no useful purpose. As defined by Schneiderman, Jecker, and Jonsen, (1990) a medical regimen can be termed futile when physicians conclude (from personal experience, or published experimental data) that in the last 100 cases a medical treatment has been useless, that treatment is futile. A treatment with less than a 1% probability of reversing 'permanent' unconsciousness and/or dependence on intensive medical care is futile (Schneiderman et al., 1990). In practice, the actual incidence of futility has been subject to debate with some investigators noting a low frequency in intensive care (Halevy et al., 1996), while others endorse the concept of futility as a practical guide for efforts at resuscitation (Ebell, 1995).

Nephrologists must regularly respond to the request for dialysis in patients with no hope of recovery. Ebbing renal function is a uniform component of multiorgan failure. Families wanting the health care team to 'do something' as life slips away accept the concept that a hemodialysis machine may accomplish a magical reversal in the downward course of a loved one. Resisting this call for intervention may be more difficult than adding one more machine with its tubing to the complex life sustaining systems already in place. Not applying a therapy that is inappropriate is a logical and defensible action. Interpreting a specific age, diagnosis, or social circumstance (non-citizenship) as justification for not providing dialysis or a kidney transplant may require 'justification' or explanation including resort to legal advice or consultation with hospital administration's risk-management officer. Extreme caution is appropriate when sentencing an ESRD patient to death by non-treatment on the basis of a futile prognosis. Projection of the patient's course can be tricky and unreliable. It is the outside change of recovery that drives initiation of dialysis in some seemingly hopeless patients. Sometimes, an entire disease category moves from exclusion to acceptability because intrepid investigators opted to go against mainstream thinking. For example: (1) totally blind diabetic individuals initially denied dialytic therapy were shown not only to attain substantial life prolongation on CAPD but to be capable of self-care with a low rate of peritonitis (Flynn, 1982); and (2) similarly, dismal survival reported as limited to days to weeks in HIV positive hemodialysis patients (Rao et al., 1985) is now the exception as antiviral regimens and appropriate application of antibiotics have been employed to extend life on dialysis to months to years with mean survival of 11.8 months in one series (Perinbasekar et al., 1996). The point extracted is that nephrologists opting to push the vanguard of therapy beyond what is conventional should be denied such opportunity only after full realization that the limits of uremia therapy are not fixed but are continuously evolving.

Non-compliant patients

Non-compliance, a vaguely defined concept when applied to the medical course of dialysis patients, means: skipping one or more dialyses in a month, shortening by 10 or more minutes one or more dialyses in a month, an interdialytic weight gain of more than 5.7% of dry weight, or a serum phosphate (PO_4) of greater than 7.5 mg/dL (Leggat et al., 1998). Alternatively, non-compliance may be reflected by antisocial or combative behavior in any chronic illness in which the doctor–patient relationship is fractured reflecting the patient's admixture of fear, fatigue, and anxiety (Anderson and Matthews, 1981).

As regimens grow in complexity, it becomes nearly impossible to 'comply' with all of their components and demands. In our outpatient renal clinic, for example, patients receive a mean of 8.3 medications but few are able to identify each drug or explain its actions and major side effects. Both dialysis and transplant patients regularly skirt full compliance with dietary and/or medication prescriptions. For example, at least one in five surveyed recipients of solid organ allografts admit to omitting one or more doses of immunosuppressive medications (Greenstein and Siegal, 1998). For ESRD patients, creating an atmosphere of antagonism and conflict transforms therapy into a struggle that may defeat the physician's primary obligation to beneficence. Faced with a belligerent, threatening and law-suit-minded patient who frustrates efforts to proffer ordinary treatment, the sometimes bewildered nephrologist seeks to break the patient–physician bond by any legitimate means. The main ethical issues in considering belligerent and threatening patients for dialysis have been set forth (Sermon, 1996). The types of conflict that may arise in a nephrology program are:

1. Missing visits, payments
2. Non-adherence to diet
3. Non-adherence to medications
4. Late arrival for scheduled visit or treatment
5. Omitting dialyses, terminating hemodialyses early
6. Proscribed behavior in treatment unit (eating on dialysis)
7. Verbal threats/abuse to health care team or support staff
8. Filing unsubstantiated complaints to State Health Department
9. Initiating unsubstantiated 'nuisance' lawsuits against health care team
10. Disruptive action in treatment unit or clinic
11. Physical assault on health care team

Non-compliance by dialysis patients, most frequently by non-adherence to diet, medications, or the dialysis schedule, disrupts unit function and frustrates well-meaning staff. By better teaching and communication, as well as through attention to patient needs the prevalence of non-compliance can be sharply reduced (Lundin,

1995). Younger men have been the most likely to reject their prescribed diet. Procci (1981) interprets ignoring dietary restrictions, despite adverse consequences as an attempt to regain control of one's person in a dependent situation. Lundin, a physician and dialysis patient observes that 'When the dialysis staff rises to the challenge of making the treatment comfortable as well as efficiently fitting it into the patient's life outside the unit there should be fewer intratreatment complications and premature signoffs.'

By answering the following six questions an evaluation of the genesis and possible resolution of a kidney patient's defiance and challenge to the health care team should become evident:

1. Does the patient realize the genesis of his kidney failure?
2. Does the patient grasp the intent of renal therapy?
3. Does the patient have the necessary intellect and motor skills to comply with treatment?
4. Can support figures assist in reasoning with the patient?
5. Is the patient psychotic?
6. Is there secondary gain by non-compliant behavior?

Once a formulation of the problem is constructed, a remedy may appear obvious. To assist, I recommend the guidance in evaluating and managing non-compliant and abusive ESRD patients developed by Alvin H. Moss at West Virginia University. Moss co-authored a manual for End-Stage Renal Disease network 5 on *Working with noncompliant and abusive patients* (Mid Atlantic Renal Coalition, 1994).

Does the patient realize the genesis of his kidney failure?

Inner-city residents lacking comprehensive medical care may present with advanced irreversible renal insufficiency late in the course of disease and pre-empt psychological preparation for ESRD (Ifudu et al., 1998). For patients lacking a physician, any perceived connection between harmful conduct (heroin injections) and renal disease may be remote. Learning that the need for dialysis derives from either hepatitis C or narcotic drug toxicity may be sufficient to cause a disruptive patient to go along with the treatment plan.

Does the patient grasp the intent of renal therapy?

Frequently, dialysis patients lack understanding of how dialysis works or why it must be performed. Only a minority are able to recite the most recent results for their serum albumin, hematocrit, or dialysis efficiency (urea reduction rate or KT/V), though these numbers govern their present and forecast their future.

Does the patient have the necessary intellect and motor skills to comply with treatment?

Severe mental deficiency obviously interdicts performance of a complicated treatment plan in the absence of support from family or a partner. Likewise, a blind diabetic stroke patient cannot be expected to perform peritoneal dialysis exchanges.

Can support figures assist in reasoning with the patient?

Interjecting a helpful spouse, parent, child, friend or member of the clergy can bridge the gap between the renal team and the non-compliant patient.

Is the patient psychotic?

Schizophrenia, bipolar disorders, and some rare enzyme deficiencies (McGuffin et al., 1987), like brain tumors may alter personality and precipitate aggressive and/or antisocial behavior.

Is there secondary gain by non-compliant behavior?

Homeless individuals may posture as antisocial in order to obtain lodging and food during a cold northern winter. An otherwise neglected sibling may 'raise a ruckus' in order to be noticed. By refusing occupational therapy and other rehabilitation programs, a dialysis patient may secure monthly disability checks that amount to a greater sum than might be earned at a low paying job for the unskilled.

A pragmatic approach to resolution of kidney patient–staff confrontation is given below:

1. Remove 'communication spoilers', such as criticizing, name-calling, moralizing, threatening, ordering and psychologic diagnosing persons.
2. Employ 'reflective listening', to show that the patient has been 'heard'.
3. Deal directly with problem behaviors: small steps, involve the patient, build on patient's strengths, be clear on who is to do what and when.
4. Devise new approaches to 'old problems', such as lateness and complaints.
5. Detail the consequences of aberrant behavior in terms that are comprehensible.
6. Prepare a behavior contract that specifies what is to be done by patient and renal team.
7. Prepare in advance to manage anger.
8. Anticipate for the staff a step-by-step coping with agitated and disruptive patients.
9. Establish and publicize a grievance procedure.
10. Appoint a patient representative.

Without preparation for 'incidents', confused and flustered team members may react in ways that inflame and accelerate rather than calm and ameliorate patient agitation.

In my experience, all ten items listed above can be distilled down to a single admonition: 'Carefully listen to the patient's complaints and wants.' Theodore Reich (1983) entitled one of his incisive psychoanalytic texts *Listening with the third ear*, conveying the necessity to be receptive to more than the words being spoken by a suffering individual. The listener's receptive posture and body language will prompt the patient to reveal what is really wrong. For example, repetitive lateness for dialysis treatments may be due to the patient's wait for a school bus for a disabled child before departing for the dialysis facility. Remedy: schedule the patient for a later shift. Likewise, an insensitive remark by a staff member may have been interpreted as racial bias inducing smoldering resentment that surfaces as hostility. Remedy: find out who said what and talk it through. By employing the technique of 'reflective listening' the therapist signals having 'heard' what another has said.

When reasoning misfires and the intensity of patient anger increases, the following sequence is suggested:

1. Inventory potential third-party problem solvers (spouse, family, friend, clergy, others).
2. Carefully document incidents and staff responses in the patient's chart.
3. Involve the unit social worker and obtain psychiatric consultation if indicated.
4. Report the growing problem to the unit or hospital 'risk management' service.
5. Advise the patient *in writing by certified mail* that a limit in toleration of the patient's action has been defined. Establish a date for compliance.
6. Should the abusive behavior continue beyond the time limit, notify the patient of termination of services *in writing by certified mail* permitting sufficient time for the patient to seek and obtain alternative dialysis care (at least 30 days). Include in the notification a list of proximal dialysis units and the directors' phone numbers.

Sussman and Spinal (1997) focus specifically on the abusive dialysis patient, concluding that for competent individuals who 'behave in dangerous ways . . . suspension of dialysis would, in our judgment, have been ethically defensible'. In an advisory bulletin to physicians, the American Medical Association's counsel states: 'The obligation to treat non-compliant patients should not be an absolute one' (Orenlicher, 1991). On the other hand, the AMA's counsel warns: 'Patients should not have to pay for their non-compliance with their lives.' Thus, like King Solomon approaching two alleged mothers claiming the same baby, the patient must not be cut in half in order to restore peace to a dialysis unit. As a last resort, an abusive non-compliant dialysis patient can be discharged to another facility providing that the patient's welfare is protected.

Sometimes, although unwanted and embarrassing to the responsible nephrologist, patient problems in non-compliance reach the courts. The most notable example in the United States is that of *Brown* v *Bower*, a case that reached the Circuit Court of Appeals in New Orleans provoking national media attention. A dialysis pioneer, Dr John Bower, Chief, Division of Nephrology and Professor of Medicine, University of Mississippi Medical Center (UMMC), was sued by Michael Brown in Mississippi. Brown sought an injunction to require Dr Bower, UMMC, and/or Kidney Care, Inc., a private dialysis provider, to deliver dialytic therapy after being refused acceptance because of prior experience with Mr Brown as an abusive, disruptive patient who had missed scheduled dialysis sessions, threatened to kill his nephrologist, and shoot the hospital administrator (Miller, 1995). Bower successfully argued that a physician and/or private dialysis facility may refuse treatment under such difficult circumstances. To compel treatment by Bower, the Court ruled, would violate the XIIIth Amendment to the Constitution of the United States, which prohibited slavery, for it would constitute, for Bower, involuntary servitude (Bower, 1995). Negating this victory for Bower, because equivalent therapy was unavailable for the complaining patient, UMMC was ordered to continue to provide dialysis care.

Despite being dismissed by a hospital's dialysis unit, the patient on a dialysis regimen who is in need of treatment (fluid overload, hyperkalemia) must be dialyzed on appearance at that hospital's dialysis unit. Diligent application of the principles enumerated above will, in practice, minimize the number of times that actual discharge letters are required. In our inner-city dialysis program, in which serious socio-economic problems confound uremia therapy, only rarely have we had to carry our exasperation to the limit of resorting to a protective police presence during dialysis sessions. With further reflection, I wonder if even these catastrophes in health care delivery were avoidable.

Conclusions

Renal care must be delivered under the umbrella of: (1) respect for autonomy; (2) nonmaleficence; (3) beneficence; and (4) justice (Beauchamp and Childress, 1994). Spital (1998) addressed these concerns in planning for a kidney transplant from a living donor (Spital, 1998). Employing Beauchamp and Childress's concept of justice as contingent on 'fair, equitable, and appropriate treatment in light of what is due or owed to persons', how should a nephrologist weigh the ethical aspects of individual patient care? As listed below, there are concerns that should be reviewed whenever complex life support (dialysis or kidney transplantation) is to be given or withheld:

1. Has all relevant medical information been reviewed?
2. Is the patient capable of making medical decisions?
3. If not, who is the appropriate decision maker?
4. Were decisions made by a surrogate? Justification?
5. Have advance directives been signed?
6. Have key parties met to discuss case?
7. Are there legal constraints?

Resort to an Ethics Committee consultation is appropriate whenever the complexity of issues surrounding delivery of care remain unresolved by the usual discussions between patient and renal team. As outlined by Freer (1998), an ethics consultation consists of collecting data and then finding the best solution. Success is contingent on preparation in which 'involved' parties should have been convened, advance directives reviewed, and any legal constraints appreciated. Freer (1998) notes: 'The goal of committee consultation is to facilitate sound decision making by the appropriate parties (patient/surrogate and physician/other health care providers). Whenever possible, the consultant should act primarily as a catalyst in that process. Outright questions like, "what should we do?" need to be reflected back onto the principal parties so they can work out the answer themselves.'

Admittedly, there have been no prospective controlled trials of the value of Ethics Committees or ethics consultations. Some critiques raise difficult questions about the worth of ethics committees even suggesting that they may result in more harm than good (Jamrozik and Kolybaba, 1999). Nevertheless, devoid of alternative mechanisms for problem solving, the prudent nephrologist will include the hospital risk-management and ethics consultation procedures in the formulation of regimens that apply or withhold life-maintaining renal therapy whenever the decision is likely to incite patient or family discontent or challenge.

References

Anderson, R. J., and Matthews, C. (1981). Non-compliance: failure of the therapeutic partnership. *Cardiovascular Medicine*, **2**, 464–70.

Beauchamp, T. L., and Childress, J. F. (1994). *Principles of biomedical ethics*. Oxford University Press, New York.

Berlyne, G. M. (1982) Over 50 and uremic equals death. The failure of the British National Health Service to provide adequate dialysis facilities. *Nephron*, **31**, 189–90.

Bower, J. D. (1995). The issue: the role of the professional in the management of noncompliant or problem dialysis patients. *Dialysis and Transplantation*, **24**, 173, 196.

Bruns, F. J., Seddon, P., Saul, M., and Zeidel, M. L. (1998). The cost of caring for end-stage kidney disease patients: an analysis based on hospital financial transaction records. *Journal of the American Society of Nephrology*, **9**, 884–90.

Cecka, J. M., and Terasaki, P. I. (eds) (1999). *Clinical Transplants 1998*. pp. 443–7. UCLA Tissue Typing Laboratory, Los Angeles.

Chandna, S. M., Schulz, J., Lawrence, C., Greenwood, R. N., and Farrington, K. (1999). Is there a rationale for rationing chronic dialysis? A hospital based cohort study of factors affecting survival and morbidity. *British Medical Journal*, **318** (7178): 217–23.

Channel 4000 (1997). James Michener Dies at 90. Internet Broadcasting Systems, Inc.

Chantrel, F., Enache, I., Bouiller, M., Kolb, I., Kunz, K., Petitjean, P., Moulin, B., and Hannedouche, T. (1999). Abysmal prognosis of patients with type 2 diabetes entering dialysis. *Nephrology, Dialysis, Transplantation*, **14**(1), 129–36.

Corley, M. C., Westerberg, N., Elswick, R. K. Jr, Connell, D., Neil, J., Sneed, G., and Witcher, V. (1998). Rationing organs using psychosocial and lifestyle criteria. Research in Nursing and Health, **21**(4), 327–37.

Ebell, M. H. (1995). When everything is too much. Quantitative approaches to the issue of futility. *Archives of Family Medicine*, **4**, 352–6.

Edvardsson, V. O., Kaiser, B. A., Polinsky, M. S., and Baluarte, H. J. (1995). Successful living-related renal transplantation in an adolescent with Down syndrome. *Pediatric Nephrology*, **9**, 398–9.

Flynn, C. T. (1982). The diabetic on CAPD. In *Diabetic renal-retinal syndrome. Prevention and management* (eds E. A. Friedman, and F. A. L'Esperance, Jr.) pp. 321–30. Grune 8 Stratton, Inc, New York, New York.

Freer, J. (1998) How to perform an ethics consult. Ethics Committee Core Curriculum. Online Edition. UB Center for Clinical Ethics and Humanities in Health Care, 10/18/98. http://wings.buffalo.edu/faculty/research/bioethics/man-case.html

Friedman, E. A. (1994). Revelations behind a fallen curtain: Dialysis restriction and the Berlin Wall. *Dialysis Transplant Nephrology*, **9**, 242–3.

Friedman, E. A. (1995). Facing the reality: The world cannot afford uremia therapy at the start of the 21st century. *Artificial Organs*, **19**, 481–5.

Friedman, E. A. (1996). ESRD therapy: An American success story. *JAMA*, **275**, 1118–22.

Friedman, E. A. (1999). Hemodialysis for French diabetic patients. Nephrology, Dialysis Transplantation, **14**, 30–31.

Friedman, E. A., and Delano, B. G. (1981). Can the world afford uremia therapy? *Proceedings of the 8th International Congress on Nephrology.* pp. 677–83. Karger, Athens.

Gladman, J. R., and Sackley, C. M. (1998). The scope for rehabilitation in severely disabled stroke patients. *Disability and Rehabilitation*, **20**(10), 391–4.

Glover, J. J., and Moss, A. H. (1998). Rationing dialysis in the United States: possible implications of capitated systems. *Advances in Renal Replacement Therapy*, **5**, 341–9.

Greenstein, S., and Siegal, B. (1998). Compliance and noncompliance in patients with a functioning renal transplant: a multi center study. *Transplantation*, **66**, 1718–26.

Halevy, A., Neal, R. C., and Brody, B. A. (1996). The low frequency of futility in an adult intensive care unit setting. *Archives of Internal Medicine*, **156**, 100–104.

Hauptman, P. J., and O'Connor, K. J. (1997). Procurement and allocation of solid organs for transplantation. *New England Journal of Medicine*, **336**, 422–31.

Hestin, D., Frimat, L., Hubert, J., Renoult, E., Huu, T. C., Kessler, M. (1994). Renal transplantation in patients over sixty years of age. *Clinical Nephrology*, **42**(4): 232–6.

Ifudu, O., Dawood, M., Homel, P., and Friedman, E. A. (1998). Excess morbidity in patients starting uremia therapy without prior care by a nephrologist. *American Journal of Kidney Disease*, **28**, 841–5.

Jacobs, C., Broyer, M., Brunner, F. P. Brynger, H., Donckerwolcke, R. A., Kramer, P., Selwood, N. H., Wing, A. J., and Blake, P. H. (1981). Combined report on regular dialysis and transplantation in Europe, XI, 1981. *Proceedings of the European Dialysis and Transplant Association and European Renal Association*, **18**, 4–58.

Jamrozik, K., and Kolybaba, M. (1999). Are ethics committees retarding the improvement of health services in Australia? *Medical Journal of Australia*, **170**, 26–8.

Kjellstrand, C. M. (1996). High-technology medicine and the old: the dialysis example. *Journal of Internal Medicine*, **239**, 195–210.

Klapheke, M. M. (1999). The role of the psychiatrist in organ transplantation. *Bulletin of the Menninger Clinic*, **63**, 13–39.

Kupferman, J. C., Stewart, C. L., Kaskel, F. J., Katz, S. P., and Fine, R. N. (1994). Chronic peritoneal dialysis in a child with Down syndrome. *Pediatric Nephrology*, **8**, 644–5.

Leggat, J. E. Jr, Orzol, S. M., Hulbert-Shearon, T. E., Golper, T. A., Jones, C. A., Held, P. J., and Port, F. K. (1998). Noncompliance in hemodialysis: predictors and survival analysis. *American Journal of Kidney Disease*, **32**, 139–45.

Laurent, G., Calemard, E., and Charra, B. (1983). Long dialysis: a review of fifteen years experience in one centre 1986–1983. *Proceedings of the European Dialysis and Transplant Association*, **20**, 122–35.

Lundin, A. P. (1995). Causes of noncompliance in dialysis patients. Dialysis and Transplantation, **24**, 174–6, 202.

Maghlaoua, M., Halimi, S., Cordonnier, D., Zmirou, D., Balducci, F., Benhamou, P., and Zaoui, P. (1997). Les diabétiques traités en France pour insuffisance rénale chronique terminale. Enquête épidémiologique. UREMIDIAB 2. Résultats prélimninaires. Symposium Gambro 18–19 Septembre 1997, Reims, France.

Mallick, N. P. (1997). The costs of renal services in Britain. *Nephrology, Dialysis, Transplantation*, **12** Suppl 1, 25–28.

Maxwell, R. J. (1995). Can we do better? *British Medical Bulletin*, **51**, 941–8.

McGuffin, P., Murray, R. M., and Reveley, A. M. (1987). Genetic influence on the psychoses. *British Medical Bulletin*, **43**, 531–6.

McKenzie, J. K., Moss, A. H., Feest, T. G., Stocking, C. B., and Siegler, M. (1998). Dialysis decision making in Canada, the United Kingdom, and the United States. Am J Kidney Dis; **31**(1): 12–18.

Mendelssohn, D. C., Kua, B. T., and Singer, P. A. (1995). Referral for dialysis in Ontario. *Archives of Internal Medicine*, **155**, 2473–8.

Mid Atlantic Renal Coalition (1994). *Working with noncompliant and abusive patients.* End-Stage Renal Disease network 5, Midlothian, VA.

Miller, R. B. (1995). Treating the disruptive patient. *Nephrology News and Issues*, **9**, 39–40.

Morris, G. E., Jamieson, N. V., Small, J., Evans, D. B., and Calne, R. (1991). Cadaveric renal transplantation in elderly recipients: is it worthwhile? *Nephrology, Dialysis, Transplantation*, **6**, 887–92.

Neves, P. L., Sousa, A., Bernardo, I., Anunciada, A. I., Pinto, I., Bexiga, I., Aniceto, J., and Amorim, J. P. (1994). Chronic haemodialysis for very old patients. *Age and Ageing*, **23**, 356–9.

Nilstun, T., and Ohlsson, R. (1995). Should health care be rationed by age? *Scandinavian Journal of Social Medicine*, **23**, 81–4.

Orenlicher, D. (1991) Denying treatment to the noncompliant patient. *Journal of the American Medical Association*, **266**, 1579–82.

Oxford English Dictionary (1971) Oxford University Press, Glasgow.

Ozminkowski, R. J., White, A. J., Hassol, A., and Murphy, M. (1998). What if socioeconomics made no difference?: access to a cadaver kidney transplant as an example. *Medical Care*, **36**, 1398–406.

Payne, S. K., and Taylor, R. M. (1997). The persistent vegetative state and anencephaly: problematic paradigms for discussing futility and rationing. *Seminars in Neurology*, **17**, 257–63.

Perinbasekar, S., Brod-Miller, C., Pal, S., and Mattana, J. (1996). Predictors of survival in HIV-infected patients on hemodialysis. *American Journal of Nephrology*, **16**, 280–6.

Procci, W. R. (1981). Psychological factors associated with severe abuse of the hemodialysis diet. *General Hospital Psychiatry*, **3**, 111–8.

Rao, T. K. S., Manis, T., and Friedman, E. A. (1985). Dismal prognosis despite maintenance hemodialysis in AIDS nephropathy and chronic uremia. *Transactions of the American Society for Artificial Internal Organs*, **31**, 160–3.

Reich, T. (1983). *Listening with the third ear: The inner experience of a psychoanalyst.* Farrar, Straus & Giroux, New York.

Schena, F. P. (1997). Report on the first meeting of the Chairmen of the National and International Registries. *Kidney International*, **52**, 1422.

Schneiderman, L. J., Jecker, N. S., and Jonsen, A. R. (1990). Medical futility: its meaning and ethical implications. *Annals of Internal Medicine*, **112**, 949–54.

Spital, A. (1998). Ethical issues in living organ donation. 1998 Nephrology Ethics Forum. *American Journal of Kidney* Disease, **32**, 676–91.

Sussman, B., and Spinal, A. (1997). Risky business: managing dangerous dialysis patients. *Seminars Dialysis*, **10**, 282–5.

United States Renal Data System (USRDS) (1999). *Annual data report.* The National Institutes of Health, National Institute of Diabetes and Digestive and Kidney Diseases, Bethesda, MD.

5
Equity and patient autonomy in dialysis
Norman G. Levinsky

Which patients with end-stage renal disease (ESRD) should receive chronic dialysis? Perhaps the question is better formulated as: Should any patients with ESRD who want the therapy not receive dialysis? This chapter explores these questions with respect to a number of patient criteria: age, comorbidities, terminal illnesses, persistent vegetative state, diminished mental status, non-compliance, and destructive behavior. Broader issues of societal allocation of resources for costly ESRD programs in nations at various economic levels are discussed in several other chapters.

Age

The general consensus among nephrologists (Kilner, 1988; McKenzie *et al.*, 1998) is that age should not be a criterion for withholding dialysis. Of the various proposals for guidelines by committees or by individual nephrologists (summarized in Moss, 1995), only one (Lowance, 1993) recommends using age to advise patients against dialysis, if 'the patient is . . . chronologically old with an estimated life expectancy of under two years'. However, the consensus assumes that there is no explicit limit on resources, which requires choices among patients. In response to a hypothetical scenario in which total dialysis resources are insufficient to dialyze all patients who can benefit, nearly 90% of directors of US dialysis programs considered age a moderately important criterion for selecting those who would receive dialysis (Kilner, 1988).

Nilstun and Ohlsson (1995) provide an ethical framework that supports this distinction, arguing that use of age as criterion violates principles of equality and patient self-determination. However, these are overridden in a situation of scarcity by an obligation to give primacy to the right of younger individuals to reach a reasonably normal lifespan. As Kjellstrand (1996) has pointed out, however, rationing by age would sacrifice several older persons to offer treatment to one younger person. This is because the lifespan of a 30-year-old on dialysis would be expected to be several times as long as that of a 70-year-old. If the 30-year-old survives 30 years on dialysis, he or she would use as many dialysis treatments as six 70-year-old patients who survive 5 years each. It is doubtful whether many analysts who support age as a criterion for rationing dialysis have considered this equation.

It is well recognized that variation in health status at any age is much greater among the elderly than among younger individuals. Hence, chronological age is a poor predictor of the ability of an individual to benefit from dialysis. 'Physiological age' and comorbidities may reduce the potential benefit of dialysis and are more suitable bases for discussing with a patient on an individual basis whether the benefits to him or her are anticipated to outweigh the burdens.

Callahan (1987), Daniels (1988), Veatch (1988) and other ethicists (see also chapter 4) have set out the ethical arguments supporting the use of age as a criterion for rationing medical care, especially advanced technology such as dialysis. They argue that limits on health care of the elderly—especially 'hi-tech' care, which is disproportionately expensive—are justifiable because all citizens would share equally in the risk that treatment to extend life at its outer limits would be denied. They also would benefit equally if the conserved resources were redirected to health care at earlier stages of life or for that matter to other socially useful purposes. Callahan (1987) has argued that citizens should be educated to substitute communalism for individualism and to accept limited health care towards the end of life for the sake of society as a whole. On this basis, the use of expensive technology such as dialysis for older persons (about one-half of patients started on chronic dialysis in the US in 1997 were over 65) is ethically inappropriate.

In my opinion, the counter-arguments are more persuasive. It is hard to predict how well any elderly person will do on dialysis. At the least, a trial to determine the quality of life is appropriate, since dialysis can be withdrawn if the burdens prove to outweigh the benefits. Life expectancy has increased markedly in Western countries; many elderly persons have good health and are able to undergo major surgery or dialysis without excessive morbidity or mortality. Moreover, previous experience in the US (Evans *et al.*, 1981) and UK (Aaron and Schwartz, 1984) when dialysis facilities were limited contradicts the belief of the philosophers that equity can be preserved if a life-sustaining treatment is rationed. Before Medicare made dialysis affordable for nearly all Americans, those who obtained it were disproportionately younger well-educated white males (Evans *et al.*, 1981). Those older persons in the UK who could 'work the system' often managed to obtain dialysis when it was informally restricted to those under 55 (Aaron and Schwartz, 1984).

Often quoted is a conclusion of a US Institute of Medicine (1991) committee on the Medicare ESRD program: 'Chronological age was considered and explicitly rejected by the committee as a criterion for patient acceptance, since it does not measure the ability of an individual to benefit from treatment'. I was chair of that committee and continue to support that viewpoint.

Comorbidities and terminal illness

Is it reasonable to dialyze patients with serious comorbidities or those with illnesses that are judged to be terminal? In answering this question, one must start by recognizing that the limited ability of physicians to determine survival accurately or to predict reliably which patients with serious comorbid conditions will have a good quality of life (as judged by the patients themselves) on chronic dialysis. Mistakes in prediction, which lead to treatment of those who do not benefit, are less serious than those that cause treatment to be withheld without a trial of dialysis. In the former case, dialysis can be stopped, although I concede this is often difficult in practice. In the latter, the decision is irreversible because the patient will die.

It is also important to remember that medical advances may alter the likelihood that patients will benefit from dialysis. Early in the use of chronic dialysis, diabetic patients usually were not treated on the grounds that they did poorly, since dialysis did not prevent complications such as coronary heart disease, stroke, blindness and neuropathy. Experience with and improvement in various aspects of dialysis and diabetic care has shown that many diabetic patients achieve benefits from dialysis which outweigh the burdens. Diabetic patients with ESRD are now routinely accepted for chronic dialysis; they made up about one-third of the population on chronic dialysis in the United States in 1997. Early in the evolution of the AIDS epidemic, dialysis of patients with AIDS nephropathy was considered inappropriate by many nephrologists because the patients survived only weeks or a few months. With the advent of protease inhibitors as therapy for AIDS, survival has increased and dialysis for patients with ESRD due to AIDS nephropathy has become routine.

A key issue is whether some minimum anticipated life expectancy is required to justify initiating treatment. Lowance (1993) suggests that patients should be advised not to begin dialysis if their life expectancy is less than two years because of co-existing disease such as advanced diabetes or heart or vascular disease. It is unclear why the line should be drawn at two years rather than one year or three. There is no medical or moral justification for selecting any specific anticipated survival as determinative. Most people no doubt would value one added year of life highly if it is of reasonable quality in their own judgment.

The SUPPORT (an elaborate Study to Understand Prognoses and Preferences for Outcomes and Risks of Treatment) investigators present a cost-effectiveness argument in favor of withholding dialysis from seriously ill patients (Hamel et al., 1997). They studied patients who had an estimated 50% 6-month probability of survival due to acute and chronic respiratory failure, heart failure, cirrhosis, sepsis, malignancies and other serious illnesses. Of the patients in whom dialysis was initiated for renal failure, 27% were alive after 6 months. The majority of the survivors rated their quality of life as 'good' or better. The cost per quality-adjusted life-year of extending life by dialysis was $128 200, which the authors note is above the $50000 that is 'many experts' standard for cost-effective medical care'. It is beyond the scope of this chapter to discuss the ethical basis for such a calculation but the criterion certainly is arguable and in my opinion indefensible. More relevant than the cost per life-year is the total cost to society in patients with anticipated short survival due to serious comorbid illnesses who benefit from brief extensions of life by dialysis. It will be low, since the duration of dialysis will be very limited.

A limited prognosis is certain in the great majority of patients with widespread cancer. Even in such persons, as Epstein (1993) states, prognosis may vary from days to months and some will be comfortable, without uncontrollable pain or symptoms. Even additional life of short duration may be valuable to patients who wish to complete some task or to participate in a family event such as a wedding or the birth of a child or grandchild. If such patients develop renal failure, dialysis is not futile. As Epstein (1993) writes, the appropriate approach is to decide whether the benefits of dialysis outweigh the possible burdens. This determination cannot be made in the abstract. It requires a dialogue between the patient, the family and the physician but the decision ultimately should be that of the patient.

A number of professional groups and individual practitioners have offered guidelines about patients for whom dialysis may be considered inappropriate (Lowance, 1993; Hirsch et al., 1994; Moss, 1995). The consensus (Moss, 1995) includes patients who are terminally ill from a non-renal disease. 'Terminally' is defined as less than 60 days in one formulation (Moss, 1995), but as already noted, Lowance (1993) recommends that nephrologists consider advising patients with serious diseases whose prognosis is less than two years that they should not be dialyzed. In my opinion, discussion by the physician with the patient and family about what can be anticipated from dialysis in such patients is appropriate, but this is always the case whenever dialysis is under consideration. It is not appropriate for physicians themselves to make the decision to withhold dialysis without such open discussion and patient agreement, based on the doctors' personal beliefs (Hirsch et al., 1994) or guidelines (Moss, 1995).

This does not imply that all such patients should be dialyzed or that a physician who anticipates that burdens will exceed benefits for a specific patient should not present his or her views and try to influence the patient to accept them. For example, in patients with multiple organ failure of 72 hours duration, anticipated mortality is 98%; the physician is not obligated to maintain dialysis in such patients (Paris and Moss, 1993). However, when the prognosis is less grim and certain—as is usually the case—a trial of dialysis is appropriate if the patient wishes.

Diminished mental status

Persistent vegetative state (PVS)

Available evidence (Multi-society Task Force on PVS, 1994) indicates that patients in a PVS rarely recover consciousness after it has persisted for more than 6 months. The exact definition of 'rarely' is uncertain but the frequency of recovery is no more than 1 or 2%. After one year, reports of recovery are limited to isolated cases. Only a fraction of those who recover consciousness achieve normal or nearly normal mental status. There appears to be a general consensus among neurologists, directors of nursing homes who often care for patients in a PVS (Payne et al., 1996) and nephrologists (Moss et al., 1993; Paris and Moss, 1993) that dialysis should be withheld from patients in a PVS. However, this opinion is not unanimous. Seventeen per cent of nephrologists (Moss et al., 1993) and 9% of neurologists and nursing home directors (Payne et al., 1996) would offer dialysis if the family requested.

Futility is often raised as justification for withholding dialysis or other 'aggressive' treatment. Dialysis is not, of course, futile in a purely physiological or technical sense: it will prolong the life of a patient in a PVS who develops renal failure. However, another definition (Schneiderman et al., 1991), which reasonably can be applied to PVS, is that a treatment is 'futile' if the likelihood of recovery from the underlying state of persistent unconsciousness is less than one in one hundred. By this definition dialysis can be withheld on grounds of futility, if a patient has been in a PVS for 6 months to one year or longer. However, the ethical argument favoring this view is by no means convincing.

The key ethical principle for a physician who must make a decision to start or withhold dialysis ought to be whether the anticipated benefits to the patient outweigh the probable burdens. It is unlikely that patients in PVS will suffer any discomfort from dialysis, since such patients presumably do not feel pain (although there is no unanimity on this point (Payne et al., 1996)). In any case, they will suffer no more than conscious patients. If there is convincing evidence such as a written statement that the patient would not have wanted life to be preserved in a state of persistent unconsciousness or if a surrogate has been appointed, the physician can follow the patient's wishes. The argument that prolonging life will burden the family with the pain of seeing a loved one suffer is understandable but irrelevant. The physician is a fiduciary for the patient; the physician's first duty is to minimize the patient's suffering and it is not morally justified to withhold treatment to relieve family suffering.

On the other hand, the family may insist on treatment. I agree with Payne and Taylor (1997) that the physician lacks moral standing to withhold dialysis if the family requests it. If all active treatment (such as antibiotics) is to be withheld, dialysis should not be given. If infections and decubitus ulcers are being treated, dialysis should be provided if there is good reason to believe that the patient would want such therapy or the family desires it. This is not to imply that I favor aggressive treatment of PVS patients but only that I would not single out dialysis. If there is conflict, the physician may attempt to persuade the family of the correctness of his or her viewpoint, obtain advice from an ethicist or ethics committee, or ultimately may withdraw from the case (with due notice) in favor of another physician if resolution cannot be reached.

Dialysis of PVS patients does raise the question whether it is a justifiable use of limited societal resources. This is a legitimate issue, which must be resolved by a societal consensus openly arrived at, not by individual doctors at the bedside of individual patients. It is sobering that nearly two-thirds of physicians who were surveyed consider it ethical to use vital organs of PVS patients for transplantation (Payne et al., 1996). It is easy to descend the slippery slope from PVS to brain dead.

Dementia

There is general agreement (Lowance, 1993; Moss, 1995) that demented patients should not be dialyzed. Arguments in support of this view include inability to cooperate with dialysis procedures, leading to a psychic burden (fear, suffering) for patients, families and caregivers. Other arguments are low quality of life and unwise use of limited societal resources. The practical difficulty is in defining the severity of dementia that would justify withholding dialysis. The decision is ethically justified to withhold therapy because a thoughtful consensus of family and caregivers decides that the burden of fear and discomfort outweighs the benefit of continued survival.

However, there is the danger that factors such as difficulties for the caregivers, disruption of dialysis unit and the burden to family of dealing with a demented relative will subconsciously influence the assessment of the burdens and benefits to the patient. In my judgment, the latter is the only appropriate criterion for withholding dialysis. Careful analysis should be undertaken by an experienced consultant of the severity of the dementia and of any potential for reversibility. Quality of life is a subjective criterion, which should be applied, if at all, only by those family and caregivers who have direct and long-term knowledge of the patient's activities and mental status, including variations over time.

The issue of use of societal resources for demented patients should be resolved as suggested for PVS patients in the previous section.

Mental deficiency

The comments regarding dementia apply as well to persons with mental deficiency, retardation, autism, etc. The danger in assessing benefits versus burdens to the patient is that it is easy at least subconsciously to substitute a negative balance for family, caregivers and society. The slope in deciding about all categories of diminished mental status is steep and very slippery.

Non-compliant and abusive patients

The term non-compliance spans a broad spectrum of behavior, which stretches from non-compliance with medical regimens that harms only the patient, to patient behaviors (such as arriving late or unannounced for dialysis) that are harmful to both the patient and other patients, through verbal abuse or even physical attacks on caregivers. Failure to take medications or to comply with prescribed restriction of diet and fluid intake are common; surveys have estimated that between 20 and 70% of patients on chronic dialysis are non-compliant by this definition (Wolcott *et al.*, 1986). There is a pattern of patient characteristics that correlates with non-compliance: young adults, male, single, living alone, unemployed, family problems including decreased family communication. The dialysis staff often dislikes these patients and they are typically characterized psychologically as full of anger and hostility to others (Wolcott *et al.*, 1986). Patients with more serious behavior problems vary from those who are probably suffering mainly from fear related to chronic dialysis to sociopaths and psychopaths. All dialysis patients are subject to fear of death and of loss of control of their lives. Patients who abuse drugs or those with psychopathology may pose great problems, including danger to other patients and caregivers. All non-compliant patients pose practical, psychological, and ethical problems for physicians and other caregivers.

The core ideal of the medical profession is that physicians will place the patient's interest above self-interest. There is general agreement that this may require physicians to accept some personal discomfort, such as long hours that disrupt the physician's personal life, if required for their patients' welfare. The ideal also may involve willingness to take some risk. There appears to be a societal consensus, for example, that physicians, in return for their license to practice, are expected to accept the small risk that they may become infected while caring for patients with HIV infection or with active AIDS. Presumably, nephrologists providing dialysis to patients who are disruptive or verbally abusive have a comparable responsibility. However, few would argue that professional ethics require physicians to risk overt violence directed at them. Renal failure does not confer a license to break the law; it is appropriate to use administrative and legal mechanisms to control and punish violent behavior. In practice, the general principles of professionalism offer little guidance as to what degree of risk physicians should be willing to accept in return for the privilege of practicing medicine. In a case at my institution, a specialist refused to complete her consultation on a verbally abusive patient who was known to threaten but never carry out threats of physical harm. She stated that as a single mother, her responsibilities for her two young children took priority over her professional duty (Levinsky and Friedman, 1999). Neither the professional code of ethics nor societal expectations define the appropriate balance between the personal right to avoid harm and professional duty. Provided that the physician includes professional responsibility in his or her ethical calculus, each physician may take a personal position.

An important component in decision-making is compassion for patients (Kilner, 1990). Understandably, caregivers often are hostile when confronted by abusive behavior, especially by individuals who appear to have 'caused their own problems'. In my opinion it is dangerous and inappropriate for physicians to withhold medical care from individuals—including expensive 'high-tech' care like dialysis—based on the judgment that their illness had been caused by their own actions. In the case of ESRD, heroin addicts who develop heroin nephropathy or AIDS nephropathy are familiar examples. One must ask, however, whether addicts are free agents or victims of 'pushers' active in socioeconomically deprived areas. In other words, are patients, once addicted, really able to exert free will in deciding to stop? Should dialysis also be withheld from patients who develop ESRD due to hypertension that was poorly controlled due to non-compliance with antihypertensive regimens? From diabetics who do not rigidly adhere to their diet and insulin regimens? It is dangerous both for medical caregivers and for society to deny medical care to self-abusing patients. Medicine ought to be a compassionate profession. The expense of providing care to addicts and other 'self-abusers' may be high, but undermining the ethical foundation of the medical profession and of society by denying care would be still more costly (Jecker, 1996; Levine *et al.*, 1999).

There is another related issue. Although, theoretically, refusal by society to care for patients 'whose own actions have caused their disease' would be applied equitably, in practice such a policy is likely to target disproportionately the poor, the powerless, and minorities. As already noted, the history of United States dialysis program illustrates this point (Evans *et al.*, 1981). Before dialysis became a Medicare entitlement, individuals on dialysis were disproportionately well-educated white males. After Medicare provided payment for dialysis of nearly all Americans with ESRD, dialysis patients became representative of the demographics of patients with ESRD.

In the United States, two legal cases (*Payton* v *Weaver*, 1982; *Brown* v *Bower*, 1987) indicate that nephrologists are entitled to discontinue treatment of abusive and disruptive patients, especially if the patients fail to meet the terms of a prior agreement reached under the jurisdiction of a court. Hospitals that received federal funding for construction under the Hill–Burton Act may be prohibited from refusing dialysis treatment. Freestanding dialysis facilities, which did not receive such funds, may terminate dialysis of disruptive or abusive patients after reasonable notice. However, the legal right to refuse to dialyze abusive and disruptive patients is not synonymous with the ethical propriety of such a decision. Patients who have demonstrated that they represent a high risk to dialysis staff or to other patients, for example by an act of physical abuse or by carrying weapons, may be removed from the dialysis unit and handed over to the police and the courts (Levy, 1993). There is no ethical obligation for caregivers to accept great and immediate danger of physical injury or death.

What about patients who are verbally abusive, repeatedly fail to keep appointments or otherwise disrupt not only their own care but that of others? Caregivers realize that many such patients are reacting to the fear of their own deaths and to the loss of control inherent in chronic dialysis, in which 'one turns one's body over' to others who control it. In some cases it is possible to identify a person whom the patient trusts, such as a relative, a pastor or a nurse. Working together, the patient and that individual may be able to set reasonable goals for compliance and for discontinuation of disruptive behavior or verbal abuse. A skilled psychiatrist or other mental health professional may be able to help with this process by working with the clinical team as well as with the patient.

Some have recommended bargaining on reasonable rules of behavior. They suggest explicitly allowing patients to negotiate details of care in order to give them the feeling that they have retained some degree of control. Even formal mediation (Johnstone *et al.*, 1997; Miller, 1997) or arbitration have been recommended as a means to improve the working relationship between the patient and the caregivers. Johnson and associates (1996) have described a program in which the patient's perspective is explored and the patient's goals for treatment are identified. Explicit sharing of control and responsibility for treatment between the team and the patient is achieved by educating the patient, by involving him or her insofar as possible in the details of treatment and even by explicitly negotiating a written behavioral contract with the patient.

Deleterious effects on the care of other patients can be minimized by dialyzing the non-compliant patient in a separate room, a tactic which may require additional expenditures for personnel. In areas where there is more than a single dialysis unit, it may be possible to share the burden by arranging for care to rotate among several dialysis units. In the event that all these measures fail and, despite the team's best efforts, the patient continues to disrupt the care of others and to verbally abuse caregivers, the temptation to dismiss the patient from chronic dialysis is great and understandable. However, although it may be legal to discharge a patient from all but emergency care, I believe that it would not be ethical. Death in patients with ESRD often results from causes that the patient cannot recognize, such as hyperkalemia. Patients limited to occasional dialysis for emergencies may die from such a cause. In the final analysis, non-compliance and verbal abuse, however offensive, do not justify imposing a death penalty.

Some general considerations

This chapter deals with appropriate allocation of an expensive resource in nations that can afford, if they wish, to provide adequate dialysis capacity for all patients with renal failure. However, no national policies or ethical precepts require even a nation as wealthy as the United States to do everything it nominally can afford to do. Any nation has the right to decide to limit the amount of dialysis it offers or even not to offer dialysis at all, in order to use the resources for preferred purposes in health care or for any other social need. Such a decision must be made by open and iterative discussion at local and national levels, with widespread public information through the media. The pressure against withholding life-preserving therapy such as chronic dialysis would be very great. This is evident both from the history of the ESRD programs in several countries and a priori from the emotional resistance against allowing fellow citizens to die when a means to prolong life is available, the so-called 'rule of rescue'.

Once the decision to offer dialysis is made by a society, the question discussed in this chapter arises: are there categories of people who should not receive dialysis? I have argued that the answer to this question generally is no. Although there are persons who should not be treated, decisions by category, such as elderly, terminal, altered mental status or non-compliant/abusive, should be avoided. For each patient, the physician, in consultation with the patient, with other caregivers such as dialysis nurses, and with family and advisors selected by the family should assess the probable benefits and burdens of treatment. It is appropriate to consider limited benefits, such as survival extended for a short period to achieve a personal or family goal.

The important criterion is what the patient wants after the physician has reviewed probable benefits and burdens. All experienced physicians have encountered decisions that seem irrational to the doctor, whether these are to refuse dialysis or to insist on the treatment. Generally, in such disputes, patient autonomy trumps physician opinion. Most difficult is the situation in which the patient is unconscious or otherwise incompetent to decide. Families, because of guilt or unreasonable hopes, may demand treatments that caregivers consider irrational because the possible benefits to the patient are outweighed by probable suffering and burdens. In most cases, an agreement can be reached by repeated family-caregiver meetings or with the help of consultants and trusted family advisors who are not directly emotionally involved. Even if that fails, the parties can sometimes reach agreement on a time-limited trial, which within days or weeks demonstrates to the family that the patient is benefiting or that dialysis leads to suffering.

None of this is to imply that I oppose guidelines for the physician who must deal with these vexing problems. On the contrary, I fully support the development of comprehensive guidelines 'for evaluation of patients for whom the burdens of renal replacement therapy may substantially outweigh the benefits' (Institute of Medicine, 1991). The key, however, is that guidelines should be promulgated, with both professional and public input, as guides to physicians in evaluating individual patients, not as dicta that list categories of patients who should not receive dialysis. 'Slippery slope' arguments should not be used to summon fear and emotion against rational guidelines. On the other hand, history teaches us that guidelines for rationing are often applied inequitably by race, sex and social class (Evans *et al.*, 1981), and that quality of life judged by 'objective' criteria and by patient opinion are often discrepant (Evans *et al.*, 1985). In the extreme, legitimate guidelines can even metamorphose to ethical horrors.

References

Aaron, H. J., and Schwartz, W. B. (1984). *The painful prescription: rationing hospital care.* Brookings Institution, Washington, DC.
Brown v *Bower* (1987, December 21). SD Miss, J86–0759(B).
Callahan, D. (1987). *Setting limits. Medical goals in an aging society.* Simon and Schuster, New York.
Daniels, N. (1988). *Am I my parents' keeper? An essay on justice between the young and the old.* Oxford University Press, New York.
Epstein, A. C. (1993). Should cancer patients be dialyzed? *Seminars in Nephrology*, 13, 315–23.
Evans, R. W., Blagg, C. R., and Bryan, F. A., Jr. (1981). Implications for health care policy: a social and demographic profile of hemodialysis patients in the United States. *Journal of the American Medical Association*, 245, 487–91.
Evans, R. W., Manninen, D. L., Garrison, L. P., Jr., *et al.* (1985). The quality of life of patients with end-stage renal disease. *New England Journal of Medicine*, 312, 553–9.
Hamel, M. B., Phillips, R. S., Davis, R. B., Desbiens, N., Connors, A. F. Jr., Teno, J. M., Wenger, N., Lynn, H., Wu, A. W., Fulkerson, W., and Tsevat, J. (1997). Outcomes and cost-effectiveness of initiating dialysis and continuing aggressive care in seriously ill hospitalized adults. *Annals of Internal Medicine*, 127, 195–202.
Hirsch, D. J., West, M. L., Cohen, A. D., and Jindal, K. K. (1994). Experience with not offering dialysis to patients with a poor prognosis. *American Journal of Kidney Diseases*, 23, 463–6.
Institute of Medicine (1991). Rettig, R. and Levinsky, N. G. (eds). *Kidney failure and the federal government.* National Academy Press, Washington, DC.
Jecker, N. S. (1996). Caring for 'socially undesirable' patients. *Cambridge Quarterly of Healthcare Ethics*, 5, 500–10.
Johnson, C. C., Moss, A. H., Clarke, S. A. D., and Armistead, N. C. (1996). Working with non-compliant and abusive dialysis patients: Practical strategies based on ethics and the law. *Advances in Renal Replacement Therapy*, 3, 77–86.
Johnstone, S., Seamon, V. J., Halshaw, D., Molinari, J., and Longknife, K. (1997). The use of mediation to manage patient-staff conflict in the dialysis clinic. *Advances in Renal Replacement Therapy*, 4, 359–71.
Kilner, J. F. (1988). Selecting patients when resources are limited: A study of US medical directors of kidney dialysis and transplantation facilities. *American Journal of Public Health*, 78, 144–7.
Kilner, J. F. (1990). Ethical issues in the initiation and termination of treatment. *American Journal of Kidney Disease*, 3, 218–27.
Kjellstrand, C. M. (1996). High-technology medicine and the old: the dialysis example. *Journal of Internal Medicine*, 239, 195–210.
Levinsky, N. G., and Friedman, E. (1999). What is our duty to a 'hateful' patient? Differing approaches to a disruptive dialysis patient. *American Journal of Kidney Disease*, 34, 775–89.
Levy, N. B. (1993). The assaultive patient. *Dialysis and Transplantation*, 501–03.

Lowance, D. C. (1993). Factors and guidelines to be considered in offering treatment to patients with end-stage renal disease: A personal opinion. *American Journal of Kidney Diseases*, **21**, 679–83.

McKenzie, J. K., Moss, A. H., Feest, T. G., Stocking, C. B., and Siegler, M. (1998). Dialysis decision making in Canada, the United Kingdom, and the United States. *American Journal of Kidney Diseases*, **31**, 12–18.

Miller, R. B. (1997). Mediation for challenging patients—A promising approach. *Advances in Renal Replacement Therapy*, **4**, 372–6.

Moss, A. H. (1995). To use dialysis appropriately: The emerging consensus on patient selection guidelines. *Advances in Renal Replacement Therapy*, **2**, 175–83.

Moss, A. H., Stocking, C. B., Sachs, G. A., and Siegler, M. (1993). Variation in the attitudes of dialysis unit medical directors toward decisions to withhold and withdraw dialysis. *Journal of the American Society of Nephrology*, **4**, 229–34.

Multi-Society Task Force on PVS (1994). Medical aspects of the persistent vegetative state. *New England Journal of Medicine*, **330**, 1572–79.

Nilstun, T., and Ohlsson, R. (1995). Should health care be rationed by age? *Scandinavian Journal of Society and Medicine*, **23**, 81–84.

Paris, J. J., and Moss, A. H. (1993). Guidelines on use of renal dialysis. *Clinical Ethics Report*, **7**, 1–5.

Payne, S. K., and Taylor, R. M. (1997). The persistent vegetative state and anencephaly: Problematic paradiagms for discussing futility and rationing. *Seminars in Neurology*, **17**, 257–63.

Payne, K., Taylor, R. M., Stocking, C., and Sachs, G. A. (1996). Physicians' attitudes about the care of patients in the persistent vegetative state: A national survey. *Annals of Internal Medicine*, **125**, 104–10.

Payton v *Weaver* (1982). *California Reporter*, **225**, 182.

Schneidermann, J. J., Jecker, N. S., and Jonsen, A. R. (1991). Medical futility: its meaning and ethical implications. *Annals of Internal Medicine*, **112**, 949–54.

Veatch, R. M. (1988). Justice and the economics of terminal illness. *Hastings Center Report*, **18**, 34–40.

Wolcott, D. L., Maida, C. A., Diamond, R., and Nissenson, A. R. (1986). Treatment compliance in end-stage renal disease patients on dialysis. *American Journal of Nephrology*, **6**, 329–38.

6
End-of-life care in dialysis

Kerry W. Bowman and Peter A. Singer

Dialysis has given many patients with renal failure a chance to live longer and more productive lives. But the medical ability to prolong the lives of these patients also poses some difficult ethical questions: When should dialysis be withheld? When should it be continued? And, finally, when should it be stopped? Much of what we know about end-of-life care comes from nephrology in the context of dialysis, but there is still much to learn.

Patients on long-term dialysis who stop the treatment account for 22–26% of deaths among patients with renal failure (Neu and Kjellstrand, 1986; Sehgal *et al.*, 1996). While there are no death rate statistics for patients who choose not to start dialysis, this rate is likely higher than the rate of withdrawal (Neu and Kjellstrand, 1986; Port *et al.*, 1989; Mailloux *et al.*, 1991; Singer and End Stage Renal Disease Network of New England, 1992). Ultimately, many patients with end-stage renal disease and their loved ones must make decisions regarding withdrawal from long-term dialysis.

Nephrologists and families generally agree about the management of requests to withdraw dialysis from competent patients, or from incompetent patients with clear prior wishes. They disagree, however, about the management of requests from incompetent patients with unclear prior wishes (Singer and End Stage Renal Disease Network of New England, 1992). In this situation, discontinuation of dialysis is often an ethical dilemma and can be a significant source of conflict for families and health care providers (Bajwa *et al.*, 1996).

When dialysis can no longer promise to enhance a patient's quality of life, the choice to discontinue it should not be marked by confusion, inconsistency or conflict. Rather, patients and their loved ones should be able to expect that health care professionals—and the health care system itself—will provide reliable, supportive and humane care consistent with their wishes.

This chapter reviews the critical issues in end-of-life care for dialysis patients, including:

1. quality end-of-life care: understanding the patient's perspective
2. pain and symptom management
3. consent and substitute decision-making
4. advance directives and advance care planning
5. do-not-resuscitate orders
6. conflict in end-of-life decision-making
7. cultural considerations

Issues raised in this chapter aim to answer the practical question, 'What should the nephrologist do?' As common themes arise throughout, it becomes clear that answering this question relies primarily on understanding the perspective of patients and their families, and on continually striving for balanced and open communication.

Quality end-of-life care

Published literature reveals that end-of-life care is not always satisfactory. In their survey of health care professionals, Solomon *et al.* found that 78% said they sometimes felt that the treatments they offered patients were overly burdensome (Council on Scientific Affairs, 1996). Another study revealed that bereaved family members found communication about end-of-life care to be poor (Lynn *et al.*, 1997). Commenting about quality of care generally, Berwick notes, 'evidence is mounting that the excellence of the status quo is a sentimental illusion' (Berwick and Nolan, 1998).

What is quality end-of-life care and how do we promote it? Quality care has been defined as 'good outcomes for patients at a cost that society can afford' (Ahronheim *et al.*, 1996). To more adequately define quality in end-of-life care, several expert groups—including the Institute of Medicine (Institute of Medicine, 1997), the American Geriatrics Society (1997), and Emanuel and Emanuel (1998)—have developed taxonomies (see Table 6.1).

These three taxonomies have been determined from the medical 'expert' perspective, rather than those of patients and families (Cleary and Edgeman-Levitan, 1997). As a result, they have several problems, including:

- the taxonomic labels are often general or vague (e.g. 'patient perception of care');
- the taxonomy seems bound by established concepts for which measurement scales are available (such as quality of life);
- the expert-derived taxonomies are focused on processes (such as 'advance care planning') or time periods (such as 'bereavement') that are only loosely connected with patient-centred outcomes (Singer *et al.*, 1999).

One could argue, then, that quality end-of-life care is most appropriately viewed from the perspective of patients. The patient's concerns—and those of their families—should rightfully be the central focus in determining quality care because, ultimately, only *they* are facing the life-and-death decisions that dialysis brings. Health care providers and organizations must better understand this perspective in order to improve the quality of care they offer to dying patients.

Beginning with this assumption, we analyzed qualitative data from three groups of patients—those receiving dialysis, those living with HIV, and those undergoing long-term care—to derive a taxonomy of quality end-of-life care from the patient's perspective. What we found were five criteria that were important to patients:

1. receiving adequate pain and symptom management;
2. avoiding inappropriate prolongation of dying;
3. achieving a sense of control;
4. relieving the burden on loved ones;
5. strengthening relationships with loved ones.

Table 6.1 'Expert-derived' taxonomies of quality end-of-life care

Journal of the American Geriatrics Society Statement[a]	Institute of Medical Committee[b]	Emanuel and Emanuel[c]
• Physical and emotional symptoms	• Overall quality of life	• Physical symptoms
• Support of function and autonomy	• Physical well-being and functioning	• Psychological and cognitive symptoms
• Advance care planning	• Psychosocial well-being and functioning	• Social relationships and support
• Aggressive care near death	• Spiritual well-being	• Economic demands and care giving needs
• Patient and family satisfaction	• Patient perception of care	• Hopes and expectations
• Global quality of life • Family burden • Survival time • Provider continuity and skill • Bereavement	• Family well-being and perceptions	• Spiritual and existential beliefs

[a] *American Geriatric Society* (1997).
[b] Institute of Medicine (1997).
[c] Emanuel and Emanuel (1998).

Compared with the expert-derived taxonomies, the patient-derived taxonomy of quality end-of-life care is much more specific. It is less bound by established concepts for which measurement scales are available, and more focused on outcomes rather than processes. We have collapsed the patient-derived taxonomy of quality end-of-life care into three simple categories that can guide physician practice at the bedside of patients dying from renal failure: (1) pain and symptom management, (2) decisions about the use of life-sustaining treatments, and (3) support of patients and families (Singer and MacDonald, 1998).

Measurement is also required to identify opportunities for improving end-of-life care, and to hold institutions accountable for the quality of care given to the dying. Developing reliable measures of quality of care in any arena of health care is very challenging, and measures appropriate to the complex domain of caring for dying patients and their loved ones is particularly difficult (Solomon *et al.*, 1993; Ahronheim *et al.*, 1996). Yet quality end-of-life care is increasingly recognized as a health care issue that deserves more attention (The SUPPORT Investigators, 1995; Cleary and Edgeman-Levitan, 1997; Hanson *et al.*, 1997a; Berwick and Nolan, 1998; Emanuel and Emanuel, 1998; Singer *et al.*, 1998, 1999). After years of inconsistency and debate, more systematic, evidence-based approaches to caring for the dying are evolving. Three approaches hold particular promise.

Report card

Quality measurement has been impeded by an insufficient number of publicly accessible, valid indicators that reflect the breadth of medical services. In recent years an increasing number of hospitals and health care programs are developing what are referred to as *report cards*. These are explicit reports on the process and outcomes of health care services to the public. The rationale for report cards is the belief that external market forces and public demand will drive quality. Recent studies report trends of decreasing mortality after coronary artery bypass graft surgery since the introduction of report cards, or outcome studies (O'Connor *et al.*, 1996).

Despite initial problems of consistency in measurement, substantial progress has recently been made in developing acceptable quality indicators and standardizing data collection. The use of explicit reports on clinical outcomes has been shown to be effective in quality improvement (Hannan *et al.*, 1994). Although report cards represent an excellent mechanism for providing quality information to the public in the realm of end-of-life care, they are not a direct change strategy and are perhaps best combined with other initiatives. While not current practice, report cards would ideally be filled out by next of kin in order to rate the overall quality of end-of-life care according to the five criteria identified in the patient-derived taxonomy above.

Rapid cycle change

In rapid cycle change, a small yet significant element of practice is selected and tested. For example, a single medical ward may decide to sample response time for patients who indicate they are in pain. An intervention for improving response time may be as simple as having a resident, rather than a staff doctor, sign for medication. New response times are then charted on a board visible to all staff members. If the change is considered an improvement, it is integrated into practice and further elements of practice are tested. Donald Berwick and Tom Nolan (1998) ask three questions when designing and applying such a model: What are we trying to accomplish? What change can we make that will result in an improvement? How will we know that a change is an improvement? Rapid cycle approaches are best used when either: inaction will lead to the unacceptable status quo, current practice is incongruous with scientific knowledge, or action without measurement is unacceptable (Berwick and Nolan, 1998).

For many health care systems, rapid cycle changes are more practical, appropriate, and informative than either formal studies with protracted baselines, or the more common implementation of changes without evaluation. When teams endeavour to implement change they often either stall, identify problems but are unsure of how to rectify them, or design elaborate changes that are difficult to test and involve more change than that with which people are comfortable (Berwick, 1998).

End-of-life improvement strategies based on family feedback

What is often missing—and so very necessary—in end-of-life care is the more in-depth perspective of patients and families (Ware and Hayes, 1988; Roach, 1996; Byock, 1997; Cleary and Edgeman-Levitan, 1997; Hanson *et al.*, 1997a; Institute of Medicine, 1997; Jacobson *et al.*, 1997; Lynn *et al.*, 1997; Institute for Health Care Improvement, 1998; Singer *et al.*, 1999). In order to effectively change practice, we need a method for generating valid, survivor-based, quality end-of-life care data and integrating it into the health care setting. Jacobson *et al.* (1997) are an excellent example of such an initiative. They arranged a dialogue between the families of patients who had died in the hospital and the members of the hospital ethics committee, with a view to applying family suggestions to practice. The results were surprising, particularly the degree of contrast between what the committee members expected the families' concerns would be and what they actually were. This kind of initiative represents a relatively efficient and effective means of building improvement strategies directly from patient and family feedback.

Pain and symptom management

A crucial element in quality end-of-life care is adequate pain and symptom management. Making decisions about life-sustaining treatment or bringing closure to lifelong relationships can be extremely difficult, particularly in the face of pain, debilitating nausea, or fatigue.

The symptoms of uremia are familiar to every nephrologist, but the management of these symptoms in the context of caring for a dying patient is not as simple. There is a growing body of palliative care literature on managing pain and other symptoms in dying patients. While a full review of the literature is beyond the scope of this chapter, the following points may be helpful.

First, pain is only one of several symptoms that can prove debilitating for dying patients. Other symptoms include fatigue, breathlessness, nausea, diarrhoea, and delirium. Because the model for palliative care was based on the treatment of cancer, pain—a common symptom for cancer patients—was a critical focus. Although dying patients with renal failure also experience pain, it is likely that these other symptoms pose more significant problems.

Second, the management of these symptoms is poorly taught in medical school and in residency. Consequently, most practising nephrologists are likely to be unfamiliar with palliative care methods for effectively managing these symptoms. Continuing education or self-education is therefore required to provide adequate pain and symptom management. Useful resources for pain and symptom control, as well as other palliative care issues, can be found in the *Oxford Textbook of Palliative Medicine* (Hanks, 1999) and the American Medical Association's Education of Physicians on End-of-Life Care (EPEC) Project. Third, the fear that the nephrologist is hastening death may impede adequate management of pain and other symptoms. Although many believe that treating pain with opioids shortens life, whether opioids—used in this context—shorten, lengthen, or have no effect on the duration of life is controversial. It is also important to distinguish the use of opioids for palliative analgesia and sedation from lethal injection euthanasia. The Chief Coroner of Ontario helps make this distinction clear by outlining some definitive criteria. An act is considered palliative care, and not euthanasia, if: (1) it is intended solely to relieve the person's suffering; (2) it is administered in response to symptoms or signs of the patient's suffering and is commensurate with that suffering; and, (3) it is not the deliberate infliction of death (Dr James Young, Chief Coroner of Ontario: personal communication, 1997).

Finally, palliative care consultation is an under-utilized resource, particularly in patients suffering from something other than cancer. Although as many as 50% of patients with cancer may have access to palliative care, only about 25% of deaths in developed countries result from cancer. For the other 75% of deaths, including most patients with renal failure, the rate of access to palliative care specialists is much lower. Therefore, it is critical that physicians caring for these patients, including nephrologists, develop basic skills for caring for dying patients, and consult with palliative care physicians when specialized expertise is needed.

Consent and substitute decision making

Capable people have the ethical and legal right to accept or reject treatments proposed by physicians. The appropriate framework for treatment of dialysis is consent, which has three elements: disclosure, voluntariness, and capacity, all of which are legal requirements.

Disclosure

In the context of patient consent, 'disclosure' refers to the provision of relevant information by the clinician and its comprehension by the patient. Both elements are necessary for valid consent. The patient should be adequately informed about: (1) the treatment and its expected effects; (2) relevant alternative options and their benefits and risks; and (3) the consequences of declining or delaying treatment. The clinician's goal is to disclose information that a reasonable person in the patient's position would need in order to make an informed decision (Etchells *et al.*, 1996a).

When deciding whether or not to stop dialysis, the patient must fully understand that discontinuing dialysis will result in death, and he or she must also be well informed about the nature of that death. It is important that clinicians be sensitive to cultural and religious beliefs (discussed latter in this chapter) that can affect disclosure.

Voluntariness

Voluntariness refers to a patient's right to make treatment decisions free of any undue influence, and it is grounded in several related concepts, including freedom, autonomy and independence (Faden and Beauchamp, 1986). A patient's freedom to decide can be impinged on by internal factors arising from his or her condition or by external factors. Coercion involves the use of explicit or implicit threats (by anyone involved in the decision-making process—be it a doctor, lawyer, family member, etc.) to ensure that a treatment, or withdrawal of a treatment, is accepted. Manipulation involves the deliberate distortion or omission of information in order to encourage the patient to accept or reject a treatment (Pendleton and Bochner, 1980; Shapiro et al., 1983). Voluntariness must be carefully assessed—both by family members and health care staff—in decisions to discontinue dialysis. There is an inherent power imbalance in the physician–patient relationship, and clinicians should strive to minimize this imbalance by fostering autonomous decision making by their patients (Etchells et al., 1996b).

Capacity

Capacity refers to the patient's ability to understand information relevant to a treatment decision and to appreciate the reasonably foreseeable consequences of a decision (Etchells et al., 1996c).

A person may be 'capable' with respect to one decision but not with respect to another. Although refusal of recommended treatment may cause a clinician to question a person's capacity (Mebane and Rauch, 1990), refusal of treatment should not be considered evidence of incapacity (Katz et al., 1995). Most refusals are caused by factors other than incapacity (Appelbaum and Roth, 1983).

Clinicians can usually identify patients who are clearly capable or incapable, but in marginal cases a clinical capacity assessment is required. Marginal cases may be common in relation to deteriorating health or consciousness. The Aid to Capacity Evaluation (ACE) is a reliable and valid clinical tool that has been developed to guide the clinician's assessment of patient capacity (Etchells website). If the clinician is uncertain about the assessment or if the patient challenges the finding of incapacity, further expert assessment is recommended. Expert assessments can be conducted by individual practitioners (e.g. psychiatrists and psychologists), hospital ethics committees, or legal review boards. If there is doubt about the assessment, consultation from a psychiatrist, hospital attorney, or bioethicist may be helpful. In cases of conflict, the ultimate judge of a patient's capacity is a court.

If the patient is deemed incapable, he or she should be informed of this evaluation and notified that someone else will be making decisions on his or her behalf. This should be done in a sensitive manner that is appropriate to the clinical circumstances.

Incapable patients have the same right to consent to diagnostic tests or treatment as capable patients. But, because they cannot exercise this right *themselves*, policy makers, judges and legislators have developed a system known as 'substitute decision making' to permit others to make decisions on an incapable person's behalf (Buchanan and Brock, 1989; Lazar et al., 1996).

Substitute decision-making poses two important questions: Who should make the decision for the incapable person? How should the decision be made? The legally appropriate answer to these questions varies from one jurisdiction to another, and physicians are encouraged to become familiar with the legal standards in their place of practice. However, the overall goal of substitute decision making is to approximate the decision the patient would make if he or she were still capable of doing so.

The most appropriate person to make such decisions is someone appointed by the patient him- or herself, while capable, through a proxy advance directive (discussed shortly). Other substitute decision-makers, in their usual order of priority, may be: a court-appointed guardian, spouse, child, parent, sibling, any other relative, or a concerned friend. In some jurisdictions, a public official will serve as substitute decision maker for a patient who has no substitute decision maker available. This situation often occurs with elderly, socially isolated patients.

The standards for making decisions are based, in decreasing order of priority, on: wishes, values and beliefs, and best interests. Wishes are prior expressions by the patient, while capable, that seem to apply to the actual decision that needs to be made. Sometimes patients will have recorded their wishes in an instruction advance directive. Values and beliefs are less specific than wishes, but give a general indication of a patient's stance on an issue or course of treatment. Best interests are 'objective' estimates of the benefits and burdens of treatment to the patient.

Both the 'who' and the 'how' questions of substitute decision making may be addressed through advance care planning and advance directives, discussed in the next section. Unfortunately, there are a considerable number of cases in which patients are clearly incapable and their wishes are either unknown, in dispute, or viewed in substantially different ways between families and health care teams. In these cases, discontinuation of dialysis often becomes a negotiated event. Conflict in these cases is often exacerbated by the lack of consensus about when to continue with, and when to terminate, life-sustaining care.

Advance care planning and advance directives

Advance care planning (ACP) is a process of communication between patients, their families and significant others, and health care providers regarding the kind of care deemed appropriate when the patient can no longer make decisions. In the context of this process, an advance directive (AD) is an optional document, written when a patient is still capable, that stipulates what his or her wishes are should he or she become incapable. 'Proxy directives' specify who should ultimately make decisions on his or her behalf, and 'instruction directives' specify a patient's wishes with respect to treatment. Proxy and instruction directives are often used in combination.

ADs are driven primarily by a patient's state of health, rather than by types of treatment, and do not usually extend to treatments in worsened states (Holley et al., 1989; Singer et al., 1995). For example, approximately 90% of patients would want treatment for a potentially reversible problem if they were in their current state of health, but only 10% of patients would opt for treatment if they were in a permanent coma. Severity of illness also has an important influence on preferences. About 80% of patients wish treatment in mild dementia, while only 15% wish treatment in severe dementia. The specific treatment has a relatively modest effect on these choices. Consequently, nephrologists should focus primarily on providing information about health states rather than treatments, and should distinguish between levels of severity of a diagnostic condition (e.g. dementia) in eliciting a patient's specific wishes for life-sustaining treatment.

Studies of ACP in dialysis have shown that:

- Written ADs have been completed by 7–35% of chronic dialysis patients (Holley *et al.*, 1993b, 1997; Perry *et al.*, 1995; Cohen *et al.*, 1997)
- Providing written material on advance directives can increase the rate of completed AD forms (Holley *et al.*, 1993a)
- Dialysis staff discuss ADs with 30% of patients on average, and this figure is influenced by professional discipline (social workers, 60%; physicians, 38%; nurses, 25–30%) (Perry *et al.*, 1996)
- Although 67–77% of dialysis patients have discussed their wishes about life-sustaining treatment with their family or someone close to them, only 14–17% have had such discussions with their doctor (Holley *et al.*, 1993a, 1997)
- The main reason people do not complete written advance directives is that their family knows what they would want (Holley *et al.*, 1997)
- Completion of written advance directives is associated with improved communication between patients and families about preferences for end-of-life treatment, but does not enhance communication of preferences to physicians (Doukas and McCullough, 1991)

In this context, we wondered if an advance directive designed specifically for people on dialysis would be helpful (Singer, 1994). We tried to design one based on two important courses of treatment: cardiopulmonary resuscitation and continuation of dialysis (Frankl *et al.*, 1989; Mendelsohn and Singer, 1994). Surprisingly, when we evaluated dialysis patients' preferences for a dialysis-specific or generic directive, we found that a dialysis-specific directive was not preferred. While further analysis confirmed our theory that people who do not want dialysis would also reject other life-sustaining treatments (e.g. tube feeding), we found that people who *want* dialysis may *still* reject other life-sustaining treatments. A dialysis-specific advance directive would therefore not capture this choice. Again, it is health states—rather than specific treatment preferences—that drive these choices. Consequently, we recommend that nephrologists offer dialysis patients generic advance directives (Mendelsohn and Singer, 1994).

Despite their value, ADs are not essential to an effective ACP process. It is commonly found that, although people have positive attitudes towards ADs, they rarely complete them, and efforts to increase the rate of completed advance directive documents are only modestly successful (Lo *et al.*, 1986; Shmerling *et al.*, 1988; Holley *et al.*, 1989; Mendelsohn and Singer, 1994; Singer, 1994; Teno *et al.*, 1994; Blackhall *et al.*, 1995; Carrese and Rhodes, 1995; Singer *et al.*, 1995, 1998; Hanson *et al.*, 1997b;). More recent research has revealed that the written advance directive form is only a piece of the puzzle, and traditional assumptions about advance care planning are incomplete (Lo *et al.*, 1986; Shmerling *et al.*, 1988; Frankl *et al.*, 1989; Stolman *et al.*, 1990; Teno *et al.*, 1990, 1994; Gamble *et al.*, 1991; Joos *et al.*, 1993; Hanson *et al.*, 1997b; Singer *et al.*, 1998).

To explore these issues from the perspective of the patient, we interviewed dialysis patients using a qualitative research method known as grounded theory. In contrast to the traditional assumptions, the patients told us that:

- The purpose of ACP is not only to prepare for incapacity, but also to prepare for death.
- ACP is not based solely on autonomy and the exercise of control but also on personal relationships and relieving burden on others.
- The focus of ACP is not only on completing written AD forms but also on the social process.
- ACP does not occur solely within the context of the physician—patient relationship, but also within relationships with close loved ones (Singer et al., 1998).

In a subsequent study on people with HIV, we learned that the primary meaning of ACP for patients was preparing for death, which involves three important elements: achieving a sense of control, relieving the burden on family, and strengthening relationships with loved ones (Martin et al., 1999).

The advance directive is therefore much more than a vehicle for the patient to transcribe his or her wishes. The nephrologist should think of it as a decision aid for patients and their loved ones to engage in the process of ACP and prepare for the patient's death together. The 'main event' in ACP does not occur between patients and their nephrologists, but rather between patients and their loved ones. Nephrologists should introduce the topic of ACP, provide information resources (including AD documents), and then counsel and support patients and families through the ACP process. Of course, there must also be a way to communicate the patient's preferences to the dialysis team. Dialysis units need to encourage communication between patients and families about end-of-life issues and ask that they be informed of ultimate decisions. Dialysis units might also want to suggest that patients and their families discuss treatment preferences for various health states; and providing an AD form will help guide and document these discussions.

Ultimately, the success of ACP programs should not be judged by the number of completed AD forms, or the impact of the program on length of stay, health care costs or utilization of life-sustaining treatments. Completing AD forms is a small part of the overall ACP process, and successful ACP can occur without them. ACP should not force people to choose one particular way of expressing themselves, but should instead provide patients with a variety of options that can allow them to bring life experiences and cultural or religious views to the process of advance care planning (Blackhall et al., 1995; Carrese and Rhodes, 1995).

Do-not-resuscitate orders

Patients with renal failure are believed to have a poor survival rate following cardiopulmonary resuscitation, and evidence suggests that the same is true of dialysis patients. Moss et al. (1992) conducted an eight-year study of cardiopulmonary resuscitation in dialysis patients on a university dialysis program, and then compared outcomes during the same time period with those of a control group of non-dialysis patients undergoing cardiopulmonary resuscitation (CPR) in the same hospital. Of 221 dialysis patients experiencing cardiopulmonary arrest, 74 had CPR (34%) compared with 247 of the 1201 control patients (21%). Six months following CPR, two of 74 dialysis patients were still alive (3%), compared with 23 of the 247 control patients (9%) ($P = 0.044$). This difference was not explained by age or comorbid conditions. Twenty-one of the 27 successfully resuscitated dialysis patients died a mean of 4.4 days later (78%); and 95% of these patients were on mechanical ventilation in an intensive care unit at the time of death. Moss concludes that cardiopulmonary resuscitation is a procedure that rarely results in extended survival for dialysis patients, strengthening the need for advance care planning that has a strong emphasis on communication.

Not surprisingly, do-not-resuscitate orders are common in dialysis patients. In certain situations, however, these orders may raise some difficult ethical questions for nephrologists. One particularly troubling circumstance occurs when cardiac arrest is caused by an iatrogenic complication in a patient with a do-not-resuscitate order.

Casarett and Ross reviewed various justifications for overriding a patient's refusal for treatment after an iatrogenic complication (listed below), and concluded that none had merit (Casarett and Ross, 1997), for the following reasons:

- The principle of non-maleficence—which is the physician's duty to do no harm—does not outweigh the obligation to follow the patient's wishes.
- The argument of proximate cause—which is the idea that the primary cause of an event is the cause that is closest in time—'ignores the fact that one action or omission is seldom either necessary or sufficient for an iatrogenic event to occur'.
- The argument of physician error—which is the notion that physicians should accept responsibility for an iatrogenic event and reverse the complications—is insufficient because 'physicians may need to perform additional procedures and provide additional therapies, each of which has its own benefits and risks. The occurrence of an iatrogenic complication does not give physicians the right to perform these interventions without the patient's consent.'
- Finally, the argument of efficacy of resuscitation—which is the claim that treatment should be permissible simply because resuscitation is likely to be successful—is insufficient because:
  (a) the iatrogenic complications are not always so easily reversed;
  (b) predictions based on groups of patients cannot be applied easily to individual patients;
  (c) resuscitative efforts often cause precisely the type of harm people commonly wish to avoid, and;
  (d) 'it is not logical for physicians to override prior directives after an iatrogenic complication when they are morally and legally obligated to respect the refusal by a competent patient to undergo other treatments that may have similar rates of efficacy.'

This justification is incomplete precisely because, in certain circumstances, resuscitation after an iatrogenic complication may *not* have similar rates of efficacy to resuscitation in different circumstances. The likelihood of resuscitation has a marked influence on whether patients would want to accept it (Murphy *et al.*, 1994).

The more general question is: How should the patient's wishes resulting from ACP—and perhaps captured in an AD document—be applied to a treatment decision? Ultimately, the nephrologist must exercise his or her best judgement. People do not generally engage in ACP to micro-manage the precise clinical decisions that are made when they become very ill, but rather to achieve a sense of control, to relieve their loved ones of burden, and to strengthen their personal relationships. These goals are all consistent with—and in some cases require—decisions that seem, at face value, to contradict the patient's expressed wishes.

A person's wishes are embedded in the fabric of his or her life and, as such, are always somewhat ambiguous and subject to change. When the nephrologist can honestly argue that the patient, if capable, might not want his or her previous wishes applied to the current situation, the wishes should not simply be applied. Clinical judgement is particularly important if the patient is facing an easily reversible, life-threatening situation from which a full recovery is likely with a relatively simple treatment. Of course, taken to an extreme, this view can be used to undermine patients' important autonomy rights and return to the era of paternalistic decision-making by physicians. Ultimately, clinical judgement is essential for making ethical and appropriate treatment decisions at the end of life. The prudence of this judgement will determine the quality of patient care.

Conflict in end-of-life decision making

The discontinuation of dialysis brings families into unfamiliar territory. Although we can easily acknowledge the medical and ethical complexities of end-of-life decisions, we have barely begun to acknowledge the psychological and socio-cultural complexities. In the past, several factors—including the absence of life-sustaining technology, a far shorter life expectancy, a higher child mortality rate, and a closer geographic proximity for many families—made death a more frequent, home-based experience that had little to do with choice. But today, end-of-life decisions abound; and the stakes are high. These decisions involve life or death, views about the quality and meaning of life, finance, moral principles, and legal rights (Neveloff Dubler and Marcus, 1994). Not surprisingly, such decisions can generate intense emotions and increase the potential for conflict.

To exacerbate this problem, substantial differences in gender, age, culture, social class and education often exist between physicians and families. What is known or valued by health care workers may be illusive or irrelevant to families. When differences exist, so too will perspectives on various issues, creating a greater opportunity for conflict. Conflicting perspectives become increasingly obvious when major decisions must be made. Large health care teams with shifting and inconsistent members —each trained in separate professions with separate working cultures—often fracture communication and make for an environment that is not conductive to balanced discussion and negotiation. Moreover, all of these factors occur within a climate of endless change that defines the contemporary health care system.

Given these various factors, it is not surprising that conflict in end-of-life decisions arises. And disagreements over in the termination of dialysis will only become more common as the number of people receiving dialysis increases. It is therefore best to anticipate conflict and develop mechanisms and policies to address it before it erupts. The most important task for renal health care workers is to focus on consistency, balanced communication, and negotiation.

When dealing with end-stage renal failure, a family's perception of the meaning and severity of an illness does not always correspond to the doctor's diagnosis and prognosis. When substitute decision makers request treatments that health care providers believe is inappropriate, these situations may be labeled as 'futility' cases. Although uncommon, futility cases exact a tremendous cost, and can lead to a breakdown in the physician—patient/family relationship. For health care workers it can lead to frustration, tension, and caregiver burnout, as well as intra-team conflict due to the polarization of opinion. Prolonged disputes can leave patients receiving treatment they may not have wanted, or missing treatments they might have chosen.

A key problem for incompetent patients in futility cases is that there is presently no consensus on ethical and legal approaches to dealing with them. During the 1990s, the primary focus concerning such cases was to define 'futility' in hopes that the right definition would clarify the most difficult and conflicted situations. However, declaring 'futility' is rarely useful in end-of-life conflict, as no broadly accepted definition has been established. In any event, a clear definition would do little to deal with a family's fears and beliefs.

More recent research has focused on the process of communication to address 'futility' cases (Halevy and Brody, 1996). This is likely a more realistic direction, given that these cases often involve fundamental differences in values between providers and patients or families (Weijer *et al.*, 1998). Two promising approaches to such situations come from the Council on Ethical and Judicial Affairs (1999) and Model Policy on Appropriate Use of Life Sustaining Treatment developed by the University of Toronto Joint Centre for Bioethics (Joint Centre for Bioethics website). These approaches focus on process rather than futility definitions. The latter policy includes the following essential factors for balanced communication and supportive care at the end of life: achieving interprofessional team consensus; enhancing communication and negotiation; offering psychosocial/spiritual support for patients and families; obtaining a second opinion; transferring the patient; and engaging in mediation and arbitration/adjudication.

Policies that offer substantive definitions of futility are therefore being replaced by policies that encourage a process involving clear and open communication as a means of containing conflict. In practice, this means providing health care workers with negotiating skills and access to formal mediation. Because this kind of conflict takes place in an environment of intense emotions—and can also evoke unresolved losses and conflicts within the family—it is important to offer the assistance of support services, such as Chaplaincy or Social Work, to the family.

Mediation, defined as the principled resolution of disagreements by a knowledgeable and neutral third party, is a useful tool (Slaikeu, 1989). Mediation promotes good health care by creating a forum that fosters respect for family perspectives while allowing for a comprehensive examination of the medical, ethical and legal elements of a situation.

Mediation can also create an environment in which multi-disciplinary teams can learn to integrate the psycho-social, cultural, ethical, legal and medical concerns in a case (Hoffmann, 1994).

While mediation can be beneficial, health care professionals should strive to achieve balanced communication *before* the need for outside consultation arises. The current necessity for mediation largely reflects a failure within our existing systems.

Culture and end-of-life decisions

Culture has been thoroughly discussed elsewhere in this book, yet it is well worth considering that attitudes toward the termination of treatments, including dialysis, may be highly influenced by cultural perspectives that are rarely acknowledged (Bowman, 1997). Cultures are maps of meaning through which people understand the world and interpret the things around them. When patients and health care workers have different cultural backgrounds, they frequently follow different 'maps', which can hinder effective communication. For example, health care workers may expect patients to: hold a biomedical perspective of illness, be punctual, be future-oriented, be willing to work on therapeutic goals, and value direct communication about their condition, regardless of its severity.

Culture is a strong determinant of people's views of the very nature and meaning of illness and death (Kleinman, 1980), of how much health—or end-of-life decisions—can or should be controlled (Rotter, 1966), how bad news should be communicated (Blackhall *et al.*, 1995), and how decisions—including end-of-life decisions—should be made (Hall, 1981).

When weighing decisions about the termination of dialysis, it is important to consider that Western and non-Western cultures hold sharply divergent views about autonomy. Autonomy is generally a Western concept reflecting a belief in the importance, uniqueness, dignity and sovereignty of each person, and the sanctity of each individual life. Accordingly, every person is entitled to self-determination. This stands in bold contrast to non-Western cultures in which interdependence is often valued over independence. Profound social and moral meaning rests in these interrelations.

Western health care teams may therefore assume that the person experiencing the illness is the best person to make health care decisions. However, many non-Western cultures vest in the family or community the right to receive and disclose information, and to make decisions about and organize patient care. Applying the concept of autonomy cross-culturally will therefore mean accepting each person's terms of reference for their definition of self. Specifically, we should respect the autonomy of patients and families by incorporating their cultural values and beliefs into the decision-making process.

The most effective way to address cultural differences in termination of dialysis is through open and balanced communication. When health care workers are uncertain about how a patient or family perceives a situation, it is best simply to ask. Frequently, differences can be easily negotiated. Many people now living in Western cultures already hold blended views of culture, illness and death. The mere acknowledgement of such differences will usually lead to improved communication.

When dealing with termination of dialysis decisions, it is important to consider the following questions: Do patients value individuality and personal choice, or do they focus more on family and collective choices? Do they value open communication, or do they tend to draw cues from the context of the situation? Do they believe a person can and should influence their health or their death? Do they believe in a Western biomedical view of illness, or do they hold an alternative, or blended, view of illness?

Conclusion

Nephrology was one of the earliest disciplines in medicine faced with end-of-life care. Because of the extended relationships between dialysis workers and their patients, nephrology provides a good model within the health care system to develop policies and practices related to end-of-life care.

To that end, our goal is to ensure that every patient who dies in dialysis receives quality end-of-life care; and that the quality of that care is reflected in patient- and family-based evaluations of the caregiving experience. As the issues raised in this chapter reflect, we can best achieve quality end-of-life care by focusing primarily on understanding the perspectives of patients and their families, and continually striving for balanced and open communication at all stages of the caregiving process.

During the past 10 years we have learnt 10 things about quality end of life care. The points build on and extend beyond the concepts discussed in this chapter, and are meant to provide guidance to nephrologists.

1. 'Aggressive' and 'palliative' approaches to treatment are not mutually exclusive. Pursue goals related to quality end of life care at the same time as goals related to treating reversible illnesses.
2. Ask yourself three questions when you are at the bedside of a dying patient: Have I adequately treated the patient's pain and other symptoms? Have I addressed issues related to use of life-sustaining treatment? Have I done what I can to support this patient and family?
3. No patient should die in pain or with other untreated symptoms, such as breathlessness, fatigue, nausea, diarrhea, etc.
4. Patients have the right to make decisions with respect to the use of life-sustaining treatments.
5. Advance care planning can help patients face death in the context of their families.
6. Approach conflict in end-of-life care as a negotiation.
7. Support patients and families as much as you can. Religious and cultural factors may arise here.
8. There is plenty of room for improvement in quality end-of-life care without recourse to euthanasia.

9. Quality end-of-life care is an essential clinical competency that every practising physician should have.
10. Quality end-of-life care requires teamwork and organizational strategies for improvement.

The authors would like to thank Dr Ed Etchells and Dr Douglas Martin for their helpful discussions, and Ms Althea Blackburn-Evans for editing the chapter.

References

Ahronheim, J. C., Morrison, S., Baskin, S. A., Morris, J., and Meier, D. E. (1996). Treatment of the dying in the acute care hospital. *Archives of Internal Medicine*, **156**, 2094–100.

American Geriatric Society (1997). Measuring quality of care at the end-of-life: A statement of principles *Journal of the American Geriatric Society*, **45**, 526–7.

Appelbaum, P. S. and Roth, L. H. (1983). Patients who refuse treatment in medical hospitals. *Journal of the American Medical Association*, **250**, 1296–301.

Bajwa, K., Szabo, E., and Kjellstrand, C. M. (1996). A prospective study of risk factors and decision making in discontinuation of dialysis. *Archives of Internal Medicine*, **156**, 2571–7.

Berwick, D. (1998). Developing and testing changes in delivery of care. *Annals of Internal Medicine*, **128**, 651–6.

Berwick, D. M. and Nolan, T. W. (1998). Physicians as leaders in improving health care: A new series in Annals of Internal Medicine. *Annals of Internal Medicine*, **128**, 289–92.

Blackhall, L. J., Murphy, S. T., Frank, G., Michel, V., and Azen, S. (1995). Ethnicity and attitudes toward patient autonomy. *Journal of the American Medical Association*, **274**, 820–5.

Bowman, K. W. (1997). Bioethics and cultural pluralism. *Humane Health Care International*, **13**, 31–4.

Buchanan, A. E. and Brock, D. W. (1989). *Deciding for others: The ethics of surrogate decision making*. Cambridge University Press, New York.

Byock I. (1997). *Dying well: Peace and possibilities at the end of life*. Riverhead Books, New York.

Carrese, J. A., and Rhodes, L. A. (1995). Western bioethics on the Navajo reservation: Benefit or harm? *Journal of the American Medical Association*, **274**, 826–9.

Casarett, D., and Ross, L. F. (1997). Iatrogenic complications: Do physicians have a right to override a patient's refusal of treatment? *New England Journal of Medicine*, **336**, 1908–10.

Cleary, P. D., and Edgeman-Levitan, S. (1997). Health care quality: Incorporating consumer perspectives. *Journal of the American Medical Association*, **278**, 608–12.

Cohen, L. M., McCue, J. D., Germain, M., and Woods, A. (1997). Denying the dying—Advance directives and dialysis discontinuation. *Psychosomatics*, **38**, 27–34.

Council on Ethical and Judicial Affairs, American Medical Association (1999). Medical futility in end-of-life care: Report of the Council on Ethical and Judicial Affairs. *Journal of the American Medical Association*, **281**, 937–41.

Council on Scientific Affairs, American Medical Association. (1996). Good care of the dying. *Journal of the American Medical Association*, **275**, 1740–2.

Doukas, D. J., and McCullough, L. B. (1991). The values history: The evaluation of patients' values and advance directives. *Journal of Family Practice*, **32**, 145–53.

Emanuel, E. J. and Emanuel, L. L. (1998). The promise of a good death. *Lancet*, **351** (suppl II), 21–9.

Etchells, E. *Aid to Capacity Evaluation (ACE)*. Website: www.utoronto.ca/jcb/_ace/ace.htm; visit May 12, 2000.
Etchells, E., Sharpe, G., Burgess, M. M., and Singer, P. A. (1996a). Bioethics for clinicians: 2. Disclosure. *Canadian Medical Association Journal*, 155, 387–91.
Etchells, E., Sharpe, G., Dykeman, M. J., Meslin, E. M., and Singer, P. A. (1996b). Bioethics for clinicians: 4. Voluntariness. *Canadian Medical Association Journal*, 155, 1083–6.
Etchells, E., Sharpe, G., Elliott, C., and Singer, P. A. (1996c). Bioethics for clinicians: 3. Capacity. *Canadian Medical Association Journal*, 155, 657–61.
Faden, R. R. and Beauchamp, R. L. (1986). *A history and theory of informed consent*, pp. 256–7. Oxford University Press, New York.
Frankl, D., Oye, R. K., and Bellamy, P. E. (1989). Attitudes of hospitalized patients toward life-support: A survey of 200 medical inpatients. *American Journal of Medicine*, 86, 645–8.
Gamble, E. R., McDonald, P. J., and Lichstein, P. R. (1991). Knowledge, attitudes and behavior of elderly persons regarding living wills. *Archives of Internal Medicine*, 151, 277–80.
Halevy, A., and Brody, B. A. (1996). A multi-institution collaborative policy on medical futility. *Journal of the American Medical Association*, 276, 571–4.
Hall, E. T. (1981). *Beyond culture*. Doubleday, New York.
Hanks, G. W. C. (1999). Oxford Textbook of Palliative Medicine. Oxford, Oxford.
Hannan, E. L., Kilburn, H. Jr., Racz, M., Shield, S. E., and Chassin, M. R. (1994). Improving the outcome of coronary artery bypass surgery in New York State. *Journal of the American Medical Association*, 271, 761–6.
Hanson, L. C., Danis, M., and Garrett, J. (1997a). What is wrong with end-of-life care? Opinions of bereaved family members. *Journal of the American Geriatric Society*, 45, 1339–44.
Hanson, L. C., Tulsky, J. A., and Danis, M. (1997b). Can clinical interventions change care at the end of life? *Annals of Internal Medicine*, 126, 381–8.
Hoffmann, D. E. (1994). Mediating life and death decisions. *Arizona Law Review*, 36, 821–77.
Holley, J. L., Finucane, T. E., and Moss, A. H. (1989). Dialysis patients' attitudes about cardiopulmonary resuscitation and stopping dialysis. *American Journal of Nephrology*, 9, 245–51.
Holley, J. L., Nespor, S., and Rault, R. (1993a). The effects of providing chronic hemodialysis patients written material on advance directives. *American Journal of Kidney Disease*, 22, 413–8.
Holley, J. L., Nespor, S., and Rault, R. (1993b). Chronic In-Center Hemodialysis Patients' Attitudes, Knowledge, and Behavior Towards Advance Directives. *Journal of the American Society of Nephrology*, 3, 1405–8.
Holley, J. L., Stackiewicz, L., Dacko, C., and Rault, R. (1997). Factors influencing dialysis patients' completion of advance directives. *American Journal of Kidney Disease*, 30, 356–60.
Institute for Health Care Improvement (1998). Improving care at the end of life breakthrough series National Congress, 22–22 July 1998, St Louis, MI.
Institute of Medicine (1997). *Approaching death: Improving care at the end-of-life* (eds Field, M. J. and Cassel, C. K.). National Academy Press, Washington, DC.
Jacobson, J. A., Francis, L. P., Battin, M. P., Green, G. J., Grammes, C., VanRiper, J., and Gully, J. (1997). Dialogue to action: lessons learned from some family members of deceased patients at an interactive program in seven Utah hospitals. *Journal of Clinical Ethics*, 8, 359–71.

Joint Centre for Bioethics, www.utoronto.ca/jcb/ccm_policy.htm; May 12, 2000.
Joos, S. K., Reuler, J. B., Powell, J. L., and Hickam, D. H. (1993). Outpatients' attitudes and understanding regarding living wills. *Journal of General Internal Medicine*, **8**, 259–63.
Katz, M., Abbey, S., Rydall, A., and Lowy, F. (1995). Psychiatric consultation for competency to refuse medical treatment. *Psychosomatics*, **36**, 33–41.
Kleinman, A. M. (1980). *Patients and healers in the context of culture*. University of California Press, Berkley.
Lazar, N. M., Griener, G. G., Robertson, G., and Singer, P. A. (1996). Bioethics for clinicians: 5. Substitute decision making. *Canadian Medical Association Journal*, **155**, 1435–7.
Lo, B., McLeod, G. A., and Saika, G. (1986). Patient attitudes to discussing life-sustaining treatment. *Archives of Internal Medicine*, **146**, 1613–5.
Lynn, J., Teno, J. M., Phillips, R. S., Wu, A. W., Desbiens, N., Harrold, J., Claessens, M. T., Wenger, N., Kreling, B., and Connors, A. F. (1997). Perceptions by family members of the dying experience of older and seriously ill patients. *Annals of Internal Medicine*, **126**, 97–106.
Mailloux, L. U., Bellucci, A. G., Wilkes, B. M., Napolitano, B., Mossey, R. T., Lesser, M., and Bluestone, P. A. (1991). Mortality in dialysis patients: Analysis of the causes of death. *American Journal of Kidney Disease*, **18**, 326–35.
Martin, D. K., Thiel, E. C., and Singer, P. A. (1999). A new model of advance care planning: Observations from people with HIV. *Archives of Internal Medicine*, **159**, 86–92.
Mebane, A. H., and Rauch, H. B. (1990). When do physicians request competency evaluations? *Psychosomatics*, **31**, 40–6.
Mendelssohn, D. C. and Singer, P. A. (1994). Advance directives in dialysis. *Advances in Renal Replacement Therapy*, **1**, 240–50.
Moss, A., Holley, J., and Upton, M. (1992). Outcomes of cardiopulmonary resuscitation in dialysis patients. *Journal of the American Society of Nephrology*, **3**, 1238–43.
Murphy, D. J., Burrows, D., Santilli, S., Kemp, A. W., Tenner, S., Kreling, B., and Teno, J. (1994). The influence of the probability of survival on patients' preferences regarding cardiopulmonary resuscitation. *New England Journal of Medicine*, **330**, 545–9.
Neu, S., and Kjellstrand, C. M. (1986). Stopping long-term dialysis: An empirical study of withdrawal of life-supporting treatment. *New England Journal of Medicine*, **314**, 14–20.
Neveloff Dubler, N., and Marcus, L. J. (1994). *Mediating bioethical disputes: A practical guide*. United Hospital Fund of New York, New York.
O'Connor, G. T., Plume, S. K., Olmstead, E. M., Morton, J. R., Maloney, C. T., Nugent, W. C., Hernandez, F. Jr., Clough, R., Leavitt, B. J., Coffin, L. H., Marrin, C. A., Wennberg, D., Birkmeyer, J. D., Charlesworth, D. C., Malenka, D. J., Quinton, H. B., and Kasper, J. F. (1996). A regional intervention to improve the hospital mortality associated with coronary artery bypass graft surgery. *Journal of the American Medical Association*, **275**, 841–6.
Pendleton, D. A., and Bochner, S. (1980). The communication of medical information in general practice consultations as function of the patients' social class. *Social Science and Medicine*, **14A**, 669–73.
Perry, E., Buck, C., Newsome, J., Berger, C., Messana, J., and Swartz, R. (1995). Dialysis staff influence patients in formulating their advance directives. *American Journal of Kidney Disease*, **25**, 262–8.
Perry, E. C., Swartz, R., Smith-Wheelock, L., Westbrook, J., and Buck, C. (1996). Why is it difficult for staff to discuss advance directives with chronic dialysis patients? *Journal of the American Society of Nephrology*, **7**, 2160–8.

Port, F. K., Wolfe, R. A., Hawthorne, V. M., and Ferguson, C. W. (1989). Discontinuation of dialysis therapy as a cause of death. *American Journal of Nephrology*, **9**, 145–9.

Roach, M. J. (1996). Bereavement and family burden. Paper prepared for Conference on End of Life, 27–28 August, Montreal, Canada.

Rotter, J. C. (ed.) (1966). *Locus of control: Current trends in theory and research*, 2nd edn. Wiley Press, New York.

Sehgal, A. R., Weisheit, C., Miura, Y., Butzlaff, M., Kielstein, R., and Taguchi, Y. (1996). Advance directives and withdrawal of dialysis in the United States, Germany, and Japan. *Journal of the American Medical Association*, **276**, 1652–6.

Shapiro, M. C., Najman, J. M., Chang, A., Keeping, J. D., Morrison, J., and Western, J. S. (1983). Information control and the exercise of power in the obstetrical encounter. *Social Science and Medicine*, **17**, 139–46.

Shmerling, R. H., Bedell, S. E., Lilienfeld, A., and Delbanco, T. L. (1988). Discussing cardiopulmonary resuscitation: A study of elderly outpatients. *Journal of General Internal Medicine*, **3**, 317–21.

Singer, P. A. (1994). Disease-specific advance directives. *Lancet*, **344**, 594–6.

Singer, P. A., and End Stage Renal Disease Network of New England (1992). Nephrologists' Experience with and attitudes towards decisions to forego dialysis. *Journal of the American Society of Nephrology*, **2**, 1235–40.

Singer, P. A., and MacDonald, N. (1998). Bioethics for clinicians: 15. Quality end of life care. *Canadian Medical Association Journal*, **159**, 159–62.

Singer, P. A., Thiel, E. C., Naylor, C. D., Richardson, R. M. A., Llewellyn-Thomas, H., Goldstein, M., Saiphoo, C., Uldall, R., Kim, D., and Mendelssohn, D. C. (1995). Life-sustaining treatment preferences of hemodialysis patients: Implications for advance directives. *Journal of the American Society of Nephrology*, **6**, 1410–7.

Singer, P. A., Martin, D. K., Lavery, J. V., Thiel, E. C., Kelner, M., and Mendelssohn, D. C. (1998). Reconceptualizing advance care planning from the patient's perspective. *Archives of Internal Medicine*, **158**, 879–84.

Singer, P. A., Martin, D. K., and Kelner M. J. (1999). Quality end of life care: Patients' perspectives. *Journal of the American Medical Association*, **281**, 163–8.

Slaikeu, K. A. (1989). Designing Dispute Resolution Systems in the Health Care Industry. *Negotiation Journal*, **395**, 31–9.

Solomon, M. Z., O'Donnell, L., Jennings, B., Guilfoy, V., Wolf, S. M., Nolan, K., Jackson, R., Koch-Weser, K., and Donnelley, S. (1993). Decisions near the end of life: Professional views on life-sustaining treatments. *American Journal of Public Health*, **83**, 14–23.

Stolman, C. J., Gregory, J. J., Dunn, D., and Levine, J. L. (1990). Evaluation of patient, physician, nurse and family attitudes toward do not resuscitate orders. *Archives of Internal Medicine*, **150**, 653–8.

The SUPPORT Investigators (1995). A controlled trial to improve care for seriously ill hospitalized patients: The Study to Understand Prognoses and Preferences for Outcomes and Risks of Treatment (SUPPORT). *Journal of the American Medical Association*, **274**, 1591–8.

Teno, J., Fleishman, J., Brock, D. W., and Mor, V. (1990). The use of formal prior directives among patients with HIV-related disease. *Journal of General Internal Medicine*, **5**, 490–4.

Teno, J. M., Nelson, H. L., and Lynn, J. (1994). Advance care planning: Priorities for ethical and empirical research. *Hastings Center Report*, **6**, s32–6.

Ware, J. E. Jr., and Hayes, R. D. Methods for measuring patient satisfaction with specific medical encounters. (1988). *Medical Care*, **26**, 393–402.

Weijer, C., Singer, P. A., Dickens, B. M., and Workman, S. (1998). Bioethics for Clinicians: 16. Dealing with demand for 'inappropriate' treatment: Medical futility and other approaches. *Canadian Medical Association Journal*, **159**, 817–21.

7
Acquisition of kidneys for transplantation

Raymond Hoffenberg

Recognition of the benefits of transplantation has made it the treatment of choice for most patients with end-stage renal disease (ESRD). Its very success has created the problem of organ shortage; the supply of donor kidneys cannot keep up with demand. To cope with a growing waiting list, either the supply must be increased or the demand reduced. More stringent selection of patients may help to reduce demand, but this introduces difficult ethical problems of choice and is unlikely to solve the problem in the long term. The solution lies in increasing supply. Limited success has been achieved by simple measures such as enhanced education and publicity, through the appointment of more and better-trained transplant coordinators, and by more determined efforts to obtain consent from the relatives of prospective donors. Other 'less orthodox' approaches aimed at increasing the supply of kidneys tend to be dismissed on the grounds that they are unethical or offensive or both—often gut-reactions that do not stand up to critical analysis. In this chapter I examine some of these ideas and the responses they evoke in an attempt to identify genuinely rational objections and to see to what extent they are rebuttable.

I make the primary assumption that kidney transplantation is a worthy activity—patients with ESRD would die if left untreated, and transplants are cheaper and offer better quality of life than the alternative of dialysis. Therefore, any measure that aims to increase the supply of organs for transplantation deserves to be taken seriously and not dismissed precipitately; the onus is on those who object to produce valid and irrefutable arguments to support their case. However, in contrast to end-stage failure of the heart or liver, dialysis does offer an alternative to transplantation for most patients with ESRD; exchanging this for a transplant is not a matter of life or death. They can survive, albeit it with a lesser quality of life. There is thus a tension between the drive to get more kidneys to improve patients' quality of life and the risk of offending propriety by introducing measures that the public would find hard to accept. The stringent requirement of incontestability may need to be subordinated to other social, cultural or religious factors.

Among measures that have been discouraged or prohibited are:

- the sale of kidneys;
- 'presumed consent' or 'opting out';
- greater use of living unrelated donors;

- the use of organs from patients in persistent vegetative state (PVS) or with anencephaly;
- the use of organs from prisoners or those who have been executed.

I am sympathetic to the general objective of increasing the supply of organs for transplantation and I believe this can be done in several ways, including some of the above, that would not prove offensive to the public. I am more concerned with the hasty reactions and illogical arguments that are elicited whenever some of them are discussed than with peremptory advocacy of their adoption. I hope that a more rational approach might persuade some readers to see them in a different light.

The sale of kidneys[1]

Most kidneys for transplantation are obtained from cadavers. In many countries because of religious or cultural beliefs, there is no alternative source—donations from living persons are forbidden. Even where they are permitted the transfer is usually restricted to organs from spouses or blood relations of the recipient. At various times from different countries reports have emerged alleging that live donors have been selling their kidneys, and the practice has almost routinely been condemned. Despite this there is still a large international trade in organs, patients in renal failure often travelling from their home countries, in which it is forbidden, to receive organs abroad. In many instances condemnation has been justified by revelations of rampant commercialization accompanied by substandard care of both donor and recipient. In most developed countries any suggestion that a properly regulated system of trade in body organs might officially be condoned has been greeted with expressions of disgust and outrage by the media and professional bodies and, indeed, the practice has invariably been banned. This almost universal condemnation has often been an emotional rather than an intellectual response. Those who adduce reasons for their protest, as opposed to reflex unreasoning condemnation, usually express concern about possible exploitation of the would-be donor who, it is argued, needs to be protected; the way to achieve this is by stopping all sales. It is hard to see how this benefits a donor who desperately needs money and is eager to sell a kidney that may be the only asset he has. Removing this option by prohibition leaves him less well-off and, coincidentally, reduces the potential pool of organs. A ban on organ sales is thus disadvantageous to both the prospective donor and those awaiting a kidney transplant.

Many different arguments have been put forward to justify a ban; most have been rebutted in a recent article (Radcliffe-Richards *et al.*, 1998).

- Poor people driven to the extreme of having to offer a kidney for sale may be unable fully to comprehend the situation, and their consent cannot therefore be properly informed. Many wealthy people experience the same problem when faced with a complex medical decision and, conversely, many poor people are quite capable of understanding the implications of the proposal. Comprehension does not necessarily

[1] See also Chapter 16 by Jha and Chugh

develop in parallel with one's bank balance. There is unease that inordinate pressure exerted by the promise of financial reward might persuade donors to take decisions that are against their best interests, that would not have been taken had circumstances been different. Whatever the individual's economic status or level of comprehension, good medical practice demands proper counselling and explanation. If real doubt remains about the donor's understanding of the issue or ability to give valid consent, it would be better not to proceed.

- The donor is exposed to untoward risk. It is widely accepted that the risk associated with removal of a kidney is small and it applies equally to all living donors, related or unrelated. In the case of related donors, it is not considered large enough to be a deterrent. An objection on grounds of risk, therefore, is not to the risk itself but to the fact that someone is being paid to take it. Many paid occupations are much more dangerous, but do not evoke the same degree of solicitude. Examples include deep-sea diving or fishing or underground mining. (In South Africa, for instance, nearly 890 gold miners have been killed in 1998–2000.) Society appears to tolerate the exposure of paid workers to substantial occupational risk. Why the concern about far less hazardous donation of a kidney?
- Less scrupulous donors might be induced by the promise of money to lie about their health and withhold relevant medical information that might place recipients in jeopardy. This is far more likely to happen where live donations are performed outside the law and the whole process is carried out in a clandestine way. If trade in kidneys were legal and properly regulated, meticulous scrutiny and careful investigation of all prospective donors would reduce the likelihood of subterfuge.
- Donation is a gift, an expression of altruism, and this important attribute should be preserved without contamination by the passage of money. Human organs, it is argued, have no monetary value, the gift is priceless—an argument I find difficult to accept—most people would give up a kidney if offered a large enough sum of money. A parent who donates a kidney to save the life or reduce suffering of a child is normally praised for a highly altruistic and loving action. If the same parent wished to sell a kidney to pay for vital drugs to save a child suffering from a serious but treatable disease, this would be frowned on and prohibited. The motive is equally altruistic in both cases. It is never easy to establish the purity of the altruism behind any organ donation and, even if it cannot be established, lack of altruism is not a basis for forbidding an action. For many years the concept of altruism dominated the field of blood donation, for which payment was not made. In recent years declining supplies of blood have persuaded many transfusion centres to abandon the altruistic principle and to offer payment in order to sustain levels of donation. Other body parts have also been traded, including semen and ova, both admittedly renewable so donors do not suffer as a result of their actions. But if there is very little risk associated with kidney donation, the fact that the organ is not renewable is of no import. It is interesting that apart from payment of expenses to donors or their families it is now acceptable to offer incentives such as an undertaking to pay the funeral expenses when the donor dies, even if death is unrelated to the event. The step from this to full-blown and transparent payment seems very small indeed. The concept of pure altruism is becoming untenable, soon it will be obsolete.

- The slippery slope argument is frequently adduced: if kidney sales from living donors are allowed, soon it will be a vital organ such as a heart or a liver. There is little logic in this. Taking a kidney from a person is not a particularly hazardous procedure; those who have donated a kidney survive as well as those who still have two. Removing the heart would kill the subject. One is a perfectly acceptable procedure, the other would not be countenanced in civilized society. In any event, the logic behind a slippery slope argument is questionable: If action A (sale of a kidney) were to be acceptable, why should it be necessary to ban it in order to prevent action B (sale of a heart) which is not? Why not simply ban B?
- The sale of kidneys will deter donation of cadaver kidneys. There is no evidence at all for this assumption. It is more likely that sold kidneys will add to the pool, attracting organs that would not otherwise be available for transplantation.
- Trade in organs will attract criminal activity. There have been persistent rumours over many years of adults and children being abducted or simply disappearing, allegedly to provide a source of body parts. (The classic oft-repeated tale involves a young man who meets and spends the night with an attractive girl and wakes up next day to find a lengthy sutured wound of the nephrectomy that was performed while he was drugged.) Despite extensive investigation there is no evidence that such abuse has actually taken place; no alleged case of forced removal of organs has yet been substantiated. On medical grounds the practice would be almost inconceivable; the whole process of removing organs, matching them, keeping them in a viable and sterile condition and then transplanting them would involve teams of doctors, nurses, anaesthetists and technicians, as well as operating theatres and other facilities. The idea that this could all be done without question or opposition is excessively far-fetched.
- The rich would benefit unfairly from trade in organs—another example of inequality of health care. By buying organs from the poor, the rich would be able to jump the queue to the disadvantage of less fortunate people waiting for a transplant. This would only be true if the kidney provided to the purchaser were to come from a limited pool; if it would not otherwise have become available, there would be no impropriety. The argument is flawed in another way—it assumes that only the rich would be able to buy kidneys. Wealth is a relative matter. In the developed world most people can afford to own a car. A kidney is likely to cost less. If it were possible to shorten the time of waiting for a transplant, many people would easily find the money, if necessary by foregoing ownership of a car. It is likely that more kidneys would then reach the market, thereby reducing the waiting time for those who could not afford to buy one.
- It is degrading to have to sell an organ in order to get badly needed money. The real degradation, of course, is the poverty that forces donors to take the step. So long as such degrees of poverty exist, there will be people willing to make sacrifices that wealthier people would regard as offensive or debasing. If one wishes to eliminate this or other forms of degradation that poor people suffer, the answer is not to declare them illegal, but to try to alleviate the extreme poverty that spawns them.

Many of these fears and criticisms would be allayed by the insertion of an intermediary between the vendor and purchaser. The purchase of organs would be possible only through a designated agency approved by government or other legal authority that would be responsible for ensuring that potential vendors are informed as fully as possible and comprehend the step they are taking. In addition, it would monitor standards of care including screening of vendors, and their organs, and adequate aftercare. The agency would ensure that the seller was paid a reasonable price for the organ and satisfy itself insofar as possible that the would-be donor was not a drug or alcohol addict simply seeking a way to satisfy an addiction. Although normally one would not wish to dictate how a vendor should spend the proceeds of an organ sale, it would seem irresponsible to go ahead if this motive was suspected. Most important—and this answers concerns about exploitation and unwarranted privilege for the rich or unjustified profits for entrepreneurial dealers—the agency would arrange for disposal of purchased organs according to need in the same way as donated cadaver organs, preferably through the same national or international organization. It would not then be possible to jump the queue except on proper medical grounds.

An interesting variant of kidney sale is 'paired kidney exchange' (Ross *et al.*, 1997). The proposition is best illustrated by an example in the United Kingdom in which a father was willing to donate a kidney to his son with ESRD but encountered tissue incompatibility. He then offered one of his kidneys to the national cadaveric donor pool in exchange for a compatible organ from this pool being made available to his son. In terms of the British Human Organ Transplant Act of 1989 this was regarded as illegal as payment by the recipient is defined as 'money or money's worth'. It is nevertheless an idea that would probably be accepted in most European countries and is worth pursuing in the UK in the hope of inducing a change in interpretation of the Act. Daar (1998) describes the rejection of an offer from a woman in the US to donate a kidney to pay for a laparoscopic cholecystectomy, perhaps a more obvious example of 'money's worth'.

Having emphasized the safety of surgery for donation of a kidney, it would seem wrong not to mention the discomfort and even pain that many donors feel as a result of it, mostly related to the wound (Nicholson and Bradley, 1999). Modern methods of pain relief and new approaches such as the use of epidural analgesia and laparoscopic surgery promise to reduce this complication. A survey of almost a thousand donors showed that 4% of the 60% who responded to a questionnaire were dissatisfied with the procedure and regretted their decision to participate, 12% found it stressful. It is perhaps significant that a high proportion of those who regretted their participation knew that their transplanted kidney had survived less than a year (Johnson *et al.*, 1999).

In recent years there has been a discernable change of opinion in favour of some form of controlled trade in organs. A prestigious Bellagio Task Force Report recently could find no unarguable ethical principle that would justify a ban under all circumstances (Daar, 1998). Most objections to organ sales can be rebutted on logical grounds. One is left with the feeling that they mostly reflect intuitive responses that do not seriously address a potentially valuable contribution towards reducing the gap between supply and demand. To be fair, this potential itself has not been tested; as yet, no one knows whether or to what extent payment will increase the supply of organs. To borrow an intuitive response, I believe it would.

'Contracting in' and 'contracting out'

In most countries the emphasis in organ donation is on voluntarism. Those who wish to donate organs after death are expected to indicate their intention during their lifetimes. In the absence of an explicit statement, provided there is no reason to believe that the dead person would have objected, consent for removal of the organs may be sought from the relatives. A system of this sort that depends on a previously expressed declaration of a wish to donate is referred to as 'contracting or opting in'. By contrast, in some countries a system exists through which consent is presumed unless there is an advance directive to the contrary; 'contracting out' or 'presumed consent'.

In several countries, notably Spain, Austria and Belgium, a change from contracting in to contracting out has been associated with an increase in the number of organs made available for transplantation (Kennedy *et al.*, 1998). The picture is often confounded by the simultaneous introduction of other measures designed to achieve this, for instance the appointment of more transplant coordinators, enhanced publicity and provision of financial incentives. Perhaps the best evidence of an improvement resulting from a change in the law comes from Belgium where an 'internal control' was provided by a decision taken in Antwerp not to accept the change. There, organ donation rates remained unaltered whereas in Leuven where the change was adopted rates rose substantially (Michielsen, 1996). In contracting-out systems it is essential to provide simple and convenient ways for people to register their unwillingness to donate. In Belgium objectors may do this at any Town Hall.

In contracting in systems donors must either have directed in advance that they were willing to provide their organs or in, the absence of such a directive, the relatives must agree to removal. In contracting-out systems, although it is not necessary to obtain the consent of relatives, doctors are encouraged to do so in all cases, and usually desist from strict application of the law if strong objections are raised. Such a system is thought to relieve grieving relatives of the need to make what they sometimes find to be a difficult and unpleasant decision to consent to removal of the organs. Consultation also gives them an opportunity to express any undeclared objection the dead person might have held. Experience in Belgium has gained support from doctors who like the idea of more openness and from families for whom being informed of the intention to proceed with organ removal is less traumatic than a request for permission to proceed.

It has been suggested that those who wish to donate after death should be able to express a preference for the person or class of persons they would like to receive their organs—so-called 'directed donations'. This seems to be legally acceptable and might persuade some prospective but undecided donors to accede. It would probably be wise not to accept positive exclusion of groups.

The Conference of European Health Ministers and WHO have supported the Belgian model in which the views of relatives are not ignored (Kennedy *et al.*, 1997). Experience with contracting out legislation has shown that by and large the public is comfortable with it. There seems no reason any longer not to adopt it.

Unrelated living donors

The proportion of kidneys derived from living donors or cadavers varies from country to country. In most developing countries because of problems in obtaining cadaver organs living donors predominate. Elsewhere, despite better survival rates of kidneys taken from living donors, cadaver organs are still preferred. The use of living donors is widely regarded in the transplant profession as a necessary but undesirable consequence of the shortage of cadaver organs, procurement of which poses fewer difficulties (Sells, 1997).

As part of the reaction to revelations of trade in human organs, many countries have introduced regulations to control donations by living persons, which is permitted only between siblings or other close relatives including spouses. On the whole these donors are eager to offer an organ to help a loved one whatever risk there might be. Donation of a segment of liver or pancreas to a family member is not uncommon despite a substantially greater risk than donation of a kidney. Generally, transfer of organs between unrelated living persons is allowed only in rare circumstances in which the donor has to prove an exceptional interest in helping the recipient. The clinical (as opposed to ethical) argument that transfer of an organ between blood relatives is preferable because of enhanced compatibility, and therefore less rejection and improved survival rates, is not sufficient ground to discard offers of organs from unrelated donors. Evidence shows that kidney transplantation between living unrelated donors is just as successful as between blood relatives matched for a single haplotype and more successful than cadaver transplants (Terasaki *et al.*, 1995).

If the clinical argument based on compatibility falls away, what is the reason for restricting donations to close relatives? The usual answer is that the risk associated with donation should not be taken unless there is a compelling reason on the donor's part to help the recipient. Within a loving family the risk is thought to be justified by the donor's devotion to the recipient. This argument fails to impress. In the first instance, the risk to the donor of a kidney is so small as to be immaterial. An overall perioperative mortality figure of 0.03% is found in retrospective surveys and it should be possible to improve on this figure. No deaths were reported in a series of 1200 donor nephrectomies performed in Oslo (Nicholson and Bradley, 1999). The possibility of a fatal outcome is statistically remote, but if it occurred in a within-family donation the practical and emotional consequences could be catastrophic.

Second, it cannot be assumed that altruistic unselfish love of the sort evinced by those who donate organs always and only exists within a family. Blood relations may be just as corruptible or open to pressure as non-relations. Purity of motive cannot be taken for granted even within a manifestly devoted family. Strong internal pressures, amounting to coercion, may be exerted on an unwilling member to supply a kidney, casting doubt on the voluntariness of the donation. Sells (1997) has discussed in some detail the obligations of the surgeon to assess the degree of voluntarism when dealing with donations even from related donors.

Most regulations permit donation between spouses, accepting that a loving bond between them is a sufficient basis for donation. Reluctance to stretch the bounds of acceptability beyond spouses is confounded by suspicion that there may be underlying commercial interests, that one party is selling an organ to another. In order to remove this stigma it is necessary to show that an unusual caring association exists between donor and recipient. Unmarried couples, including gays, have to demonstrate the stability of their relationship. How long has it lasted? Is it 'permanent'? (One could ask the same questions about donations between married couples). Why should close and dear friends be excluded? Do people have to live together in order for one to wish to help the other? As with other medical decisions, minors and adults who are mentally incompetent are excluded from consideration because of uncertainties about consent.

From an ethical point of view, what is the objection to donation by an unrelated person, even to a complete stranger? If altruism is the desirable motive, why deny someone the opportunity to do good during his or her lifetime by giving away a kidney? A person who dives into the sea to rescue a drowning person or runs into a burning house to save a threatened child does not first check whether it is a blood relative. In both cases the risk to the rescuer is greater, but saving a life in this way is not banned by law or limited to those with genetic links. The fact that one action takes place in the heat of the moment, the other planned in cold blood, does not detract from the heroism, or altruism, of both.

In summary, it is hard to see the logic behind the 'protection' of unrelated donors apart from suspicion that there might be a hidden commercial transaction—another argument in favour of legalizing organ sales?

Organs from persistent vegetative state (PVS) or anencephaly

In the USA there are an estimated 10000–25000 adult patients and 4000–10000 children in a persistent vegetative state (Multi-Society Task Force on PVS, 1994); figures for the UK are probably much lower, perhaps 1000 in all. There is a growing consensus, popular as well as legal, that treatment may be stopped in patients who have been in this state for a prolonged period of time without any sign of cerebral recovery. Could such dying patients ever be considered as a potential source of organs for transplantation?

In most countries, subject to varying forms of consent, organs may be retrieved from the body once the diagnosis of brain death has been established. In the US, brain death is defined as irreversible death of the whole brain. In the UK, it is sufficient to demonstrate absence of brainstem function with or without loss of higher brain function—death of the brainstem is equated with death of the brain. Patients in PVS do not fall within either definition of death since they have lost higher brain function while retaining activity of the brainstem. According to both the US and UK criteria, they are still alive and removal of the organs would not be permitted. In a landmark case in the United Kingdom in 1994 it was established in the House of Lords that all treatment, including the provision of food and water, could be stopped in selected patients in a persistent vegetative state who would then be allowed to die. This applied only to those who had been in PVS for longer than a year without evidence of recovering cerebral function, on the grounds that restoration of function after this time was highly improbable. Each individual decision to withdraw treatment had to be taken by a court of law (House of Lords Report, 1994).

Most of the large number of patients in PVS quoted above would have had the condition for less than a year and would not therefore satisfy the UK requirement for withdrawal of treatment. Nevertheless, there would be a substantial prospective source of organs if it were possible to retrieve them from patients *once a legal decision had been taken to withdraw treatment and to allow them to die.* There are problems, however.

In PVS, since brainstem activity is retained, the patient is able to breathe, the heart beats spontaneously and there are reflex and other purposeless movements. Because of these recognizable elements of 'human behaviour', there is understandable opposition from some quarters to the judgment that life may be terminated. This has been fuelled by reports claiming that occasionally the first signs of recovery have taken place after the stipulated period of a year and that improvement has continued after this. In many of these cases the original diagnosis was probably incorrect or earlier signs of recovering function had not been recognized. While agreeing that the diagnosis of PVS may at times be difficult, Andrews, who has profound experience of the condition, affirms that an accurate diagnosis can be made if the patient is assessed over a period of time by a well-trained team. He asserts that fear of misdiagnosis should not constitute an argument against ending the life of a person in PVS in accordance with the House of Lords guidelines (Andrews et al., 1996).

The above arguments are essentially concerned with decisions about the withdrawal of treatment that leads to death of the patient. Once this decision has been taken why should the organs not be used to benefit those who need transplantation? In the first place, in all jurisdictions the law distinguishes between passively allowing a person to die and actively accelerating death. Removing treatment is allowing a patient to die and is permissible; removing organs while a patient is deemed to be alive, as in the case of PVS, would cause or accelerate death and is clearly against the law. This introduces an almost incontrovertible case against the use of their organs. When treatment including water and nutrition is withdrawn, the heart and lungs continue to function for 10–12 days until they fail because of inanition, electrolyte imbalance or dehydration. By this time, the organs are no longer in prime condition and are unsuitable for transplantation. To obtain viable transplantable organs death would have to be accelerated and this is unlawful. A priori it would seem that, even where a decision has been taken to allow a patient with PVS to die, there is no acceptable way of retrieving his organs.

One may ask three separate but linked questions: First, regardless of the issue of removal of organs, should patients in PVS be maintained on supportive therapy until they die 'naturally', a process that could take many years? A decision to withdraw treatment after 12 months of unresponsiveness is regarded as reasonable by both the British Medical Association (1992) and the American Neurological Association (1993). In favour of this step is the relief it would afford to families and carers faced with lengthy distress as they continue to tend someone who has no hope of improvement. There would also be a substantial financial saving; the overall cost in the US of keeping patients in PVS alive has been estimated as between one and seven billion dollars per year (Multi-Society Task Force on PVS, 1994). When there is no longer any hope, would it not be more humane to divert funds to those who have a better chance of recovery? It is not a responsibility of doctors to preserve life at all costs and treatment may be withheld or withdrawn if it is inordinately painful, damaging or futile. In such circumstances a doctor's primary duty of care to a patient may cease and be re-directed instead to the interests of the family, carers or to society as a whole.

Second, once a decision has been taken to end life (for argument's sake, in a court of law), how should this be done? Again, regardless of the issue of removing organs, could a case be made for a more speedy termination of life? This would reduce the distress of those who are obliged to nurse or otherwise care for, or simply observe, the slow process of dying by inanition once food and water have been withdrawn? One may question whether insistence on the long drawn-out process of dying sanctioned by law is really humane.

Third, could it ever be legally, morally or practically possible to procure organs for transplantation from patients in PVS who are deemed legally still to be alive but from whom it has been decided to withdraw treatment? If one has to wait for death, the organs will be unusable; any attempt to retrieve organs before this would be illegal. From a legal point of view there is no way out of this dilemma; from a moral point of view it is less critical. The crucial decision is whether to terminate life or not. Once this has been made affirmatively there is no clear ethical distinction between allowing a patient to die by omission of therapy and more actively ending life, for instance, by injection of a fatal substance. For religious, cultural and other traditional reasons it is unlikely that the public would at the present time find the latter step acceptable.

In recent years there have been cases in which the heart and other organs have been transplanted from anencephalic neonates into children with untreatable end-organ failure. This has occasioned quite heated debate (American Neurological Committee, 1993). Anencephaly is similar to PVS in that the higher brain is non-functioning (usually absent) but brainstem function is preserved. At birth anencephalics may be legally regarded as alive although, because of the gross deformity and hopelessness of the condition, few would take exception to a decision to allow them to die and this, in fact, is common practice. The reaction to a proposal from reputable medical bodies that their organs might be used for transplantation into infants or children with end-organ failure, especially of the heart, suggests that the public would not approve, since this would require removal while the heart was still beating. Looked at realistically, the number of organs that would accrue from patients with PVS or from anencephalics would not be large and it is doubtful whether an effort to change public opinion would be justified.

The use of organs from prisoners or executed persons

These are essentially different problems (Cameron and Hoffenberg, 1999). In the past *prisoners* have been used as subjects for medical research, not always carried out in accordance with the usual codes of research ethics. Objections have been raised in particular to the unreliability of any consent obtained under the circumstances of imprisonment and a suspicion that many experiments have been carried out without any consent at all or even under duress. In many instances 'volunteers' were exposed to unacceptable risk. Often they were rewarded by remission of sentence, a form of inducement that is generally regarded as unacceptable. Reports of several experiments of dubious ethical validity led to prohibition of the use of prisoners for research in most countries. It could be argued that this has removed a favourable option from prisoners who might have hoped that their willingness to be the subjects of research would be rewarded by a remission of sentence, similar to that expected for good behaviour. Removal of this option left them somewhat worse off.

Despite misgivings about the financial inducement of subjects of medical research, overt payment, especially for participation in drug trials, is now widespread. The fact that prisoners are not permitted to participate, with or without similar inducements of financial or other reward, reflects concern about their status and the special relationship that exists between them, their warders and the prison doctors. This is similar to the relationship between students and teachers, or laboratory workers and their employers, where great care is needed to ensure that undue pressure is not applied. It seems invidious to permit students or employees to take part in research projects, but not prisoners, and since payment is permitted, why not reward them in kind (remission of sentence) instead of cash? It should not be impossible to determine whether or not the agreement to participate was truly voluntarily.

The position of prisoners in relation to medical research is mirrored in relation to organ donation. Subject to similar safeguards a case could be made to allow them to donate kidneys for transplantation in return for a remission of sentence. The risk is small, the benefit substantial, measurable in days of remission rather than pounds or dollars. It is indeed possible that some prisoners might be motivated by a desire to seek expiation for their crimes rather than by the prospect of financial or other reward. Should this altruistic avenue be denied them?

Controversy about the use of organs from *executed prisoners* usually confuses two separate issues: first is concern about application of the death penalty itself and, second, whether once it has been carried out the organs of the executed prisoners might be used for transplantation. Conflation of these two elements of the debate makes logical nonsense.

The death penalty is now prohibited in most European countries. It is, however, still legally extant in more than 100 countries worldwide, including a majority of states in the US. More executions are carried out in China than in the rest of the world combined and there are reports that organs are commonly removed from executed prisoners for purposes of transplantation. At various times other countries (Singapore, Taiwan, France and the US amongst others) have also permitted removal of organs from executed persons, but all appear to have abandoned the practice in recent years.

Although there are substantial grounds for objecting to the death penalty, which I share, this chapter is not primarily concerned with the question of its global abolition. The issue here is more focused—whether it is morally acceptable to make use of the organs once a legal execution has been carried out. The role of the doctor in removing organs from someone who has just been executed is debatable; in general doctors are advised to take no part in practices such as capital or corporal punishment. Partly for this reason, most leading transplant organizations and a large number of individuals have voiced objections to the practice, even to the extent of threatening to expel any member of a society who is found to engage in it.

Behind the widespread condemnation of removal of organs from executed prisoners, mostly directed against China, are claims of frequent and serious abuse (Guttmann, 1992). These include:

- Prisoners are deliberately executed in order to provide a source of organs and China is seen as the main offender. The rumour is almost certainly unfounded, as China has no need to increase the number of executions in order to meet the demand for transplant organs—more prisoners are executed annually than would be needed to meet demand. It is not a shortage of kidneys that limits the number or transplants performed, other factors come into account such as the high cost of immunosuppressive drugs.
- The process of execution is modified in order to satisfy the requirements for transplantation. The normal practice in China is a bullet through the back of the neck, which allows organs including the heart to be removed expeditiously. The important aspect of execution—if one has to have it—is that it should be carried out as humanely as possible with least suffering to the individual. Is a bullet through the neck less humane than hanging or the electric chair?
- In the circumstances that surround executions it is unlikely that consent to removal of kidneys or other organs would be freely given by condemned prisoners; their autonomy is thus compromised. In China dominance is not accorded to individual autonomy to the same extent as in the West and it claimed that family consent is sought as a routine rather than consent of the individual. Moreover, it seems irrational to worry about the abuse of a sophisticated principle of medical ethics (autonomy) when a major breach of fundamental human rights (killing) is about to be committed.
- There is some evidence that organs taken from executed prisoners are sold for profit. The morality of selling organs in general is discussed above and it is difficult to discern why the special case of selling organs from prisoners should be censured. Critics may object to the fact that the proceeds of the sale go to the government or to entrepreneurs and not to the family of the deceased, but this point is not clearly stated when the subject is reviewed. If the money went to the family, would the sale be condoned? Chinese law prohibits the export and/or sale of organs to foreign nationals, therefore any such trade is in conflict with the law. Criticism should perhaps be directed at abuse of the system rather than the legitimate and controlled removal and use of the organs from a dead person. It is perfectly reasonable for people to buy and sell shares in the stock-market; the fact that this is occasionally abused through insider trading does not justify banning the whole enterprise.

Condemnation of China over its policy of capital punishment is almost universal in the West, yet the continuing and widespread use of the death penalty in a majority of American states is not attacked with the same vehemence. Criticism appears therefore to be aimed at some other aspect of its use in China—the inordinately high number of victims, the relatively minor nature of the offences for which the death penalty is applied or, more likely, the fact that executions are thought to be planned simply as a mechanism for obtaining organs. Criticism of the high rate of execution—indeed of all execution—is justifiable but, once this point has been made, one has to ask exactly why use of the dead person's organs is so widely condemned. The practice is not without some merit. In a country that has to limit transplants because of financial constraints it provides a source of healthy kidneys at low cost and logistical ease. Awareness that the death of their relative has been of benefit to another person might also offer some solace to the families of executed prisoners. It makes more sense to condemn continued use of the death sentence—not only in China, but wherever it is carried out—rather than the defensible practice of making use of the deceased person's organs.

In this chapter I have considered a number of initiatives that have been proposed as means of alleviating the serious shortage of organs for transplantation. I have attempted to show that most of the objections to them are quite easily rebuttable, that the responses are frequently based on emotion or intuition rather than logic. It is tempting to dismiss these responses. As Dunstan (1992) has said: 'Intuitive repugnance, moral indignation, cannot have the last word in ethics'. He goes on, however, to say, 'But the exercise would be a very cold affair without it, probably less effective; and certainly less than human'. The gap between supply and demand for kidneys is very large indeed—and growing—and even the most optimistic forecast of the improvement in supply that would follow endorsement of the ideas discussed in this chapter would not balance the equation. Many of them have sufficient merit to justify their adoption notwithstanding, but something far more radical is needed to redress the imbalance. Unless a radical solution is found a smaller and smaller proportion of those with ESRD will receive transplants. If this figure declines to 10% or 5% or less, it will become increasing difficult to justify a procedure that offers relief to such a small minority. Selection of patients fortunate enough to qualify for a transplant would generate even more invidious and ethically dubious decision making. A more radical solution to the problem of ESRD is the only real hope and one looks to two possible long-term solutions—xenotransplantation and the development of acceptable and cheap artificial kidneys. Both are on the horizon but whether or when they will come into full vision is at present conjectural. Until they do we should view with more open minds the few ideas that have been proposed to ease the shortage.

References

American Neurological Association Committee on Ethical Affairs Report on PVS (1993). *Annals of Neurology*, 33, 386–90.
Andrews, K., Murphy, L., Munday, R., and Littlewood, C. (1996). Misdiagnosis of the vegetative state: retrospective study in a rehabilitation unit. *British Medical Journal*, 313, 13–16.
British Medical Association Ethics Committee (1992). *Discussion paper on treatment of patients in PVS*. BMA, London.
Cameron, J. S. and Hoffenberg, R. (1999). The ethics of organ transplantation reconsidered: paid organ donation and the use of executed prisoners as donors. *Kidney International*, 55, 724–32.
Daar, A. S. (1998). Paid organ donation–the grey basket concept. *Journal of Medical Ethics*, 24, 365–8.
Dunstan, G. (1992). Ethics in kidney transplantation. *Journal of the Irish Colleges of Physicians and Surgeons*, 21, 189–92.

Guttmann, R. D. (1992). On the use of organs from executed prisoners. *Transplant Review*, 6, 189–93.

House of Lords. Report of the Select Committee on Medical Ethics (1994). Session 1993–94. London: Her Majesty's Stationery Office.

Johnson, E. M., Anderson, J. K., Jacobs, C., Sun, G., Humar, A., Suhr, B. D., Kerr, S. R., and Matas, A. J. (1999). Long-term follow-up of living kidney donors: Quality of life after donation. *Transplantation*, 67, 717–21.

Kennedy, I., Sells, R. A., Daar, A. S., Guttmann, R. D., Hoffenberg, R., Lock, M., Radcliffe-Richards, J., and Tilney, N. (1998). The case for 'presumed consent' in organ donation. *Lancet*, 351, 1650–52.

Michielsen, P. (1996). Presumed consent to organ donation: 10 years experience in Belgium. *Journal of the Royal Society of Medicine*, 89, 663–6.

Multi-Society Task Force on PVS (1994). Medical aspects of the persistent vegetative state. *New England Journal of Medicine*, 330, 1499–1508 and 1572–79.

Nicholson, M. L., and Bradley, J. A. (1999). Renal transplantation from living donors. *British Medical Journal*, 318, 409–10.

Radcliffe-Richards, J., Daar, A. S., Guttmann, R. D., Hoffenberg, R., Kennedy, I., Lock, M., Sells, R. A., and Tilney, N. (1998). The case for allowing kidney sales. *Lancet*, 352, 1950–52.

Ross, L. F., Rubin, D. T., Siegler, M., Josephson, M. A., Thistlethwaite, J. R., and Woodle, E. S. (1997). Ethics of a paired kidney exchange program. *New England Journal of Medicine*, 336, 1752–5.

Sells, R. A. (1997). Voluntarism and coercion in living organ donation. In *Procurement, preservation and allocation of vascularised organs* (eds Collins, G. M., Land, W., and Persijn, G. G.) pp. 295–300. Kluwer Academic, Dordrecht.

Terasaki, P. I., Cecka, M. J., Gjertson, D. W., and Takemoto, S. (1995). High survival rates of kidney transplants from spousal and unrelated donors. *New England Journal of Medicine*, 333, 333–6.

8
Xenotransplantation: An ethical dilemma
Norman G. Levinsky

There is a shortage of transplantable organs, and because of this many people who need them do not benefit from one of the major medical advances of the past 50 years. In the United States in 1999, 6448 individuals on waiting lists for an organ died before they could get a transplant (UNOS, 2000). Such preventable deaths have been the principal impetus to scientific exploration of the possible use of animal organs for transplantation into humans. Xenotransplantation was tested as early as the turn of the twentieth century. The first systematic studies, which took place in the 1960s, included xenotransplants of kidney, heart, and liver. All failed because either the transplanted organs were rejected or the patients succumbed to complications of the immunosuppressive regimen used to prevent rejection. Thereafter, although laboratory research proceeded, clinical trials generally were discontinued. Occasional exceptions in the 1980s and 1990s, including the transplant of a baboon heart into a newborn infant, of baboon livers into two patients with liver failure, and of baboon bone marrow into a patient with the acquired immunodeficiency syndrome (AIDS) also failed despite significant improvements in immunosuppression. The application of recent advances in immunology and molecular biology to xenotransplant research has raised realistic hopes that the rejection barrier can be overcome before 2010. Some enthusiastic investigators believe that experiments in animals already have reached the point at which well-designed human trials of organ xenotransplantation are justified in the near future.

There is some evidence that transplanted cells and tissues may be useful in treating a number of common illnesses, such as Parkinson's disease and diabetes mellitus. The prospect for overcoming rejection of xenotransplanted cells or tissues is even more promising than for whole organs. Hyperacute rejection, which is directed against vascular endothelial cells, is a major barrier to organ xenotransplants but not a problem with isolated cell or tissue xenotransplants, which contain no blood vessels. Moreover, in certain cases cells or tissues can be enclosed in microcapsules, which are impervious to the immune cells or antibodies that cause rejection but are porous enough to permit vital products of the cells, such as insulin, to pass out into the bloodstream of the recipient. Clinical trials of porcine pancreatic islet cells in diabetic patients and porcine neural tissue in patients with Parkinson's disease, among others, have been underway for a number of years in several countries. Although preliminary reports suggest some benefit, definitive results have not yet been published.

The unmet need for organs, the therapeutic potential of cell and tissue transplants, and promising scientific advances in transplant immunology have generated pressure to conduct more human trials. Established pharmaceutical and biotechnology companies have increased their expenditures in this area. New companies, which are focused on transplant immunology and xenotransplantation, have sprung up. The commercial agenda of industry has added to the pressure for more clinical trials of xenotransplantation. There is a danger that this agenda rather than careful analysis of benefits and risks will determine the pace at which this new technology is introduced.

The purpose of this chapter is to review certain ethical issues that require thoughtful analysis before more research in humans is undertaken. The focus is on several problems that are unique—or at least especially relevant—to xenotransplantation. Most attention is given to the balance between the possibility of risk to the entire population from infectious agents and the potential benefit to the recipients of xenotransplants. Other pertinent issues treated very briefly include tension between the right of persons to withdraw from clinical studies and the requirements for long-term surveillance of patients and their contacts for the development of infectious illnesses; problems in informed consent; equity in allocation of human and animal organs; and the effect of xenotransplantation on donation of human organs. Issues that are generic to many types of research, including the use of animals and the ethical allocation of societal resources, are noted but not analyzed in this chapter. Recent reviews of ethical issues in xenotransplantation include Hughes (1998), Vanderpool (1998, 1999), Clark (1999) and Daar (1999).

Individual benefit versus societal risks

There is no doubt that infections can be transmitted from animals to humans (zoonoses) or that, once established, such infections can spread from person to person (Chapman *et al.*, 1995; Fishman 1997). Organisms that are endemic but do not cause disease in animals may, if transmitted to humans, become pathogens that cause serious or even lethal infections resistant to therapy. The Ebola, Marburg and Crimean-Congo viruses, endemic in certain primates, have caused limited but lethal epidemics in human populations. It is generally agreed that the human immunodeficiency virus (HIV) was introduced into the human population from a primate source. Recent observations show that the genome of the pig, the likeliest transplant donor, includes endogenous retrovirus, which is capable of infecting human cells *in vitro* (LeTissier *et al.*, 1997). This strongly suggests that it will be very difficult and perhaps impossible to eliminate the risk of xenozoonoses (infections from xenotransplanted organs or tissues) by breeding pathogen-free pigs. The term 'pathogen-free' also must be used with caution because there is the possibility that other infectious agents, as yet unrecognized and hence undetectable, may be present in pigs or other donor animals. Of particular concern are agents like HIV that cause diseases with long clinical latency, which might spread silently through the human population for years before they are detected. The possibility that human recipients of xenotransplants will become infected with animal pathogens is increased because the animal organs and tissues are in intimate contact with the recipients' bloodstreams. In addition, the use of immunosuppressives to prevent rejection lowers normal immune barriers that resist infection. Hence, the risk is much greater to transplant recipients than to people who own pets or handle animals on farms or in abattoirs. Retrospective epidemiological studies of 160 patients who had been treated with various pig tissues or organs up to 12 years earlier (in many cases only for brief periods, including two whose blood was extracorporeally perfused through pig kidneys) did not detect any evidence of infection with porcine endogenous retrovirus, the virus that is integrated into the pig genome (Paradis *et al.*, 1999). However, experts—even those who disagree on policy implications—agree that introduction from animal donors into the human population of a pathogenic agent transmissible from person to person is a realistic possibility, and that although the risk cannot be quantified, it is greater than zero. There are various methods to decrease the risk but it cannot be eliminated by currently available techniques.

The risk to individual subjects is an ethical issue in all clinical trials. The hazard of introducing new infectious agents from animals into the human population is unique to xenotransplantation. However, there are partial analogies to other biomedical innovations. When recombinant DNA technology was first undertaken, there was great concern regarding potential danger from spread of genetically altered microorganisms. Investigators using recombinant technology met for intensive discussion of risks and then imposed a brief informal moratorium on research. Thereafter, in the USA a national committee was established to review every research proposal for potential benefits and risks. After two decades without untoward incidents, regulation was turned over to local institutional review boards (IRBs). Anxiety about possible dangers of genetically altered plants is a more recent example of public concern about the potential hazards of biomedical innovations to the population at large. The use of antibiotics in the treatment of patients with infectious illnesses poses a risk to the general population through the appearance of antibiotic resistant bacteria. Outside of biomedical science, new technology, for example nuclear power, regularly involves societal risks as well as benefits.

Given the danger of transmitting xenozoonses, some investigators, policy analysts, and ethicists have argued strongly that the balance between potential benefit to individuals and collective risk is so uncertain that a moratorium for extensive public discussion and debate is required before new clinical trials of xenotransplantation are authorized. One group recommended that a national advisory committee should organize 'an iterative process of analysis and deliberation involving public officials, scientists, and interested and affected parties' (Bach *et al.*, 1998). Since infections do not respect national boundaries, such efforts would have to be coordinated internationally in all countries active in xenotransplantation research. Other experts, including officers of the American Society of Transplant Physicians and Surgeons (Salomon *et al.*, 1998), have rejected calls for a moratorium, arguing that the issues have been reviewed extensively at public meetings and in numerous reports in the scientific and public media and that the consensus opinion is to proceed now 'cautiously with well-defined and highly controlled clinical trials'.

In assessing the justification for new clinical trials of xenotransplantation, I would argue that careful evaluation of the scientific base supporting potential benefit is the first requirement. For example, clinical trials of kidney xenotransplantation are justified only when there is strong evidence from animal-to-animal xenotransplants that survival of functioning kidney xenotransplants approaches the success rate of allotransplants in man. Moreover, the hurdle for trials of kidney xenotransplants should be higher than for organs such heart or liver, for which no equivalent to chronic dialysis is available as the means of preserving the life of potential recipients. Similarly, the hurdle for new trials of porcine pancreatic islet cells should be high, because current treatment of diabetes, while imperfect, is reasonably effective. If alternative therapy is available, the balance of risk and benefit requires more evidence of efficacy in experimental animals than is needed when potential human subjects have no alternative except death, as in advanced heart or liver failure. Even in the latter circumstances, the precondition to trials in humans must be substantial experimental evidence that the proposed protocol has a reasonable chance for success. A major responsibility of review groups should be expert assessment of the scientific base.

If the scientific base justifies trials in humans, they must be conducted under the most stringent requirements for reducing the likelihood of infections and for monitoring subjects and contacts for the appearance of infections. Only institutions that are willing to establish the requisite expensive programs should be eligible to conduct a trial. Various professional groups and public agencies have proposed programs for this purpose. These include prohibiting the use of primates because they are a more likely source of infectious agents capable of propagating in humans than biologically less closely related donor species (Allan, 1996). Other requirements include testing of all donor animals for the presence of infectious organisms and possibly the use only of animals bred to be free of known pathogens. Also required are: repeated testing of experimental subjects and their close contacts for evidence of infection for decades or even throughout their lifetimes; the establishment of banks containing tissue and blood samples from donor animals and from patients and their close contacts; and the creation of international registries of patients receiving xenotransplants.

Various formal proposals for oversight and regulation of clinical trials of xenotransplantation have incorporated mechanisms for assessing the scientific base for each protocol and for ensuring compliance with techniques to reduce the risk of transmitting xenozoonoses. In the UK, a national advisory committee has been established for review and regulation of individual proposals. In the USA, final regulations have not yet been issued but draft federal guidelines leave primary review of individual proposals to IRBs. There is concern about this arrangement because IRBs, the standard mechanism for oversight of other types of clinical research in the United States, are subject to pressure from prominent investigators, who may exert undue influence because of their ability to attract patients, clinical revenues, and research grants to an institution. Moreover, the key issue in xenotransplantation is the risk to public health, while IRBs are constituted to judge risks to individuals. In my opinion, it is vital that national regulatory agencies and advisory committees (which must collaborate internationally) be fully empowered to develop and oversee national regulations and to modify them as information accumulates. Initially they must also be authorized to limit the number of trials to the minimum needed to test each scientifically sound proposal. Redundant trials may have scientific value but they are ethically dubious until there has been extended follow-up for infection in early recipients. Only after several years of monitoring a limited number of trials would it be appropriate to authorize IRBs to approve greater numbers of studies locally. The national advisory committee or regulatory agency would continue to monitor IRBs to assure that they are following national regulations. This schedule is similar to that which evolved in the case of recombinant DNA research, as described above. Ideally, there should be international collaboration to enforce requirements for scientific validity and infection control and to avoid redundant protocols. Given the pressures from enthusiastic investigators, industry, and national governments eager to foster biotechnology, this may be an unattainable goal.

These pragmatic issues—whether to impose a moratorium, how to obtain public input into decision making, how to regulate clinical trials—all presuppose that at some point trials of xenotransplantation in humans will proceed. What is the moral justification for exposing the entire population to *any risk* of xenozoonoses for the potential benefit to specific individuals with serious or life-threatening diseases? Despite the delicate balance between individual benefit and societal risk, I believe it is morally justifiable to proceed with well-considered and tightly regulated clinical trials. This position assumes enforcement of all the appropriate precautions: strong regulatory mechanisms, careful review of the scientific basis for each clinical trial, limited numbers of well-chosen human trials, and full implementation of methods for reducing the likelihood of xenozoonoses. The survey of previous recipients of porcine xenotransplants cited earlier gives some weight to the viewpoint that the risk of infection is not high. However, the data do not conclusively indicate that the risk of xenozoonoses is negligible, even assuming that word can be applied at all to the risk of a lethal pandemic in the worst case scenario.

Most societies give some priority to helping those in greatest need, among whom certainly are numbered persons facing death. If, based on rigorous evaluation of the scientific base, xenotransplanting an organ or cell represents rational experimental therapy for a serious or lethal disease, it is justified to proceed with a carefully monitored clinical trial. As argued by the Committee on Xenotransplantation of the US Institute of Medicine (IOM, 1996), as a society we are morally obligated to take some risk of harm to save the lives of fellow human beings. A committee of the Nuffield Council on Bioethics (1996) reasoned that all innovation involves unknown risks and that 'it would be unacceptably conservative to restrict innovation merely by appeal to the possibility of risk'. (They emphasized, however, that the infectious disease risk of xenotransplantation required further definition before human trials begin.) I subscribe to these key arguments for proceeding.

An advisory group on the ethics of xenotransplantation (1996) established by the UK government concluded that it would be ethically acceptable to proceed with xenotransplantation after a full investigation shows that risks of infection are 'within tolerable margins'. Societies undertaking clinical trials of xenotransplantation must decide how much risk they will tolerate to achieve potential clinical benefits. There is precedent for formal involvement of the public in such decisions. The well-publicized events that led to federal control of recombinant DNA research in the United States have already been noted. Early in the development of recombinant DNA research, the city council of Cambridge, Massachusetts (USA) imposed a moratorium on research in that city, the home of Harvard University and Massachusetts Institute of Technology, until a non-scientist citizen review board approved resumption under increased requirements for safety measures. Recently a national referendum was held in Switzerland to determine whether genetic engineering research should be permitted to continue. Xenotransplantation research is active in several nations, including large countries, such as the USA, where it seems unlikely that the societal decision whether to permit this research can be made by pure democratic methods like referendums. On the other hand, wide discussion in open public forums and the media and complete transparency about risks and benefits is mandatory. Evidence that this is occurring in the US includes a website for xenotransplantation, articles in the New York Times in 1998 and 1999, and a presentation on a popular television program, *60 Minutes*, in 1998. Ultimately, elected representatives must determine whether the potential of xenotransplantation to alleviate suffering and delay death of some citizens justifies the uncertain risk of this new technology.

Informed consent and the right to withdraw

In clinical trials of xenotransplantation, as in all clinical research, the issue of informed consent is critical. The enthusiasm of clinical investigators may lead to exaggeration of benefits and understatement of risks to potential subjects and their contacts. This has occurred repeatedly in the history of organ transplantation. Potential subjects are especially susceptible to such influence if the experimental treatment is plausibly lifesaving, for example xenotransplantation of a heart or liver. In trials of kidney xenotransplantation, in which the novel treatment may be better than dialysis but will not be the only alternative to death, the susceptibility to overenthusiasm is less. At a minimum, IRBs should require that potential recipients of xenotransplants are informed in understandable terms of the state of scientific knowledge, are given a clear estimate of the risks including data on mortality and morbidity of previous human recipients, and are offered alternative therapy, such as continuation of chronic dialysis (McCarthy, 1995). In this respect, xenotransplantation poses no unusual ethical problems of informed consent beyond those typical of research in novel technology at an early state of development.

A method in use in some institutions to enhance dispassionate presentation of risks and benefits to potential subjects would be appropriate in clinical trials of xenotransplantation. The potential conflict of interest between the dual roles of a clinical investigator who also serves as the patient's physician is avoided by prohibiting the investigator and others directly involved in the clinical trial from obtaining informed consent. Instead, other well-trained personnel, such as nurses employed by the institution, present information to potential subjects and obtain their informed consent. The risk that such personnel will be less able than the investigators to communicate the detailed risks and benefits is outweighed by the reduced likelihood of an overly enthusiastic presentation by members of the research team.

Issues of informed consent more specific to xenotransplantation arise from the potential hazard of xenozoonoses to caregivers, family, and other close contacts of patients who receive xenotransplants. Investigators are obligated to inform close contacts (including medical personnel) of the risks to them. Because the magnitude of the risk is uncertain it is especially difficult to communicate to these individuals the danger that they may acquire infections, especially retroviral infections for which no curative treatment is available. Although formal consent from most contacts should not be required, it may be necessary for very close contacts such as sexual partners to participate in the trial by agreeing to periodic medical examinations and blood tests for evidence of infections. A firm principle of research ethics is that subjects may withdraw from research protocols at any time. The requirement that patients and close contacts agree to periodic surveillance and guarantee to participate in extended data collection programs is contrary to this principle. Some have suggested that it will be necessary to contract legally with subjects and their closest contacts to submit to periodic surveys for evidence of infectious diseases throughout their lifetimes. However, even if patients and their close contacts in clinical trials of xenotransplantation agree to give up the right to withdraw, how can compliance be enforced? It is hard to envision public support for civil or criminal penalties for individuals who breach their contracts. The probability that some subjects and contacts will refuse to participate in surveillance over the years or will be lost to follow-up represents a significant hazard of clinical trials of xenotransplantation.

Effect of xenotransplantation on donation of human organs

The difficult ethical dilemmas involved in organ xenotransplantation could be avoided if the number of human organs available could be increased to meet clinical needs. The various proposals to increase organ donation (see Chapter 7 by Hoffenberg) not only pose difficult ethical issues themselves but are unlikely to increase the availability of human organs sufficiently to meet need. Moreover, if cells such as pancreatic islet cells and nerve cells prove valuable in the treatment of disease, it is most unlikely that human sources will meet clinical requirements. It seems likely that human donations always will be the preferred source of organs and cells. For these reasons some transplant surgeons, among others, are concerned that overoptimistic reports in public media about xenotransplantation will diminish the already inadequate rate at which human organs currently are being donated. On the other hand, it is conceivable that success in xenotransplantation will be a mechanism for decreasing the sale of human organs in some countries, which many consider ethically repugnant (see Chapter 16 by Jha and Chugh). The interplay between xenotransplantation and donation of human organs will not become clear until scientific advances permit the routine use of xenotransplanted organs as clinical rather than experimental therapy.

Equitable access

An important ethical problem in transplantation is equitable access to the limited supply of cadaver organs. In the USA, a national system established by the federal government allocates organs according to formulas based on medical and ethical criteria. Although this system is designed to assure equity, studies have indicated that race, gender, and economic status influence access to kidney transplantation (Gaylin *et al.*, 1993). Should xenotransplants prove to be effective alternatives to human organs, a new set of ethical and policy issues will arise. It seems likely that both on psychological and on technical grounds, human organs will be preferred by most recipients. Psychologically, many individuals will be more comfortable if human organs are transplanted into their bodies than if they receive organs from animals. Technically, it seems likely that recipients of animal organs may require more intense and hence more dangerous immunosuppressive therapy than those who get human organs and that graft survival will be better for human organs. Programs for equitable allocation of cadaver and animal organs will be complex. Broad input from the professions, patients, and government will be needed to assure equitable distribution of both types of organs.

Utilization of resources

It is likely that xenotransplantation will be very expensive. Hence the issue of appropriate use of societal resources is raised. The allocation of funds for xenotransplantation will consume resources that could be used for other purposes, such as preventive medicine or primary medical care. However, it is not possible to begin cost-benefit analyses until more information is available. If kidney xenotransplants are successful, they may replace more costly chronic dialysis therapy and thereby lower the total cost of caring for patients with end-stage kidney disease. Xenotransplanted hearts or livers may increase the cost of caring for persons with terminal failure of those organs by keeping alive patients who otherwise would have died. However, if the current high cost of caring for patients in late stages of failure of those organs can be avoided by xenotransplantation, overall costs may decrease. If the potential for therapy of Parkinson's disease, Huntington's disease, and diabetes with xenotransplanted cells is fulfilled, the total cost of medical care for these chronic conditions may be decreased despite the expense of xenotransplantation. In the light of such uncertainties, it seems prudent to pursue the science and leave it to society to decide whether to allocate funds for clinical therapy when xenotransplantation of any organ or cell type is successful.

Use of animals

Xenotransplantation raises the same issues of ethical use of animals and the rights of animals that are raised by the use of animals in all types of biomedical research. For both technical and philosophical reasons, it seems unlikely that primates will be used as donors for xenotransplantation. Many experts believe that infectious agents in primates are more likely to be transmissible to and among humans than infectious agents from biologically more distant species such as the pig (Allan, 1996). Moreover, some primates such as chimpanzees are too limited in numbers to be a significant pool of donors and other primates such as baboons are so expensive to raise that they are unlikely donors. Philosophically, because of the biological and apparent psychological closeness of primates to humans, many people are very reluctant to accept them as donors for xenotransplantation. On the other hand, millions of pigs are raised for food. The use of several thousand animals as donors for xenotransplantation does not seem to pose any new ethical problems. Several major religions do not forbid the use of animals to meet human needs (Daar, 1994). However, advocates of animal rights who wish to limit the use of animals for the benefit of humans consider xenotransplantation an inappropriate expansion of suffering and death of animals. The issue of animal rights and the ethical use of animals is widely discussed but no resolution between the differing viewpoints is apparent. Xenotransplants are a very small subset of the broader issue, which is beyond the scope of this chapter.

References

Advisory Group on the Ethics of Xenotransplantation (1996). *Animal tissue into humans*, p. 74. Her Majesty's Stationery Office, Norwich.

Allan, J. S. (1996). Xenotransplantation at a crossroads: Prevention versus progress. *Nature Medicine*, 2, 18–21.

Bach, F. H., Fishman, J. A., Daniels, N., Proimos, J., Anderson, B., Carpenter, C. B., *et al.* (1998). Uncertainty in xenotransplantation: Individual benefit versus collective risk. *Nature Medicine*, 4, 141–4.

Chapman, L. E., Folks, T. M., Salomon, D. R., Patterson, A. M., Eggerman, T. E., and Noguchi, P. D. (1995). Xenotransplantation and xenogeneic infections. *New England Journal of Medicine*, 333, 1498–501.

Clark, M. A. (1999). This little piggy went to market: The xenotransplantation and xenozoonose debate. *Journal of Law, Medicine and Ethics*, 27, 137–52.

Daar, A. S. (1994). Xenotransplantation and religion: The major monotheistic religions. *Xenotransplantation*, 2, 61–5.

Daar, A. S. (1999). Animal-to-human organ transplants—a solution or a new problem. *Bulletin World Health Organization*, 77, 54–61.

Fishman, J. A. (1997). Xenosis and xenotransplantation: Addressing the infectious risks posed by an emerging technology. *Kidney International*, 51, S41–S45.

Gaylin, D. S., Held, P. J., Port, F. K., Hunsicker, L. G., Wolfe, R. A., Kahan, B. D., *et al.* (1993). The impact of comorbid and sociodemographic factors on access to renal transplantation. *Journal of the American Medical Association*, 269, 603–08.

Hughes, J. (1998). Xenografting: ethical issues. *Journal of Medical Ethics*, 24, 18–24.

IOM (Institute of Medicine), Committee on Xenograft Transplantation: Ethical Issues and Public Policy (1996). *Xenotransplantation: science, ethics, and public policy*, pp. 71–2. National Academy Press, Washington, DC.

LeTissier, P., Stoye, J. P., Takeuchi, Y., Patience, C., and Weiss, R. A. (1997). Two sets of human-tropic pig retrovirus. *Nature*, 389, 681–82.

McCarthy, C. R. (1995). Ethical aspects of animal to human xenografts. *ILAR Journal*, 37, 3–9.

Nuffield Council on Bioethics (1996). *Animal-to-human transplants. The ethics of xenotransplantation*, p. 75. Nuffield Council on Bioethics, London.

Paradis, K., Langford, G., Long, Z., Heneine, W., Sandstrom, P., Switzer, W. M., *et al.* (1999). Search for cross-species transmission of porcine endogenous retrovirus in patients treated with living pig tissue. *Science*, 285, 1236–41.

Salomon, D. R., Ferguson, R. M., and Helderman, J. H. (1998). Xenotransplants: proceed with caution. *Nature*, **392**, 11–12.

United Network for Organ sharing (UNOS) Scientific registry data as of May 6, 2000.

Vanderpool, H. Y. (1998). Critical ethical issues in clinical trials with xenotransplants. *Lancet*, **351**, 1347–50.

Vanderpool, H. Y. (1999). Commentary: a critique of Clark's frightening xenotransplantation scenario. *Journal of Law, Medicine, and Ethics*, **27**, 153–7.

9

Allocation of kidneys for transplantation

Robert A. Sells

There is general agreement that for the great majority of persons with end-stage renal failure, a kidney transplant is preferable to chronic dialysis. With the progressive expansion in the number of patients suitable for transplantation over the past several decades, the demand for kidney transplants has increased. Even though there is evidence that a significant number of suitable dialysis patients may not be referred for kidney transplantation (Tilney, 1998), the gap between supply and demand has increased relentlessly since the late 1980s. In the 1990s, the number of registrants in the United States increased by 17% annually, with a simultaneous increase in the death rate whilst waiting for kidneys, whereas the number of cadaver kidney donors available per year has expanded by only 5–6% per year (UNOS, 1996). To achieve even this rate has required loosening of the criteria for donor kidneys, so that the quality of kidneys from cadaveric donors is, on the whole, decreasing. Donors currently include individuals over 65 years of age, hypertensives, diabetics, and those with a history of hepatitis C, with a discard rate of kidneys removed and not used of about 20%.

Assuming that the selection criteria of patients for treatment are appropriate for each modality, the limitation on the availability of *dialysis* is defined mostly by cost, and also by the criterion of cost benefit. However, such resource-based limits on the number of *renal transplants* are exacerbated by the chronic lack of cadaveric kidneys available for transplantation. The allocation of a kidney to one individual, therefore, means that another patient of virtually equal suitability will be deprived of a graft. Kidney transplants are a public resource and should be used in a way commensurate with social and public goals. In virtually all countries legislation exists preventing the buying and selling of kidney transplants. Consequently, the criterion of medical suitability is the principal discriminator between competing potential recipients, not the ability to pay. Kidney distribution networks must be transparently just and equitable: all other things being equal, all patients of equivalent medical suitability should have equal access to an available cadaveric kidney.

There is great tension between the principle of equitability of distribution on the one hand and the principle of 'best medical benefit' on the other. Moreover, organ distribution agencies must ensure that the grafts are not wasted. A logical and humanitarian basis for graft allocation must, therefore, combine these criteria. The medical conditions that determine success are too numerous and variable to be able to predict exactly the prognosis of a transplant in any individual. These include: the condition of the cadaver donor; the limit of maximum ischaemic injury, which the graft would sustain during transport to the recipient; the blood group and HLA matching of the donor and recipient; co-morbidity in the recipient; and the tolerance of immunosuppression.

These variables may be quantified to a degree. With the chronic shortage of transplants, there has been an increased rigour in the selection of patients for maximum survivability, and longevity of graft function. This chapter describes systems that have been developed to distribute kidneys in as fair, and as medically useful, a way as possible to patients on lengthening waiting lists for renal transplants.

Factors in the allocation of kidneys

Compatibility, waiting time and graft ischaemic time

The ABO blood group system and the major histocompatibility complex (HLA) play a dominant role in transplant survival and therefore in allocation. Blood group ABO compatibility is now regarded as a mandatory first selection step because of the near certainty of irreversible severe acute rejection mediated through complement fixing anti-red cell iso-antibodies. Transplants between living relatives benefit from close HLA matching: HLA identical transplants (no mismatches at the HLA A, B or DR loci) between non-identical twin siblings enjoy prolonged survival in the region of 80% at 15 years. Less well-matched grafts do nearly as well with current modern immunosuppression, at least up until 10 years survival. Living *unrelated* donor kidneys fare as well as one-haplotype (three antigens) mismatched related donor kidneys, and significantly better than equivalently matched cadaver grafts, over 6 years follow-up (Foss et al., 1998), although the rejection frequency is greater than in consanguineous kidneys. With increasing awareness of their success, the use of unrelated living donor kidneys is rising.

Recipients of cadaveric kidneys obtain less rejection and better graft survival by receiving an HLA-identical graft. Despite the physiological injury of the prolonged ischaemia in transit over long distances in the USA required to effect such matches, the survival of HLA-identical grafts remains superior to that of poorly matched grafts (Terasaki et al., 1985). Transplants with a lesser degree of match may achieve reasonable success rates, and matching for Class II (DR) antigens seems to achieve most benefit, even with co-existing incompatibility at the HLA A and B loci (Ting and Morris, 1987). Of the Class I antigens, the B-locus appears more powerful than the A, providing better survival in recipients matched for B antigens on the cadaveric graft (Opelz, 1992). As the evidence in favour of HLA-matching cadaveric kidneys accrued, and successful preservation times extended to 40 hours and beyond, policies evolved that mandated the transport of kidneys to well-matched recipients. However, deficiencies became apparent in this policy: many patients waited interminably for a transplant whereas others were transplanted promptly.

The HLA system is very polymorphic and different populations reveal different frequencies in the prevalence of different antigen specificities. This difference is seen particularly in members of different races. Those patients with a common HLA antigen phenotype are usually transplanted much more quickly than those of rare HLA type. Where allocation is based on maximizing HLA compatibility, the latter patients would usually finish up at the bottom of the allocation list. In particular, where one ethnic group relies mainly on cadaveric organs from another ethnic group, its members will be disadvantaged. In the United States, black American patients have a threefold incidence of renal failure compared with white patients and a high frequency of blood groups O and B. Further, donation rates from blacks are low. These factors explain the prolonged waiting time (approximately twice that of white recipients) and the fact that a relatively low proportion of blacks receive first transplants compared with whites (Daar, 1994).

An uncomfortable question has recently been addressed (Ayanian et al., 1999): are racial differences significant determinants in the admission of patients to waiting lists for renal transplantation? In a carefully conducted survey of African-American and white American dialysis patients it appears, after adjustment for socio-demographic and co-morbid factors, that blacks are less well-informed about the possible benefits and risks of renal transplant than whites. They start with more reservations about the procedure than whites, yet are less likely than whites to be given the medical information that they desire. Black Americans were less likely to gain a place on a cadaver kidney transplant waiting list than whites, although offers from black living donors were no less numerous than in whites. The study implicates social discrimination as one cause of medical disadvantage and recommends that specialized counselling may be necessary in units where this effect is seen.

Faced with a steadily increasing list of patients who have been on the waiting lists for a long time, some physicians suggested abandoning the HLA matching scheme and favoured a system that gave higher priority to a patient who had been waiting a long time. Yet the accumulated data suggested that such a policy would be associated with a high graft failure rate, and those who rejected their grafts would frequently be very highly sensitized, making it even more difficult subsequently to obtain a crossmatch negative graft. This unsustainable situation required that factors other than HLA matching should be studied, and significant prognostic factors should be given appropriate weight in the allocation system by using scales aimed at eliminating the disadvantage attributable to rare HLA phenotype. These factors (donor and recipient age, distance between units) and other patient dependent factors were studied with a view to improving equitability and at the same time conserving benefits of good HLA matching.

Three kidney exchange programmes have gone through this exercise, with interesting results. The recently developed allocation programmes reflect the challenges of long-distance transport, balance of trade in kidneys, and differing approaches to the compromise necessary to maximize patient equality as well as graft success.

Eurotransplant

This organization co-ordinates the organ exchange in Austria, Belgium, Germany, Luxembourg, and the Netherlands. Responding to the criticisms of the system developed in 1988, a new Eurotransplant Kidney Allocation System (ETKAS) was implemented in 1996. It used a refined version of the XCOMB programme of Wujciak and Opelz (1993), the basic version of which had been used since 1994. The new

ETKAS assigned points to recipients using five allocation factors: (1) the number of HLA mismatches, (2) the chances of obtaining a well-matched kidney (mismatch probability), (3) waiting time, (4) distance between donor and transplant hospital, and (5) the national net kidney balance. This 'points' system cut in at the second stage of sorting as a discriminant between two or more potential recipients still eligible for a kidney after the preliminary allocation steps (ABO match rules, HLA mismatches, and high urgency). The points scale gave highest potential weight for HLA mismatch, lowest for mismatch probability, and intermediate weight for waiting time, distance to the transplant unit and national kidney balance. In addition, paediatric patients less than 16 years of age received a special waiting time bonus, and double HLA mismatch points.

During the first year of operation (1996–1997) there was a marked increase in the number of kidney transplants carried out in long-waiting patients, with poor matchability. Despite the abolition of the minimal HLA antigen sharing rules, there was no significant increase in the number of poorly matched grafts, and importantly the percentage of OOO HLA matched transplants increased from 21% to 23%. The kidney balance formula resulted in rapid equilibration of the national import/export balance from a range of -40 to +169 among the countries, to -10 to +10 within four months of implementing EKTAS, and more paediatric transplants were carried out. These results of applying a computer simulation study to an allocation policy revealed immediate and substantial improvements in the allocation system by bringing new patient-orientated factors into the sorting programme. In summary, waiting time was improved without significant reduction in the standards of HLA matching (Demeester et al., 1998).

UNOS

The UNOS (United Network for Organ Sharing) system in the United States was formed in 1977 as the principal agency for the distribution of kidneys between collaborating centres, and in 1986 it was awarded the federal contract to manage the national Organ Procurement and Transplantation Network (OPTN). Participation of all recognized centres in OPTN is now mandatory. Initially waiting time was the principal allocation factor, followed by HLA matching and degree of sensitization. The system favoured equitability of distribution, rather than the European bias towards favourable HLA matching (with the exception of zero-mismatched kidneys). With the realization that OOO mismatched organs do very significantly better than any other mismatched transplants (Terasaki et al., 1985), the sharing of these kidneys became mandatory, although ABO compatibility rather than identity was allowed in order to achieve the perfect HLA match. In 10 years, the number of zero-mismatched kidneys rose to 13.9% of all transplants. In descending order, the current weighting of allocation factors after selection of zero-mismatched grafts, is: waiting time; HLA match; sensitization (PRA > 80%); and paediatric recipients. Additionally, kidneys are offered on a local, then a regional, then a national basis (Pfaff, 1998). This policy gives greater weight to extended waiting time than beneficial HLA matching and favours a reduction in ischaemic time. As a result of the 'locals first' policy, geographical disparities in patients' eligibility for transplantation have arisen; in particular, a patient living near a large unit with a successful retrieving programme may receive a transplant before another patient with a greater medical need, whose unit retrieves fewer kidneys.

New regulations have recently been proposed for OPTN. These require publication of criteria for listing patients for transplantation, determining their medical status with a view to adding weight to high urgency categories, and reducing the geographic influence to improve the chances of transplantation for high urgency recipients who have a reasonable likelihood of survival. A debate is currently ensuing over the standardization of criteria for eligibility and medical status. In a legal move to protect state residents, two states have passed legislation that protects the 'locals first' step in the allocation system. Meanwhile, in the USA as in the rest of the world, the gap between the supply of kidneys and the demand for them increases relentlessly with time. The ratio of waiting list to cadaver kidney transplants rose from two to four over the 10 years to 1996. As the waiting list expands, pockets of perceived inequality of access to kidneys have appeared. Doctors fear that favouring the sickest patients will exacerbate this problem, as more kidneys will be diverted towards a few large transplant centres with the longest waiting lists and sickest patients. The chronic organ shortage has exacerbated the tension between the politician's wish to match the allocation process to patient need, and the doctors' assertion that decision making regarding urgency of need for a transplant should be a medical decision (*Lancet*, 1998).

UKTSSA

In the United Kingdom the UK Transplant Support Service Authority (UKTSSA) holds the national kidney recipient registry and has operated a distribution system, largely based on HLA matching, between all UK centres. In 1989, each centre agreed to contribute one of a pair of kidneys to UKTSSA for distribution to a beneficially matched recipient (000, 100, or 010 mismatches). In 1996, 5-year graft and patient survival data were studied to re-assess the influence on outcome of donor and recipient age, and the equitability of the system in terms of waiting time (Morris *et al.*, 1999). The audit confirmed that the best outcomes are achieved with 000 mismatched kidneys; the next best with 'favourable matches' (100, 010, or 110 mismatches); and that although prolonged cold ischaemic time had a deleterious effect on the aggregate outcome, good results in identical and favourably matched patients persist in kidneys ischaemic for <30 hours. The study confirmed previous reports that patient survival is reduced in elderly recipients, although those who survived revealed superior graft survival due to less rejection (Tesi *et al.* 1994). Beyond the age of 25 years, increasing donor age adds significantly to the risk of graft failure at 5 years, irrespective of the age of the recipient.

Following this analysis, the HLA Taskforce recommended that donor units should offer both kidneys from 000 mismatched donor to recipients in the national pool or locally, and that the definition of a favourable match should be extended to include up to 110 mismatched recipients (one kidney would be offered to the pool for these recipients). In addition, the points system was introduced to favour younger transplant recipients, avoid large differences in donor/recipient age, favour longest waiting patient, and the less sensitized patient, to favour the highest centre balance, and to improve matchability. The results of this policy change are awaited. However, during the first nine months of the scheme, the number of recipients receiving 000 mismatched kidneys increased from 7% to 13%. This was associated with commensurate drop in the number of non-favourably matched kidney transplants. During the same time period, 73% of transactions have involved the new 'points' system.

These examples from three major organ distribution agencies demonstrate that progress has been made to reconcile the need to optimize the results of a kidney transplant and at the same time to improve the equality of opportunity, which each recipient deserves. At the same time, the points system reduces the risk of bias or interference in kidney allocation by transplant physicians. This benefit is not to be underestimated. Every transplant programme will be expected to perform as many transplants as possible annually, and there is pressure from hospital executives as well as local patient groups to perform as many kidney transplants locally as possible. The responsible doctor needs a very good reason to part with a donor kidney, retrieved locally, in favour of a distant recipient who is marginally better matched for the graft than a local patient who has been waiting for years. No other surgical speciality is required to obey these highly restrictive rules of resource allocation. It speaks volumes for the prevailing mood of altruism in clinical transplantation that such allocation procedures, which require that local pressures should be ignored in favour of benefit to the whole national pool, are generally accepted. The 'payback', of course, is the expectation that the local patient's turn will eventually come by the arrival of a reciprocally-referred kidney. But the chances of a payback actually occurring depend crucially on full compliance by every collaborating centre.

Other medical factors in allocating kidneys

The most difficult factor to quantify (and allocate points for) is medical urgency. Some doctors may wish to represent their patient's interests best by maximizing the number of points attributable under this heading. Perhaps the time has come for a debate, which might further refine the points-based allocation system for medical urgency, as is happening in the USA now. The process will not be as simple as in the case of liver and heart transplantation, where long-term physiological support (the equivalent of chronic dialysis in renal patients) is not available. The expectation of imminent death, which can be defined fairly clearly in liver and heart patients, is more elusive in the renal population. But progress is possible in at least two areas of risk.

Cardiovascular complications

Of all the risk factors, the risk of cardiovascular complication in renal patients has become dominant, and accounts for 33% of deaths following renal transplantation in Europe (Sells, 1997). Of these, acute myocardial infarction is probably the most common cause of non-infective post-transplant death. Selection of patients for transplantation therefore requires careful pre-listing investigation for coronary artery disease (CAD) and heart failure. Correction of heart failure is frequently possible by more effective dialysis and scrupulous medical management. Detection of CAD is more problematic: although most centres perform stress nuclear ventriculography in symptomatic ESRD patients, the gold standard test of prompt coronary angiography is not routinely available for patients awaiting a decision about listing for transplantation. In 1995, the American Society of Transplant Physicians published a screening schedule specifically to evaluate cardiac risk (American Society of Transplant Physicians, 1995). Such a screening algorithm routinely applied in suitable cases, and converted to a 'points' system could form the basis of an objective evaluation of medical urgency and risk.

In diabetics suffering ESRD and who are particularly susceptible to CAD, there seems to be a clear case for pre-transplant surgical coronary revascularization where operable coronary stenotic lesions have been shown angiographically (Manske et al., 1992). Yet despite careful screening, the results of renal transplantation in diabetics remains poor with a high risk of death with a functioning graft. However, messages are coming through that simultaneous pancreas transplantation with a kidney reduces the mortality rate in diabetic patients compared with those who receive a kidney alone, 10 years after transplantation. In a case-controlled study, Tyden et al. (1999) compared the outcome of kidney alone versus simultaneous pancreas and kidney transplantation in a small group of diabetics, each of whom had been declared suitable for a kidney *and* a pancreas graft, but half of whom had only received a kidney. All recipients were followed up for 10 years, during which time three of the 14 pancreas/kidney recipients died compared with 12 of 15 patients receiving a kidney alone. In those countries where pancreas and kidney transplantation is not as widely practised as in the USA, perhaps pancreas plus kidney transplant programmes should be expanded to further reduce the risk in this disadvantaged group of patients.

Cytomegalovirus infection (CMV)

This remains the single most important pathogen in kidney transplantation. In CMV non-immune recipients of kidneys from a CMV-positive donor (as detected by routine anti-CMV antibody screening), there is a 60% risk of viraemia and a minority of these patients will develop parenchymal infection including the small risk of life-threatening pneumonitis. Approximately 50% of Western ESRD patients and donors are CMV negative, which gives a random chance of 50% infection vectored by the graft. The severity of the disease is proportional to the amount of interventional immunosuppression, particularly with biological anti-T-cell agents. There have been marked improvements in the routine post-operative screening of these high-risk patients and the severity of the disease has been substantially reduced by the administration of Gancyclovir and Valacyclovir (Lowance et al., 1999). Matching recipients and donors for their CMV status can avoid this risk by selecting CMV-negative donor organs for CMV-negative patients on the waiting list. The cost to the CMV-negative patient of electing to avoid a CMV-positive organ is a prolongation of the waiting time for a suitable kidney. If such patients have other disadvantageous factors (low matchability, younger patients, and low sensitization status) and if the patient persistently wishes not to incur the risk of CMV after informed consent, there would be a case for 'tuning' the allocation algorithm further to give points under the heading of CMV matching.

CMV is a useful model for the Epstein Barr Virus, an agent that may be transmitted from an EBV-positive patient to an EBV-negative recipient with the consequent risk of infectious mononucleosis and B cell lymphoma. Here the risks are much less in adult kidney recipients, 95% of whom will have EBV antibody. However, young children may not be immune. There is a risk that adjunctive immunosuppression administered to an EBV-negative paediatric kidney recipient of an EBV-positive organ may be associated with a high risk of lymphoma. In such cases the chances of obtaining an EBV-negative kidney, which is reasonably matched, are incredibly small. Perhaps the right strategy here would be to seek a favourably matched kidney to minimize the necessity for powerful adjunctive immunosuppression.

A non-medical factor: the 'signed-up donor'

In 1995, it was suggested (Jarvis, 1995) that only those patients who had agreed to their organs being donated after death should have access to the waiting list for an organ transplant and that adults who had not 'contracted in' as cadaver donors should not be allowed a place on the waiting list for a kidney transplant. There seemed little interest in this first publication, yet the principle, if not the Draconian lengths to which Jarvis wished to go with it, seems attractive on further scrutiny, if only because of the 'double benefit' that could accrue: virtue would be rewarded, and, hypothetically, the number of donors would be increased. The principle has been followed up by Gubernatis and Kliemt (2000), who present a 'solidarity' model by introducing a discriminator step in the organ allocation algorithm, which would favour an individual who had in the past agreed to donate his organs. This would put such a patient at an advantage over another patient of comparable medical status who had not opted in to organ donation. Children and high urgency patients would be excepted by omitting this discriminatory step during their allocation procedure. In its 'solidarity' form the discriminator has the added value of removing the risk of interpersonal conflict of interest further away from the doctors as well as having the potential to increase the number of organ donors. The criteria of Beauchamp and Childress (1989) of beneficence, respect for autonomy, non-malevolence, and justice seem to be satisfied. However, there are areas of ethical concern:

- 'Justice' is generally interpreted as a system that favours the well behaved. But when it comes to the administration of health care, is it fair to say that justice should put a positive premium on more responsible past behaviour? In the UK, the National Health Service in its statute makes treatment available to all comers, both the blameworthy and the praiseworthy, on an equal basis. If those who do not contract in to donate are denied a lifesaving or life-enhancing transplant, why should the same rule not apply to those who in their chosen lifestyle increase their risk of having to use NHS facilities, for example the smokers, the voluntarily obese, and the recidivist alcoholics? These free-riders could, if the solidarity principle were adopted more widely, find themselves further down the pecking order for treatment.
- A counter-argument states that the principle of solidarity is just, within the circumscribed context of organ donation and acceptance, since the benefits of donation

will be apparent to more people and organ donation is likely to rise, to the net benefit of all potential recipients, not just those who 'contract in'. However, the perceived inequality of individuals' access to transplants will be a significant political hurdle to this model being adopted in the UK.

- Members of dissenting minorities whose religious or other convictions would normally prevent them from donating organs should be exempt from the solidarity discrimination step, as should paediatric and highly urgent patients.
- A problem with this system would arise within the European Union: it would discourage individuals from travelling to another country with a high calibre transplant list, to get on the waiting list there. EU regulations were developed to encourage free movement of EU nationals throughout the community without prejudice to their health. To achieve this, EU foreign nationals have equal rights to treatment from another EU country's health service. It is highly unlikely that a foreign patient in an EU country would be able to redeem his 'solidarity points', were that system not to operate in the new host country.
- Solidarity is not strictly speaking a medical discriminator, since the points would be earned by having the right attitude, and not having a pressing medical indication to receive a priority kidney. But that does not mean that the principle should not be introduced into the kidney exchange algorithm such as EKTAS, which already allocates points to a recipient on the basis of national or regional organ import/export balance. This is not strictly speaking a 'patient specific' factor, rather, it reflects the energy of the patient's local transplant centre as well as the availability of intensive care units locally. Yet the precedent is set for using a patient-independent factor in allocating cadaver kidneys. Therefore, there can be no quibbling about including solidarity, which has such obvious hypothetical potential to increase organ donors.

The ingenious systems for organ distribution discussed above use medical and non-medical discriminators to achieve fair allocation of kidneys to medically suitable patients in a way that optimizes the prognosis for the patient's survival and the longevity of the graft. At the same time, they attempt to enhance the equality of waiting list patients to access for a kidney, in a way that reduces waiting time engendered by poor matchability or local shortage, and endeavour to minimize the risk of failure or poor graft function by prolonged storage times. So long as the global lack of donor organs persists, the proprietors of exchange programmes will continue to tinker imaginatively with their distribution systems. The only strategic answer to this problem is to increase the supply of donor organs.

These systems will always represent a compromise so long as there are insufficient kidneys to transplant. They are tactical devices aimed at reducing disadvantage to many, rather than strategic programmes based on moral values, to maximize advantage. Simple moral values may determine our actions in unconstrained areas of health provision. But in a resource-deprived specialty the clash of values is inevitable: for example, shipping a kidney to a distant, poorly-matched high-urgency patient in preference to a local perfectly-matched, medically-fit recipient may satisfy the value principle of priority determined by medical need; but that operation often carries a higher risk of death, graft failure, and higher expenditure than would the local transplant. Here, the value-based principles of minimizing harm, maximizing utility, and cost effectiveness have to be ignored or flouted; and that judgment is only real when we know the outcome of the transplant. Agencies can only be guided by estimates of the probability of risk and success in each patient group. This works well enough in conditions of plenty but can be sidelined by the dominant humanitarian appeal of the clinically urgent patient. Currently, every kidney allocated to one is a kidney denied to another. We are in the business of maximizing aggregate benefit to the recipient pool rather than offering absolute benefit to the individual. The only strategic answer to this problem is to increase the supply of donor organs.

Some authors have given up on this problem. Although the best that can be done is being done to allocate each precious kidney to the best possible recipient, the continuing rise in waiting lists means that the future for some will be a very long waiting time, or death on the waiting list. Three stark alternatives are proposed:

1. That we recognize that there is a lottery, that other than the sickest patients are not likely to be transplanted, and that renal transplants often occur only with the good fortune of a perfect match.
2. That we reduce the weight allocated to medical need, and encourage transplantation of patients who have the higher probability of success. These are also generally the less urgent patients.
3. That we invest more in increasing organ procurement (Tilney, 1998; Pfaff, 1998).

Evidence-based methods to increase the supply of kidneys

First, non-heart beating donors (NHBD) are an important and new source of organs with a great potential for growth. It has been estimated by Kootstra (1997) that the number of NHBD may be twice as many as heart beating donors. For this potential to be unleashed, it would be necessary for there to be agreement about the criteria for diagnosis of death. Also, uniform legislation will be necessary to permit the cooling of kidneys by arterial catheterization and whole body flushing, whilst waiting for family consent. The results of transplanting NHBD kidneys are improving (up to 85% of grafts surviving for more than 1 year) and compare favourably with the prognosis following transplants from heart beating donors at the same centres (Kowalski *et al.*, 1996).

Second, increasing the number of living-related and unrelated donors would increase the supply of kidneys. Living-related donor transplants accounted for 20% of the transplants in 1988 and 27% in 1995 in the USA. A more promising new source, however, is the living-*un*related transplants from spouses and friends. The realization that such transplants yield results similar to those with related donors has opened up a significant new source, which has not yet been actively recruited (Terasaki *et al.*, 1998).

A third method is presumed consent legislation. There is general agreement, endorsed by the World Health Organization (WHO, 1991), that organs may be removed from the body of a dead person if any consent required by the law is obtained and if there is no reason to believe that in the absence of any formal consent during his or her lifetime the dead person would have objected to such removal. Rules governing the removal of cadaveric organs generally either require the permission of the relatives, at the time of death, for post-mortem organ removal, or presume that consent to such removal is implicit if the individual had not 'contracted out' by recording his objection on a central national computer system. There is clear evidence that presumed consent legislation favours cadaveric organ donation compared with 'informed consent' laws. The best case to support this system comes from Belgium: since presumed consent law was introduced in 1986 there has been a substantial increase in the supply of organs independent of other donor procurement initiatives (Michelsen, 1995). In the country as a whole, donation rose by 55% within 5 years in the face of a reduction in road traffic deaths. Belgian doctors are required to ascertain from the relatives so far as possible the wishes of the donor to validate the presumption of consent. Crucially, the relatives are not asked to decide about donation on behalf of the dead relative who may not have expressed his wish in life. But, the 'soft' variant of this law employed in Belgium may still allow the doctors not to remove the organs if they perceive that it would cause unjustifiable distress to the relatives. Intensivists have found the new law favourable to donation and seem keen to refer more donors because the distress to the relatives is lessened by relieving them of the burden of making the decision on behalf of the deceased. Where contracting out legislation does not exist, the professions and their representatives should develop a case of need to encourage or facilitate organ donation by early adoption of such legislation.

Finally, transplant Coordinators have the responsibility of taking over the physiological management of the donor, to confirm the legal status of brain death, to obtain the family and legal consent and to arrange surgical removal of organs. These crucial transplant team members can, therefore, relieve the stress and strain associated with organ donation from the intensivists. They may also play a role in identifying suitable organ donors. When faced with a crisis in organ donation, the Spanish Department of Health set up a new framework of transplant coordinators and significantly increased their numbers. Rather than working in teams responsible to transplant centres as elsewhere in the West, each district general hospital with an intensive care unit is allocated a coordinator or a coordinator team responsible to the head of the hospital and working within a centralized organization, with its headquarters in Madrid. There has been a striking improvement in organ donation in Spain as a result: donor numbers rose from 14 donors per million population (pmp) in 1989 (3 years after the new arrangements were inaugurated) to over 30 donors pmp in 1999. This rise continued steadily despite the reduction by approximately 40% of the annual death rate from road traffic accidents; the waiting lists for kidney transplants fell by 15% over an equivalent time. The system operates well within a 'presumed consent' legislative framework. This remarkable result indicates that hospital units and government departments should be asked to consider the benefits of coordinators or coordinator teams working full-time in acute hospitals, rather than in transplant units.

In summary, the many ethical issues in the allocation of kidneys are a resource-dependent problem. There is convincing evidence that the number of kidney donors can be significantly expanded by joint professional and governmental efforts to inaugurate changes in the law, clinical practice, and administrative arrangements for organ donation to redress the deficit. The prediction would be that many of the ethical problems will fade as the supply increases.

References

American Society of Transplant Physicians, the Patient Care and Education Committee (1995). The evaluation of transplant candidates: clinical practical guidelines. *The Journal of the American Society Nephrology*, 6, 1–5.

Ayanian, J. Z., Cleary, P., Weissman, J. S., and Epstein, A. M. (1999). The effect of patients' preferences on racial differences in access to renal transplantation. *New England Journal of Medicine*, 341, 1661–9.

Beauchamp, T., and Childress, J. (1989). *Principles of biomedical ethics*, 3rd edn. Oxford University Press, New York, Oxford.

Daar, A. (1995). Transplantation in developing countries. In *Kidney transplantation principles and practice*, 4th edn. (ed. Morris, P. J.), pp. 478–503. Saunders, Philadelphia.

Demeester, J., Persijn, G. G., Wujciak, T., Opelz, G., and Vanrenterghem, Y. For the Eurotransplant International Foundation (1998). The new Eurotransplant kidney allocation system. Report one year after implementation. *Transplantation*, 66, 1154–9.

Foss A., Leivestad T., Brekke I. B., Fauchal P, Bentdal O., Lien B., Pfeffer P., Sodal G., Albrechtsen D., Soreide O., and Flatmark A. (1998). Unrelated living donors in 141 kidney tansplantations. *Transplantation*, 66, 49–52.

Gubernatis, G., and Kliemt (2000). *Transplantation in press*.

Jarvis, R., (1995). Join the club: a modest proposal to increase availability of donor organs. *Journal of Medical Ethics*, 21, 199–204.

Kootstra, G. (1997). The asystolic or non heart beating donor. *Transplantation*, 63, 917–22.

Kowalski, A. E., Light, J. A., and Ritchie, W. O. (1996). A new approach for increasing the organ supply. *Clinical Transplantation*, 10, 653–7.

Lancet (1998). Changing the US transplant system (editorial). *Lancet*, 352, 79.

Lowance, D., Neumayer, H-H., LeGendre, C. M., *et al.* (1999). Valacyclovir for the prevention of cytomegalovirus disease after renal transplantation. *New England Journal of Medicine*, 340, 1462–70.

Manske, C. L., Wang, Y., and Rector, T. (1992). Coronary revascularisation in insulin dependent diabetic patients with chronic renal failure. *Lancet*, 340, 998–1001.

Michelsen P. (1995) The effect of transplantation laws on organ procurement. In *Organ shortage: the solutions* (eds Touraine, J. L., *et al.*), pp. 33–39. Kluwer. The Netherlands 33–39.

Morris, P. J., Johnson, R.J, Fuggle, S. E., Belger, M. A., and Briggs, J. D. On behalf of the HLA Taskforce of the Kidney Advisory Group of the UKTSSA (1999). Analysis of factors that effect outcome of primary cadaveric renal transplantation in the UK. *Lancet*, 359, 1147–52.

Opelz, G. (1992). How unusual are the University of Minnesota HLA matching results? *Transplantation*, 53, 694.

Pfaff, W. W. (1998). Principles for allocation of cadaver organs to transplant recipients in the USA (UNOS). In *Organ allocation* (eds Touraine, J. L., *et al.*), pp. 45–50. Kluwer Academic Publishers, Dordrecht.

Sells, R. A. (1997). Cardiovascular complications following renal transplantation. *Transplantation Reviews*, 11 (3), 116–26.

Terasaki, P. I., Toyotome, A., and Mickey, M. R. (1985). Patient graft and functional survival rates: an overview. In (ed. Terasak, P. I.), *Clinical kidney transplants 1985*, pp. 1–26. UCLA Tissue Typing Laboratory, Los Angeles.

Terasaki, P.I., Cacka J. M., Jertson E. W., Cho Y., and Takemoto S. (1998). Increasing kidney supply is the best solution to the allocation problem. In *Organ allocation* (eds Touraine, J. L. *et al.*), pp. 67–72. Kluwer Academic Publishers, Dordrecht.

Tesi, R. J., Elkhammas, E. A., Davies, E. A., Henry, M. L., and Ferguson, R. M. (1994). Renal transplantation in older people. *Lancet*, **343**, 461–4.

Tilney, N. L. (1998). The crisis in transplantation: Too much demand for too few organs. *Transplantation Reviews*, **12**, 1–10.

Ting, A., and Morris, P. J., (1987). HLA matching in transfused, Cyclosporin treated patients at Oxford. In *Clinical transplants 1987* (ed. P. I. Terasaki), p. 235. UCLA Tissue Typing Laboratory, Los Angeles.

Tyden, G., Bolinder, J., Solders, G., Brattstrom, C., Tibell, A., and Groth, C-G. (1999). Improved survival in patients with insulin dependent diabetes mellitus and end stage diabetic nephropathy, ten years after combined pancreas and kidney transplantation. *Transplantation*, **67**, 645–8.

United States Department of Health and Human Services (UNOS) (1996). *Annual Report.*

World Health Organization (1991). *Human organ transplantation: A report on developments under the auspices of the WHO 1987–1991.* Geneva, WHO.

Wujciak, T., and Opelz, G. (1993). A proposal for improved cadaver kidney allocation. *Transplantation*, **56**, 1513–20.

10

Genetics: Ethical issues in kidney disease

Rita Kielstein and Hans-Martin Sass

We are witnessing a revolution of Copernican dimension in medicine and health care, which is based on the rapid and enormous progress in molecular genetics. These revolutionary forces have already entered and soon will influence even more patient care, carrier typing and consultation, and molecular genetic and pharmacogenetic research in nephrology. The new understanding of the genetic origin of some disorders and of the genetic predisposition to many diseases and health disorders creates controversies in the ethical assessment of the new forms of information and intervention; this will be controversial for some time. (Sass, 1996).

On one side there are the foes of genetic knowledge pointing out that genotyping in human genetics will do more harm than good to the individual and to the moral and social fabric of humankind. They argue that: (1) discrimination based on the individual's genetic set-up will add to many other already existing forms of discrimination; (2) genetic information cannot be kept confidential and therefore will do more harm to the individual than good; (3) fellow humans with specific genetic make-ups will find it harder, if not impossible, to gain access to certain jobs or to be accepted by health insurance companies; (4) life-style regulation in the name of health-risk management and cost reduction will be the logical consequence in predictive and preventive medicine; and finally (5) there will be a loss of solidarity towards those with known genetic disorders.

On the other side, it is argued that individuals will: (1) be able to make more educated choices in life based on their genetic risk factors; (2) get guidance for making reproductive decisions giving them for the first time the opportunity for parental responsibility via pre-implantation diagnosis and prenatal screening; (3) get more individualized medication with less side-effects based on their specific genetic set-up for drug metabolism; (4) get a better understanding of their individual risk factors in the workplace and in the environment, thus protecting health and quality of life before acute or chronic illnesses occur; (5) improve health-risk solidarity as everyone will have predictable risks in her or his genetic set-up, some more severe than others.

As with all new forms of knowledge and technology, individuals, families, societies, professionals, organizations and governments, locally and globally, have to evaluate the risks and benefits associated with genetic knowledge and capabilities. It will be a new world, but the blueprint of the story is the old one: knowledge and technology can be used both ways, for the good as well as for the bad. We are truly venturing into a new world, one that must define—so far it has not—its own moral and ethical obligations and rights and a new understanding of health literacy, genetic literacy, and responsibility. We hope that new genetic knowledge will lead to an *improved concept of autonomy* and self-determination, empowering as well as requiring the individual to take better control over her or his health care and risk protection. It also will lead to a *modified concept of health* and health care. Health cannot simply be understood anymore as 'a state of complete physical, mental and social well-being and not merely the absence of disease or infirmity' (WHO, 1958, p. 459). Rather, health is a process of challenge and response, a process of balancing, which needs understanding, protection, stewardship and prudent management by the individual person. Health is the health-literate and risk-competent care of one's own physical, emotional, and social well-being and well-feeling, achieved in competent understanding, modification and enhancement of individual genetic, social and environmental properties, with the support of health care professionals and equal access to health care information, including predictive and preventive services.

Genetics, ethics, diagnosis and treatment of hereditary renal disorders

While introduction and application molecular genetics will have broad and revolutionary effects, specific medical and ethical issues associated with the development, interpretation, and application of genotyping for renal diseases and disorders can be more narrowly focused. They include: (1) the debate about an 'obligation to know' versus a 'right not to know'; (2) ethical and medical issues associated with pre-symptomatic information about carrier status for the individual carrier's health care and life plan and the carrier–physician interaction; and (3) new responsibilities in family planning and towards members of the immediate and extended family. Of particular ethical importance is the hope to develop pharmacogenetic products capable of modifying, neutralizing or turning off undesirable enzymatic activities leading to progressive renal failure. But as long as there is no direct remedy for genetic disorders, carriers have to know how to cope with, how to postpone, and how to reduce the impact of genetic renal diseases. Denial, fear, ignorance, and accusations are well-known obstacles for individuals and families in dealing with genetically 'transmitted' diseases. We see common challenges to carriers, their partners and families, to individually and collectively develop a new understanding of the concepts of health and disease, and a new predictive and preventive partnership between pre-symptomatic and symptomatic carrier and physician in addition to the traditional roles of patients and physicians.

Hereditary kidney disorders include glomerular, tubular, and tubulo-interstitial renal diseases, as well as the rare vitamin D disorders and disorders of amino acid storage, transport, and metabolism. Carriers of polycystic renal diseases in adults (PKD-1, PKD-2), followed by patients with Alport's syndrome and various types of renal tubular acidosis (RTA) are the most widely represented in clinical practice. While the familial nature of most cases of polycystic kidney disease [PKD] is well known to doctors in developed countries, carriers of glomerular disorders and of Alport's syndrome often seek medical advice from general pediatricians. Many of these physicians may not be experienced enough in diagnosing renal disorders if a family history is not established or not known. Nephrologist and general pediatricians have to work closely together, and continuing education of pediatricians must include diagnosis and treatment of renal disorders (Coe and Satish, 1994; Chapman and Guay-Woodford, 1997; Brodehl, 2000; Ritz and Zeier, 2000).

Autosomal dominant polycystic kidney disease [ADPKD], with an incidence of 1:400 to 1:1000 within most populations, is by far the most common and best known late onset genetic disorder; it is more common than cystic fibrosis, Down syndrome, hemophilia, muscular dystrophy, and sickle cell anemia. Carriers of PKD [polycystic kidney disease] suffer from cysts in both kidneys, which lead to endstage renal disease [ESRD] requiring dialysis or kidney transplantation. They also suffer from arterial aneurysms, which may occur in any arteries, but are most clinically significant in the cerebral circulation.

The adult type ADPKD has at least two different types, the more common PKD-1 located on chromosome 16 and the less common PKD-2 associated with disorders on chromosome 4 (Murcia, 1998). There is probably a third type, which is caused by, as yet unknown, chromosomal disorders. Clusters of genetic factors within families influence onset and severity (Guay-Woodford, 1999). It is likely that a special protein diet may reduce or postpone the development of tubular epithelial cells in ADPKD by influencing the mutated polycystin-1 and polycystin-2 interaction responsible for triggering the formation of cysts (Walz, 1999; Ritz and Zeier, 2000; Ogborn et al., 1998; Ong, 1999). Among carriers of the rare recessive form [ARPDK] resulting in nephromegaly and microcystic kidney transformation prenatally and in early childhood, nearly 50% do not survive the newborn period [Guay-Woodford *et al.*, 1996, p. 15]. The US National Institute of Health estimates the incidence of ARPKD to be one in 10- to 40-thousand. PKD can be diagnosed by genetic screening, ultrasound, computed tomography (CT) or magnetic resonance imaging (MRI).

Among the forms of renal tubular acidosis (RTA), types 1 (distal) and 2 (proximal) are often autosomal dominant genetic diseases, while type 3 is a rare combination of type 1 and type 2; type 4 is not hereditary. The Fanconi syndrome is usually autosomal dominant, although in rare cases it may be autosomal recessive. Fabry's disease and X-linked nephrogenic diabetes insipidus (DI) are X-linked recessive genetic disorders, with various degrees of expression of DI in heterozygous female carriers. Bartter's syndrome can be an autosomal recessive disorder or acquired. Cystinuria is an autosomal recessive disorder of amino acid transport. Most other genetic diseases of membrane transport and vitamin D disorders are also autosomal recessive.

The Alport syndrome, with an incidence of 1 in 10000 (1 in 5000 in certain populations) is an X-linked disorder associated with sensorineural deafness and hematuria, which may progress to nephritis in late adolescence. Even though the disorder is X-linked, milder forms of deafness have been reported in females. As deafness is often recognized earlier than the renal disorder, it is important that pediatricians and otologists be knowledgeable in diagnosing Alport's syndrome as associated with renal disease.

Of particular importance is the *close cooperation* of nephrologists with general pediatricians and with clinical geneticists to guarantee early detection of hereditary renal disorders, as early treatment is important for all forms of RTA and control of hypertension is essential for all disorders because progression of disease and hypertension are interrelated. [Kielstein, 1993; Ecder et al., 1999]. The Alport syndrome and most forms of RTA are early onset disorders and require early diagnosis and treatment by an experienced nephrologist; but most likely parents will seek help first from pediatricians or, in the case of Alport's syndrome, from otologists.

Renal disorders influence blood pressure, tissue development and bone density, mineral and water balance, central and peripheral nervous systems, and immunological response. Therefore, it is important that patients in all stages of progression are well informed about lifestyle requirements, which can influence or postpone chronic disorders. Clinical experience shows that specifically designed physical exercise has a positive impact on hypertension, uremia, anemia, acidosis, myopathy, polyneuropathy, osteopathy, immunological response and mental depression. Horseback riding, step aerobics, and contact sports such as hockey, soccer, and football are not recommended for PKD patients. However, swimming, hiking, water exercises and other specifically designed training programs for carriers of renal disorders focusing on endurance training, particularly of leg musculature have been proven to result in improved blood pressure, muscle mass and strength, as well as indirect improvement of bone metabolism, nerve conductivity, and quality of life (Kielstein, 1995).

'Duty to know' versus 'right not to know'

Current molecular genetic information predicts the probability and predictability of disorders, but not severity, time of onset, severity of symptoms, lifespan, and quality of life. Preventive options and therapeutic possibilities mostly lie in the future. Genetic knowledge has to be translated into real life situations and predictions for families and individuals. Genetic risk factors alone do not predetermine the individual quality of life or the personal fate of one person. This is the clinical and ethical challenge to carriers, physicians, and society. Further progress in molecular prediction will show that everyone has her or his very personal genetic risk profile of genetically predetermined advantages and disadvantages for health, life, and happiness.

It is our thesis that there is a *categorical imperative to know* about one's genetic properties, at least about those which can be influenced, postponed, modified or someday neutralized by appropriate lifestyle, diet or various forms of health care. As hypertension control is essential in the prevention of renal diseases, how will pre-symptomatic carriers of renal genetic disorders be able to care for their health by prevention or control of hypertension, if not told of their genetic status? How can ADPKD carriers avoid hematuria, if not told about their carrier status and instructed to avoid recreational activities that might cause bleeding and rupture of vessels in cysts? How can young patients with sensorineural deafness get necessary follow-up of glomerular filtration rate and control of proteinuria, if not told that in carriers of Alport's syndrome deafness is associated with hereditary nephritis and that good lifestyle monitoring and patient management is essential to keep the progression as slow as possible? How can carriers of genetic renal disorders make career decisions, if not told that the span and strength of their productive occupational or professional life will be influenced by the probability of earlier or later renal replacement therapy? The claim of a 'right' not to know about the existence of hereditary renal disease seems to be a claim of a right to ignorance, to give up on autonomy and self-determination.

Renal disorders represent severe diseases, burdensome to patients and their families. However, unlike many other degenerative chronic diseases, these disorders can be treated medically, and even for endstage renal disease there are well established forms of renal replacement therapy. Because of the slowly degenerative nature of developing renal diseases, nephrologists often have experience in following and advising pre-symptomatic and symptomatic patients. Over relatively long periods of time, they can become trusted partners—and sometimes friends—in maintaining their patients' health. Therefore, the fact that genetic origins for many renal diseases now can be known long before the onset of symptoms or complications does not represent a totally new medical or moral scenario in patient–physician interaction in nephrology.

Clinical experience teaches us that pre-symptomatic knowledge about renal genetic disorders translates into very different individual life stories. For example, consider the story of Mrs Winters, a 55-year-old ADPKD patient who became a dialysis patient in 1981, soon after she was diagnosed as a carrier. At that time, her four sons underwent testing for the first time, which showed that all the sons were pre-symptomatic carriers of ADPKD, and, at that time, still living healthy lives. The following were the reactions of the sons after they learned about their carrier status. First, the sons criticized their mother for having as many as four children even though she knew that a renal disease was present in the family. Her father and his two brothers had died of ESRD prior to the availability of dialysis treatment. One son, Albert, 32, married and father of a 6-year-old son, committed suicide when he developed first symptoms of pain and renal dysfunction three years later. Otto, 30 and married, sold a house when he learned about the diagnosis. He did not want to make long-term plans for his life and burden his family with a mortgage. Karl, 25, and his fiancée dissolved their engagement because Karl did not want to have children nor burden his fiancée with his own genetically predictable renal failure. Paul, 21, did not complete his studies but rather took a job in order to make money and enjoy life while it lasted. The Winter family story demonstrates very clearly different ways of translating DNA prediction into real-life situations. Also, this story exemplifies how lay people without sufficient professional advice and consultation by experienced nephrologists in trust-based communication and cooperation might jump into premature or unnecessary life-style decisions. The Polycystic Research Foundation is one of the leading institutions providing education, advice and support for carriers and families of PKD disorders (homepage: www.pkdcure.edu; see also Gabow and Grantham, 1994; Chapman and Guay-Woodford, 1997).

It would be a return into the dark ages of dependency on the cruel fate of nature, of ignorance and personal illiteracy, if culture, society, the medical community and individual physicians were to withhold from carriers information that would empower those carriers to take control of their life plans and the care of their health. We see a *societal and medical duty to inform* and an *individual obligation to know* about carrier status, if such knowledge can change the course or the speed of the disease. We do not see a right of society or of the health care system to require carriers to live a life based on rigid control of diet and lifestyle at the cost of individually defined quality of life and life goals. It would be against the concept of respect for persons and for the dignity of personal choice to regulate lives paternalistically and to control the actions of carriers of renal and other genetic disorders. The individual obligation to know does not include a requirement to behave according to the prevention textbook; but knowing is the only available basis to make educated choices (Kielstein and Sass, 1992). Ignorance does not give a basis for any kind of choice. If genetic information is without relevance for influencing the probability or course of the disorder, then it should be the right of the potential carrier to ask or not ask for such information. We also see a corresponding right of carriers of all types to have equal and free access to testing information, and to consulting and counseling services. Society and the medical establishment are obligated to make these services available and as supportive and effective as possible.

The new interactive counseling model

We see a newly extended role for the nephrologist as a medical expert in renal genetic disorders: the trusted and responsible partner in a model of interactive counseling, in addition to the traditional role of prevention specialist in pre-symptomatic diagnosis and intervention specialist in renal replacement therapy. The new requirements in genetic renal diseases exceed the traditional competence of the classical human geneticist.

Traditionally, it has been the role of the human geneticist to diagnose genetic disorders and to offer advice to carriers. The time has passed for one medical discipline, human genetics, to accept full medical and moral responsibility for assisting carriers in understanding and applying genetic information in their lives, health care and life goals. Only an experienced nephrologist can be a trusted and responsible partner for educating and advising pre-symptomatic or symptomatic renal disorder patients, just as only a specialized oncologist would be the ideal discourse partner for carriers of genetic oncological risk (Kielstein, 1995). For assistance and consultation in making good health-care decisions and in pondering reproductive choices or at the crossroads of occupational and professional planning, the renal specialist would be the partner of choice (Kielstein, 1996; Fouser, 1998; de Almeida *et al.*, 1999; Fick-Brosnahan *et al.*, 1999; Tanner and Tanner, 1999). Also, as we already discussed, nephrologists should work closely with general pediatricians, to assist them in early diagnosis and treatment of renal disorders, some of which are rare and not easy to diagnose and to treat. Traditional principles in medical ethics such as truth-telling and confidentiality will need to be re-emphasized and prioritized in the age of molecular genetic prediction of progressive and late-onset renal diseases.

In consultation in human genetics, it has become the gold standard of modern bioethics to avoid paternalism and directive counseling in favor of non-directive counseling. Given the severity of most renal genetic disorders and the importance of good symptomatic and pre-symptomatic patient–physician interaction in communication and cooperation, we feel that the controversy between directive and non-directive counseling should be replaced by new and more appropriate models of patient–physician interaction, an interactive counseling model of discourse and evaluation.

An *interactive model of counseling*, respecting the patient's or client's self-determination and actually empowering autonomy, would require that the physician: (1) inform and educate the carrier, depending on the carrier's capacity to understand information and to make judgments and decisions; and (2) assist and support the carrier to make medically important decisions such as compliance with routine check-ups, dietary regimen, physical training, and hypertension control. There will be other very personal challenges and decisions related to the carrier status that do not belong in the realm of medical responsibility and involvement. The new model of neither directive nor non-directive counseling has also been called 'interpretive ethics' (White, 1999). The interactive discourse-and-evaluation based dialogue model will work differently depending on the individual case and the carrier's or patient's quest for guidance or value statements by the consultant. Of course, the discourse model will have to make it clear, as is true of all models of non-directive counseling, that paternalism in decision making cannot be accepted and that carriers have to make final decisions and accept final responsibility for those decisions. There are patients who for various reasons are unable to accept responsibility or to follow a strict regimen. For those patients traditional forms of paternalism might still be appropriate, but one must not pressure fellow humans into regimens they do not like and do not want.

We have developed an interactive *Action Guide* for the discourse model, outlining challenges and responsibilities for both the carrier and the consultant.

Action guide

There are six challenges for the carrier:

1. Understand and accept your individual predispositions for health and understand your individual genetic set-up, which will allow you to define your very specific quality of life and goals in life, taking your genetic heritage into account.
2. Become health literate and define your individual challenge to happiness and health within the parameters of your genetic heritage and your challenges in the social and natural environment.
3. Live a happy life and protect your health and happiness by appropriate and prudent rules for diet, exercise and relaxation, work and love, social activities and self-determination.
4. Expect from the health care professional and the health care system individualized prediction, advice for prevention, guidance in health care and in acute care intervention, and a trust-based interactive professional and personal partnership in dealing with carrier status, chronic illness and suffering.
5. Understand that no health care professional can relieve you from being the prime caretaker of your health, happiness, and life.
6. Discuss your concept of health and disease, long-term care plans, and advance care documents with health care professionals you trust and with family and friends.

There are also six challenges for the consultant:

1. You are responsible for your patient as a person, not just for her or his symptoms.
2. Inform and educate your patient about her or his individual predisposition for health and health risks and help the patient to understand individual challenges and opportunities.
3. Help the patient to find her or his individual way to respond to the technical details of dealing with the processes of degeneration and the possibilities of postponement of onset of more severe stages of her or his disorder.
4. Be a professional expert for your patient and do not discriminate against those patients who do not exercise their right to care for their own health in an appropriate manner.
5. You cannot expect any patient to become a medical expert. Therefore you have to continuously and patiently educate your patient and keep yourself up-to-date with the best available options for prevention and treatment. You must stay in close contact with medical developments and the experts in your field.
6. Help your patient to find her or his own way to cope with disorders, to develop long-term care plans and to execute and review care directives in advance.

Ethics challenges and limits of modifying genetic properties

As molecular genetic knowledge progresses, cooperation of nephrologists and geneticists is a high medical and moral priority in order to better understand abnormal enzymatic processes and to modify, neutralize or stop them. This acceptance of a new role in molecular genetics and pharmacogenetics, identifying the actual workings of the genetic disorders of enzyme function in protein metabolism, is of highest ethical importance. Treatment based on a better understanding of enzyme disorders will not necessarily require the development of new medication by strategic drug design. As the case of phenylketonuria demonstrates, enzyme defects can already be neutralized or treated by appropriate diet, in this case by providing for phenyalanine-free or -reduced nutrition for the first few months after birth. In most cases this effectively avoids neurological symptoms and physical disorders causing lifelong suffering and dependency. It is at the molecular genetic level that dietary or pharmacological interventions will have to be developed to modify or to stop the development of hereditary kidney disorders. Already, the disorderly functioning of polycystin metabolism (Adelsberg, 1999) has been identified as the cause for late-onset ADPKD. Successful modification of polycystin metabolism resulting in the non-development of cysts has already been reported in PKD rats (Cowley et al., 1996).

It has been suggested that the repair of genetic disorders and the fight against genetic diseases will discriminate against already existing carriers or patients suffering from these diseases. We do not accept those arguments as valid or ethically authoritative, even though we share the concern that discrimination against disabled fellow humans can and indeed does occur for a variety of unacceptable reasons. In our argument for fighting genetic disorders at their very roots, we follow Kamm's reasoning: 'If certain traits are genuinely impairments, this will mean that individuals having those traits must accept that their natures are rightly to be discouraged in future generations, other things being equal. But this does not mean that they as persons *already in existence* have fewer rights than others; indeed they may have greater rather than fewer claims on social efforts on their behalf' (Kamm, 1996, p. 94).

When and if direct modification of disorderly functioning enzymes and proteins becomes possible, a 'direct' therapy of genetic renal disorders will be possible. The ethical advantages of those developments will not only benefit the carrier. It also will avoid hard choices of selective abortion in family planning and the multitude of ethical problems associated with germline therapy; that is, the direct modification of DNA controlling enzymatic functions which lead to the development and progression of renal disorders and finally to endstage renal disease.

Breakthroughs in pharmacogenetics of renal disorders will also solve the currently unsolvable ethical problem of justice and equal access to all or any of extremely expensive renal replacement therapies on a global level, especially for carriers born into less fortunate social and economic societies. It is our thesis that research in pharmacogenetics for renal disorders is of the highest ethical priority. Well-intended discussions of sharing health-care costs and allocation with those less fortunate in poor countries unfortunately will not lead to ethically acceptable solutions.

Family planning and responsible parenting

Ethical complexities associated with making responsible reproductive choices by carriers of genetic renal disorders are manifold. Most of them are related to the unsolved ethical controversy regarding the moral status of unborn human life. If, one day in the future, there are opportunities for direct 'therapy' of DNA disorders on the enzymatic level, we will be able to avoid uncomfortable debates about selective abortion or other hard choices in parenting. We are not there yet.

The ethical parameters of responsible parenthood of carriers of severe genetic diseases are well illustrated in the case of Anita M. Anita had been diagnosed as a carrier of ADPKD at the age of 16 when she was a subject in a research project, which studied the family history of patients with this disease. Five years later she was 21 years old and pregnant. Her mother, 45 and divorced, is on repeated dialysis treatment [RDT]. Her grandmother has just died due to liver complications after being in dialysis treatment for 14 years. Anita requests prenatal testing, which now can be done by genetic screening. She expresses an obligation not to give birth to a baby with a definite diagnosis of ADPKD, as this means dialysis dependency in later years, decreased quality of life, other complications, pain, hypertension, and a way of suffering and dying she just had witnessed in her grandmother's last years. The test identifies the fetus positively as a carrier. Anita schedules a counseling session prior to setting a date for elective abortion, but she misses this appointment and never calls back; she probably moved somewhere else and gave birth to her child.

In Anita's case there are at least four different values at conflict: respect for life, self-determination, responsible parenthood, and family planning. As in most cases of reproductive ethics Anita faces a special challenge in balancing the respect for unborn life and responsible parenthood. This is a different situation than normal conflicts between right to choose (self-determination of the mother) and right to live (i.e., a potential interest of the fetus). Anita's fetus carries a severe genetic disorder which forecasts, if nothing else happens, dialysis treatment or transplantation, which are uncomfortable and reduce quality of life, plus all other associated burdens and symptoms of ADPKD (Kielstein, 1993).

Aborting the fetus might be an ethical option of responsible parenthood and, indeed, it was the original choice of Anita. The fact that she did not have the abortion might have been caused by (1) emotional stress, (2) situational ethical uncertainty, (3) a desire to have a baby disregarding its carrier status, (4) avoidance of making any decisions, or finally (5) trust in progress of ADPKD treatment over the next 30 years, i.e., the time of probable first onset of her fetus's acute symptoms (Kielstein and Sass, 1992). We see at least nine scenarios of decision making in reproductive ethics for severe genetic renal disorders of various kinds in cases similar to Anita's situation, all more or less ethically complicated.

1. Give birth: Giving birth and establishing a family by having children is a very normal individual and cultural goal in a woman's life. An ADPKD carrier most likely will be 'healthy' and happy for a long period of life and might even die of other causes a long time before the onset of severe symptoms. The offspring might have a family of his or her own and, over the next few decades, progress in medicine might develop new methods of prevention by diet or medication, of healing or other forms of efficacious treatment of many disorders. On the other hand, the mother knowingly decides to give life to a carrier of a very severe genetic disorder. This is particularly burdensome in rare cases of recessive disorders causing death shortly before or after birth. As for late onset disorders, can she responsibly give birth being aware of many future risks and uncertainties including expensive and uncomfortable dialysis treatment or transplantation? Moreover, accusations of irresponsible parenthood may come from the offspring, the spouse, the family at large, the society and the insurance companies.
2. Abortion: Anita could have chosen abortion as her preferred means of contraception because she did not want to give birth to a child having the same disease as her mother, grandmother and herself. However, higher moral acceptance would attach to family planning methods such as sterilization, the use of contraceptives, or elective abortion after prenatal diagnosis of ADPKD.
3. Abortion after prenatal diagnosis: Selective abortion would value the principle of responsible parenthood higher than the principle of respect for early unborn human life. If parents have responsibilities for their children, then there is a prime parental duty to not harm the unborn by an unhealthy life-style, such as smoking cigarettes or drinking alcohol excessively. Similarly, one could argue, that there might be a duty not to give birth to a child 'harmed' by one's own severe genetic disorder.
4. Pre-implantation diagnosis: Carriers of severe hereditary diseases might for medical, ethical, and emotional reasons prefer pre-implantation diagnosis over elective abortion. Pre-implantation diagnosis has been reported to be successful in cystic

fibrosis (Handyside *et al.*, 1992) and might become the ethical instrument of first choice in responsible parenthood decisions.
5. Not having children: This might be a choice for those who, for religious or ethical reasons, do not accept pre-implantation or prenatal diagnosis or selection of unborn human life by abortion.
6. Having no heterosexual partners: Preference for and within homo- or heterosexual activities predominantly are based on other than reproductive decisions. However, choices in sexual activities can have the additional 'side effect' that carriers will not implant their own severe disorder into other, unaffected people. In the modern world, however, carrier status also could be used as an excuse for a responsibility-free singles' life-style.
7. Adoption of a non-carrier would allow for having a child of one's own who would not be a carrier. Family planning by adoption would come within the well-known parameters of ethical and emotional 'pros and cons' of adoption.
8. Surrogate motherhood, oocyte 'donation', cloning: The list of modern fertility technologies, mostly developed in veterinary medicine, gets longer every day and includes the 'use' of oocytes from a non-related non-carrier party and also, probably in the not too distant future, cloning from a non-carrier partner. Ethical benefits of having children who are not carriers of renal genetic disease, of course, is a laudable goal in responsible parenting, but the other ethical, medical, and financial costs associated with any of these technologies seem rather high and must be balanced against the expected goal by those making reproductive decisions. We do not see valid arguments that one or the other method should be criminalized. We see, however, no societal or moral obligation to allocate public funds or group funds of health insurance providers. The ethical complexities seem too high and the acceptability by the public or the solidarity group most likely will be too low for the support of these and other individual decisions.
9. Give birth and offer child for adoption: This would be the worst case scenario for responsible parenthood. But in individual cases of heavy moral-theological, ethical, familial, or social stress on pregnant women, such a scenario cannot be excluded.

Anita was left alone for one of most crucial decisions a woman is challenged to make. She could have been helped by organizations such as the US Polycystic Kidney Research Foundation by the nephrologists who had cared for her grandmother and mother. Nephrologists should feel challenged to provide adequate information and be available for repeated interactive counseling. (www.pkdcure.org; www.zysten-nieren.de).

The fact that some or all insurers might put pressure on pregnant women carrying an ADPKD carrier to abort or discriminate otherwise against parental decisions they do not like is unfortunate. But issues of insurers accepting or rejecting patients are ethical issues of political, regulatory or oversight responsibility. They are not the responsibility of the physician, even though consulting nephrologists and patients have to take those unfortunate, sometimes unethical circumstances into account. The ethical difference between health insurance and life insurance should be the difference between the principle of solidarity in health care matters and the principle of insurance against risk based on specific personal risk factors.

New responsibilities towards family

New genetic knowledge causes complex ethical issues, which extend beyond individual responsibilities in making reproductive choices. As carriers share DNA disorders and the certainty of carrier status with their immediate and wider family, how can these new broader responsibilities be defined, or are there none? Of course, information about the probability of carrier status for a specific genetic renal disorder does not necessarily depend on the decision of a known carrier whether or not to inform her or his family. However, since early diagnosis is important, if other means of getting access to such personal information cannot be relied on, whatever the carrier decides will have far-reaching effects on each individual of the larger family. In most cases, the likelihood that a member of the family of a carrier will also be a carrier is 50% or less. To know that one is not a carrier is medically and ethically highly beneficial and welcome information. If the carrier does not tell, should the physician do so? Has a physician an obligation, or even the right, to tell strangers about a patient's status as a carrier?

Are there obligations of the medical community to guide the public discourse or individual carrier's attitudes in a particular direction? We favor disclosure of information, as we have argued that only clear and reliable information can be the basis for exercising fundamental human and civil rights of self-determination, health care, and the prudent planing of one's life. However, we see that family traditions and cultural attitudes differ and that individuals have the right to accept or not accept responsibility for others (that is, members of the wider family). Some might make a very personal deliberate decision not to inform those who are not close, who are unfriendly or even personal enemies.

Are there some genetic disorders that warrant a more active approach by carriers, their physicians or the medical community to inform potential carriers about these severe disorders? Will insurance funds be ready or even eager to pay for information on pre-symptomatic carrier status? Which consequences will the public or the community of the insured allow the insurance companies to draw from such knowledge? These are examples of the many general and new ethical questions for which we do not have general answers. Most answers will and should be determined by personal experience, cultural tradition or philosophical or religious conviction. Such a situation will make it extremely difficult to formulate definite and concrete public policy rules and to define quality standards in nephrology.

What we do know is this: family relations will be influenced by new sources of information, which may generate—mostly unfounded—feelings of guilt and shame, accusations, self-denials, divorce, suicide, and the break-up of families and familial relations. Nevertheless, the golden rule for future family ethics in renal genetic disorders must be not to hide behind traditional attitudes towards secrecy and privacy, but to inform openly and aggressively, to educate, teach and support dialogue and discourse in the families and in society. This should be done, however, not against the grain of traditional familial forms of communication and cooperation or against the will of the diagnosed carrier, but by seeking her or his support and by making the best use of sometimes dormant principles of family responsibility and solidarity. A discourse model, as we described for the carrier–physician interaction, will still have to be developed in different forms for different families based on tradition and attitude.

Given these complex issues of privacy, disclosure, the right not to know, and the duty to know, we suggest that individual patients should be legally empowered and morally supported in making individual choices: (1) for mandating disclosure of individual predictive, preventive, or therapeutic knowledge; (2) for refusal to disclose all or some information; and (3) for postponing such a decision until a later time with the decision based on then existing individual circumstances or clinical results. Moral issues of informing and protecting family members can be handled similarly by allowing (1) the diagnosed carriers to choose for themselves among a number of procedures by which family members of various degree may or not be involved, informed, or invited, and then (2), based on the options chosen, informing family members about genotyping issues. The degree to which intimate and other relationships within families will change as a result of genotyping for carrier status is beyond the control—and the responsibility—of physicians and insurers. Attitudes, virtues and vices associated with genetic information must be left to the family. Only the support and encouragement of public education and discourse and the financial and institutional support of genetic screening, consulting, and educating services should be within the realm of political and social responsibility.

Identifying and encouraging the appropriate moral agent

Genotyping provides an entire set of new tools for humankind to better understand the human condition, to better care for health, and to fight against and avoid sickness and disease. But like all tools, new and old, genotyping and identification of a carrier can be used in a virtuous or in a vicious way. Public discourse and education and the appropriate protection of human and civil rights will be needed to steward and accompany the transition into a new millennium of health literacy and health care and to deal with the associated ethical issues of family planning and family ethics. Our charter into the new territories of self-understanding and self-destination, of better health care and improved quality of life for all will not be made easier if we hold on to old models of regulation and control by bureaucracies of various kinds. These may intend to protect people from the dangers of progress, but in fact prevent progress from happening and prevent people from finding their own way to use and to enjoy the new properties of genetic knowledge for more liberty, more justice and for the pursuit of happiness.

The new challenges require different virtues and ethical commitments from a diverse group of individuals, different from rules, which were appropriate during periods of limited medical knowledge and lay ignorance. The new world of health care in the age of identifiable genetic disorders of one or the other kind also will have to call more for lay ethics than physician's ethics in health-care matters, since carriers will be given more and better information to take care of their health. New ethical challenges do not call for a different ethics, but for a different priority of traditional ethical principles, among which self-determination and self-understanding, the right and duty to know and to learn about one's own genetic properties and risk profiles, and genetic solidarity with other fellow humans will have to play the most important roles. There are different ethical challenges for different types of moral agents and their personal, professional, or political responsibilities:

- Educated and responsible people have a moral duty to learn about their genetic properties and how to make the most out of these properties; they also have a moral duty to help fellow humans in taking care of their individual genetic properties, in particular to help members of their families.
- Health care professionals are obligated not to suppress or withhold genetic information from patients; they have the duty to do their utmost to educate their patients and to guide and to accompany them in caring for their health.
- Lay persons and health-care professionals should feel bound by an invisible contract of communication-in-trust and cooperation-in-trust, sharing responsibilities, rights, and obligations, also in the care of the less fortunate, less healthy, and less competent.
- Governments, national and international institutions and organizations must provide legal, regulatory, and information networks for the protection of human and civil rights, for the development and improvement of health literacy, and for protection against exploitation and discrimination. Regulatory ethics in human genetics should be based on the ethics of information and education, and also on the promotion of predictive services and the protection of privacy.

References

Adelsberg van, J. (1999). Peptides from the PKD repeats of polycystin, the PKD1 gene product, modulate pattern formation in the developing kidney. *Developmental Genetics*, 24, 299–308.

de Almeida, A., Martins Prata, M., de Almeida, S., and Lavonha, J. (1999). Long follow-up of a family with autosomal dominant polycystic kidney disease type 3. *Nephrology, Dialysis, Transplantation*, 14, 631–4.

Brodehl, J. (2000). Primäre und hereditäre Tubulopathien. In *Klinische Nephrologie* (ed. Koch, K. M.) pp. 467–88. Urban und Fischer, München.

Chapman, A. B., and Guay-Woodford, (1997). *The family and ADPKD. A guide for children and parents*. Polycystic Research Foundation, Kansas City, MO.

Coe, F. L., and Satish, K. (1994). Hereditary tubular diseases. In *Harrison's principles of internal medicine*, vol. II (eds Isselbacher, K. J., Wilson, J. D., Martin, J. B., Fauci, A. S., and Kasper, D. L.), 13th edn, pp. 1323–9. McGraw-Hill, New York.

Cowley, B. D., Grantham, J. J., Muessel, M. J., Kraybill, A. L., and Gattone, V. H. (1996). Modification of disease progression in rats with inherited polycystic kidney disease. *American Journal of Kidney Diseases*, 27, 865–79.

Ecder, T., Edelstein, C. L., Brosnahan, G. M., Johnson, P. A., Gabow, P. A., and Schrier, R. W. (1999). Progress in blood pressure control in hypertensive patients with autosomal polycystic kidney disease (ADPKD). *Journal of the American Society of Nephrology*, vol. 10 Sept. 1999 [Program and Abstract Issue], p. 415A [abstract A2096]

Fick-Brosnahan, A. M., Duley, I. T., Johnson, A. M., Strain, I. D., and Gabow, P. A. (1999). Patterns of disease in siblings of children with very early onset (VOE) of autosomal polycystic kidney disease (ADPKD). *Journal of the American Society of Nephrology*, vol. 10 Sept. 1999 [Program and Abstract Issue], p. 416 [abstract A2099]

Fouser, L. (1998). Consultation with the specialist. Familial nephritis; Alport syndrome. *Pediatric Review*, 19, 265–7.

Gabow, P. A., and Grantham, J. J. (for the Polycystic Kidney Research Foundation) (1994). *Q&A on PKD*. Polycystic Kidney Research Foundation, Kansas City, MO.

Guay-Woodford, L., Cole, B. R., and Stapleton, F. B. (1996). *Your child, your family, and autosomal recessive polycystic kidney disease*. Polycystic Kidney Foundation, Kansas City, Mo.

Guay-Woodford, L. M. (1999). Phenotypic variability in PKD1: the family as a starting point. *Kidney International*, 56, 344–6.

Handyside, A. H., Lesko, J. G., Taris, J. J., Robert, M. L., and Winnton Hughes, M. R. (1992). Birth of a normal girl after in vitro fertilization and preimplantation diagnostic testing for cystic fibrosis. *New England Journal of Medicine*, 327 (13), 905–9.

Kamm, F. M. (1996). Genetic therapy, disability and enhancement. *Jahrbuch fuer Recht und Ethik/Annual Review of Law and Ethics*, 4, 81–91, 93–98.

Kielstein, R. (1993). *Klinik, Genetik und Ethik der Autosomal Dominant Polyzystischen Nierenerkrankung*. Zentrum für Medizinische Ethik, Bochum.

Kielstein, R. (1995). *Goals and results of exercise training in ESRD patients*. University Verlag Brockmeyer, Bochum.

Kielstein, R. (1996). Clinical and clinical-ethical aspects of genetic prediction. The case: hereditary kidney disorders. *Jahrbuch fuer Recht und Ethik/Annual Review of Law and Ethics*, 4, 81–91.

Kielstein, R., and Sass, H. M. (1992). Right not to know or duty to know? *Journal of Medical Ethics and Philosophy*, 17(4), 395–405.

Murcia, N. S., Woychik, R. P., and Avner, E. D. (1998). The molecular biology of polycystic kidney disease. *Pediatrics Nephrology*, 12, 721–6.

Ogborn, M. R., Bankovic-Calic, N., Shoesmith, C., Buist, R., and Peeling, J. (1998). Soy protein modification of rat polycystic kidney disease. *American Journal of Physiology*, 274 (3 Pt 2), F541–F549.

Ong, A. C. M. (1999). Cyst formation in ADPKD: new insights from natural and targeted mutants. *Nephrology, Dialysis, Transplantation*, 14, 544–6.

Ritz, E., and Zeier, M. (2000). Polyzystische Nierenerkrankungen. In *Klinische Nephrologie* (ed. Koch, K. M.), pp. 447–52. Urban und Fischer, München.

Sass, H. M. (1995). Some cultural and ethical reflections on moleculargenetic risk assessment. *Proceedings of the International Bioethics Committee 1994*, vol II. UNESCO, Paris.

Sass, H. M. (1996). Copernican challenge of genetic prediction in human genetics. *Jahrbuch fuer Recht und Ethik / Annual Review of Law and Ethics*, 67–79.

Tanner, G. A., and Tanner, J. A. (1999). Potassium citrate/citric acid intake prevents a decline in renal function in Han:SPRD rat, but not in pcy/pcy mice with polycystic kidney disease [PKD]. *Journal of the American Society of Nephrology*, vol. 10 Sept. 1999 [Program and Abstract Issue], p. 234 [abstract A2153].

Walz, G. (1999). Signaling in polycystic kidney disease. *Kidney Blood Pressure Research*, **22**, 412–13.

White, M. T. (1999). Making responsible decisions. An interpretive ethic for genetic decision-making. *The Hastings Center Report*, **29**(1), 14–21.

World Health Organization (WHO) (1958) *The first ten years of the WHO*. WHO, Geneva.

11
Special issues in the care of children

*Howard Trachtman, Mark Grijnsztein, Rachel Frank,
and Bernard Gauthier*

Introduction

Ethical conduct is mandatory in all medical disciplines and it must be exercised in all patients regardless of their underlying disease or their age. Therefore, it might appear superfluous to discuss ethical issues specifically in pediatric patients with renal disease. However, this entire volume reflects the fact that special ethical problems occur in the practice of nephrology. Some of these difficulties reflect the variable nature of medical progress in different areas, for example the development of renal transplantation, and the impact of political developments, for example the decision to reimburse the costs of end-stage renal disease (ESRD) therapy in many countries with national funds. This chapter is written based on the premise that children under 18 years of age with kidney disease differ from their adult counterparts. As a consequence of this distinction, there are particular questions that are often asked about how to handle certain clinical dilemmas in children with renal problems in an ethically sound and coherent manner. The following discussion does not aim to be exhaustive but instead it focuses on three distinct topics: (1) informed consent and surrogate decision making in children; (2) kidney donation for transplantation; and (3) screening for genetic renal diseases.

Informed consent

General

The requirement for informed consent animates all decisions to provide medical care. It is based on the presumption that each person is an autonomous individual and, as such, he or she is empowered to make all decisions about care. In practice, this translates into the obligation to provide every patient with the relevant information that a reasonable person would request about prognosis, the anticipated outcome of treatment, alternative therapies, and potential risks in order to make a meaningful decision before instituting a therapeutic intervention. This standard applies just as much in day-to-day medical practice as it does in clinical research. In order to satisfy the requirements for informed consent, the patient must be of legal age, of sound mind and body, and capable of making rational judgements. Only under these circumstances can one be sufficiently confident that the decision represents a truly informed choice by an individual who has competently weighed all of his or her options.

Children cannot satisfy the requirements for informed consent. Therefore, questions about and recommendations for medical care are directed at the child's parents or guardian. Nonetheless, in recognition of the substantive position of the child in the actual scheme of things, serious consideration must be given to the child's developmental status and his or her potential role in the decision-making process (Committee on Bioethics, 1995). It is now a governmental requirement that the assent or permission of the minor 9 years of age and older be obtained prior to commencing medical or surgical treatment. This may be especially relevant in providing 'standard medical care', where safeguards such as the Institutional Review Board are not in place (Truog et al., 1999). Parents can overrule a child's refusal of standard treatment or enrollment in a clinical trial of experimental therapy under circumstances where the child may inappropriately reject a potentially helpful therapeutic modality. The following paragraphs describe clinical scenarios that are unique to pediatric patients with serious kidney disease in which the adequacy of the informed consent process is open to question.

Dialysis and/or transplantation

For many serious pediatric illnesses, such as progressive genetic disorders there may be no effective therapy. In others such as liver failure there may be only one method to sustain life; that is, liver transplantation. Finally, in children with oncologic disease, there may be a legitimate choice between two equally credible clinical protocols to eliminate the malignancy. ESRD represents a singular situation in which three entirely disparate treatment modalities are available for long-term use in the management of a problem that would be fatal if left untreated. Hemodialysis (HD), peritoneal dialysis (PD) and transplantation (living-related or cadaveric) are three viable solutions to the patient with irreversible kidney failure.

Adult patients with ESRD can be given the relevant information and be asked to make an informed decision about the treatment that he or she thinks is best. The three options for treatment of ESRD may not be considered equally feasible in a given case and adult patients presumably have well-defined preferences and expectations regarding ESRD therapy. In general, the consensus is that most adult patients are receiving their preferred treatment. However, confounding factors such as race and socioeconomic status may influence this choice. Compared with whites, a smaller percentage of non-white patients on dialysis undergo transplantation (Kasiske et al., 1991). A recent study indicates that black patients are somewhat less likely to want a kidney transplant and to be less certain about this preference. However, a more conspicuous reason why transplantation rates may be lower in blacks is that black patients on dialysis are less likely to be placed on a transplant list (Ayanian et al., 1999). Thus, even for adults, physician practices may compromise the free exercise of informed consent by patients with ESRD.

In children there may be other issues and problems that hinder the family from making an informed decision about ESRD care. There may be competing claims on 'the best treatment' for the child. None of them may adequately take the child into account and seek consent or assent for the therapy. From the pediatric nephrologist's perspective, renal transplantation is almost always presented as the optimal long-term solution for the child with ESRD because it has the highest likelihood of restoring a regular life style, normal growth, and intact neurocognitive development (Potter et al., 1991). Children who received a kidney transplant before 18 years of age and who maintained graft function for at least 10 years had a favorable social and professional outcome (Morel et al., 1991). This expert bias generates pressure on apprehensive parents in favor of a decision that may overlook the child and family's readiness for the procedure. It may understate the potential hazards and discomforts associated with this surgical treatment. When a recommendation is made to initiate dialysis, the pediatric nephrologist may be anxious to protect his or her professional domain against unwanted intrusions by internal medicine nephrology counterparts. Many regional nephrology advisory councils, at the urging of pediatric nephrologists, have adopted the position that pediatric patients who require dialysis achieve the best outcome with PD. Pediatric nephrologists, in turn, may claim special expertise in this procedure and oversell PD as the next best alternative therapy for children with ESRD. Pain caused by medical treatment is a factor whose importance is magnified in children. Because HD necessitates repeated needle punctures and is associated with disquieting symptoms secondary to osmotic and hemodynamic changes, it may be inappropriately avoided without giving due consideration to the child's wishes or expressed preference for HD. This decision-making process may unfold even though indwelling catheters are available for long-term use in children, eliminating much of the pain and distress involved in the HD procedure. If HD is selected, it may be chosen solely because of parents' reluctance or outright refusal to be trained in PD. A negative assessment of the home environment or by the renal team may disqualify PD as an option. This decision may be reached without even soliciting the input of the parents or the child.

The low incidence of ESRD in children (1–2 new cases/million population/year) (Warady et al., 1997) introduces several other variables that are not factors when treatment is offered to adults with kidney failure. Expertise and clinical experience in the care of pediatric patients with ESRD may not be universally available at all medical facilities. Therefore, children may not be treated by the most qualified sub-specialist. The option of transfer to a center with a larger group of affected children may be withheld. Financial incentives and the specific treatment setting may influence the choice of treatment without the child or family even being aware of a bias. A recent study indicates that children who are treated in non-profit facilities are nearly three times as likely to receive PD *versus* children who are dialyzed at for-profit centers (Furth et al., 1999). It is important to acknowledge that being dialyzed in a for-profit facility may have an adverse effect on clinical care regardless of the age of the patient. In a recent analysis based on a representative sample of 3681 adult patients, using data that had been compiled by the US Renal Data System, dialysis in a for-profit facility was associated with a 20% higher mortality rate and a 26% lower rate of placement on a waiting list for a kidney transplant (Garg et al., 1999).

The assessment of risks and benefits of ESRD treatment is never a straightforward process. There is a paucity of rigorous quantitative data on clinical outcomes, for example survival, rehabilitation, and quality of life that physicians can rely on in presenting the options in ESRD care. A recent study from the Netherlands attempts to rectify this shortcoming in adult patients. The physical quality of life was assessed in 230 new chronic dialysis patients recruited from 13 centers. This outcome measure was better if HD was prescribed compared with PD (Merkus *et al.*, 1999). Similar investigations are urgently needed in pediatric ESRD. In the words of the National Commission for the Protection of Human Subjects of Biomedical Research and Behavioral Research, 'It is commonly said that benefits and risks must be "balanced" and shown to be "in a favorable ratio". The metaphorical character of these terms draws attention to the difficulty of making precise judgements' (National Commission for the Protection of Human Subjects of Biomedical Research and Behavioral Research, 1978).

There is currently no standardized method of evaluating the available therapeutic options and asking children their feelings and preferences about impending ESRD treatment. Because this therapy is viewed as highly technical and the complications of treatment are serious, pediatric patients are routinely disenfranchised when a particular therapy is selected. ESRD treatment is demanding on patients and their parents, and can consume a great proportion of the family's financial and emotional resources (Reinhart and Kemph, 1988). All three parties to the decision—the child, the parents, and the medical team—should be encouraged to reach a common ground about treatment. The standards of ethical decision making are violated if any one member of the triad is systematically excluded, ignored, or benignly neglected. Poor compliance with treatment is a frequent cause of therapeutic failure in pediatric patients with ESRD. It is no wonder that this problem exists if children and adolescents are not routinely involved when informed consent is obtained prior to embarking on a management regimen.

Treatment of ESRD in infancy

A distinguishing feature of ESRD in children *versus* adults is the prominent role of congenital anomalies such as renal dysplasia, obstructive uropathy, and reflux nephropathy as causes of kidney failure. As a consequence, the disease can present in the neonatal period or early infancy. The difficulties of ESRD treatment are compounded greatly in infants during the first year of life. Somatic growth and neurocognitive development may be profoundly disturbed by uremia during this period because of the enhanced susceptibility of growing child to the deleterious impact of chronic azotemia. In the past, the lack of suitable equipment limited the capability of treating infants with severe congenital renal disease. These patients invariably died of unremitting azotemia. However, during the 1990s, nutritional therapy of these children was refined and new medications, such as erythropoietin and recombinant human growth hormone, were introduced. Dialysis supplies and equipment have been dramatically downsized so that chronic dialysis can be performed even in neonates. Furthermore, techniques in renal transplantation have made it feasible to consider this procedure as a long-term 'cure' for children weighing less than 10 kg.

Is aggressive medical treatment of ESRD in infancy the correct ethical choice? The requirements for adequate PD treatment in an infant, the number of medications that are prescribed to these patients, the possible complications that can occur, the frequent visits to physicians, add up to an overwhelming burden on parents. That families perform as well as they do under these trying circumstances is nothing short of miraculous. However, to the parent who cannot endure this regimen, is refusal of treatment an ethically justified choice? In 1987, one could view dialysis and transplantation in infancy as 'innovative and experimental treatment', thus, enabling parents to opt not to provide renal replacement therapy (Cohen, 1987).

More than a decade has passed and a great deal of valuable experience has been compiled in the treatment of infants with ESRD. There are centers with recognized expertise in transplantation for children during the first 2 years of life. The outcome at these centers is nearly as good as in patients over 2 years of age (Nevins, 1987). At the University of Minnesota, 37 children who underwent early kidney transplantation before 30 months of age and whose allograft functioned for at least 1 year displayed gratifying improvements in somatic growth, cognitive development, and psychomotor function (Davis *et al.*, 1990). Many pediatric nephrologists at institutions across the United States have been successful in providing long-term PD to infants as small as 2 kg, beginning in the immediate neonatal period (Bunchman, 1995). Do these centers of excellence set the bar and define the ethical minimum standard line for the rest of the nephrology community? The awareness of favorable results motivates the majority of pediatric nephrologists to sincerely attempt to treat any infant with ESRD (Geary, 1998). The principle of beneficence, or trying to help patients in need, suggests that this is a valid response by the physician (Moskop, 1987). However, prolonging life is not always a benefit to the child. Constant reassessment of the outcome in the particular infant and review of the performance of the entire pediatric nephrology community with these patients are mandatory. Large databases such as the North American Pediatric Renal Transplant Cooperative Study (NAPRTCS) represent invaluable sources of unbiased information about the changing outcome of ESRD treatment in infants (Harmon *et al.*, 1991). Patient support groups and educational programs run by private foundations can assist families as they wrestle with their decision. These efforts will ensure that parents are making a truly informed decision about the care of their young child. Everyone involved must keep in mind that the patient will be silent and will be unable to request that treatment be withheld. The conundrum in infants who commence treatment for ESRD contrasts sharply with the situation in children and adolescents who can articulate a desire to discontinue renal replacement therapy (Doyal and Henning, 1994).

Screening of eligible children for treatment

Paternalism is a venerated model to describe the interaction between physicians and patients. Since 1980, increased emphasis on patient autonomy and informed consent has led to the formulation of alternatives paradigms in which the doctor is seen as acting as an educator or a facilitator. Despite these important and useful developments, the ease of acting in a paternalistic manner is an alluring posture for pediatric nephrologists who care for children with ESRD. As mentioned above, this disease is very complex and it has multiple interrelated effects on virtually every body system. The management of the child with ESRD necessitates the administration of numerous medications and requires the implementation of various dietary and life-style changes. Finally, families are confronted with decisions about procedures, such as dialysis and transplantation, for which their prior experience provides no precedent or guidance.

Faced with this reality, pediatric nephrologists often rely on their own judgement and preferences in prescribing a treatment plan. They may tacitly assume that the decision is too complicated to be left to the family and the child. There are many new sources of information about ESRD that are accessible by computer and via the Internet. However, pediatric nephrologists may consider parents unable to assimilate this plethora of, often, conflicting information in a meaningful way. Thus, they may deem it proper and justified to make the right decision that is in the best interests of the child and the parents and completely circumvent the process of informed consent.

This stance, namely, taking the decision out of the patient's hands out of fear that they will come to a flawed judgement, is more pronounced when caring for children. However, it is not confined to pediatrics. It has been advocated in the context of adults who participate in clinical research projects. For example, the use of sham surgery during the evaluation of fetal nigral transplantation for Parkinson's Disease has been condemned even in patients who sign an informed consent (Macklin, 1999). It is asserted that patients must be protected against the risks of placebo-surgery despite their professed willingness to proceed with the trial. Informed consent is not adequate and should be superceded by the ethical imperative on the physician to minimize risk and to safeguard patients against medical injury.

This ethical stance is more susceptible to abuse when caring for children with ESRD. Pediatric nephrologists may arrogate to themselves the right to make all important decisions because they consider themselves the only ones capable of balancing the pros and cons of treatment and choosing the best option. The choice of medical *versus* surgical treatments, conservative *versus* aggressive approaches to medical problems, enrollment into research protocols, may be made unilaterally by the doctor because the parents, and certainly the child, are considered incapable of contributing to the decision-making process. One might assume that parents, as adults, would be treated the same by pediatric nephrologists as adult patients by internist nephrologist. However, the parents are not the pediatric nephrologist's patient. Moreover, pediatric nephrologists may question the 'independent' judgement of parents and be suspicious about whose interests are paramount in finalizing decisions regarding therapy. These temptations must be strenuously resisted if children and their parents are to be credible partners in the design of a feasible therapeutic regimen.

Compliance

In pre-adolescent children, the onus of treatment is placed squarely on the shoulders of the parents. They are held accountable for administration of medications and adherence to the therapeutic plan. However, as children grow and mature, even though adolescents are not of legal age to assume full responsibility for their care, they should play a significant role in medical decision making and implementation of treatment. Under optimal circumstances, the adolescent is empowered and made into an integral part of the team together with their parents.

What happens when an adolescent patient disagrees with medical instructions? The usual outcome is failure to comply with the medical regimen. Patients may articulate a variety of reasons for not adhering to treatment including an unwillingness to acknowledge the presence of a serious illness, inconvenience of the therapy, physical discomfort arising from treatment, perceived disturbances in body image and self-esteem, and outright rebellion against any external control or supervision.

In more mundane clinical circumstances, where the stakes are not so high, pediatricians live with the consequences of adolescent non-compliance by downgrading treatment objectives, altering drug regimens, or begrudging surrender. In the context of pediatric patients with ESRD, these are not options and the net result of non-compliance can be catastrophic. Failure to take the prescribed immunosuppressive medications, specifically corticosteroids, is the most common cause of delayed renal allograft failure in adolescent patients (Foulkes et al., 1993).

In view of the significant shortage of available cadaveric kidneys relative to the pool of prospective renal transplant recipients, strategies have been designed to assess the compliance of potential adult renal allograft recipients in order to avoid loss of a precious medical resource. This appraisal is considered part of the routine evaluation of an adult patient with ESRD and a complete psychosocial assessment cannot be performed without the full consent of the individual. In pediatric patients, the situation is considerably less straightforward. The clinical impressions of the nephrologist and nurse, interviews with parents, data compiled by the social worker can become surrogates for face-to-face meetings with the adolescent. Intra-family difficulties, for which the child cannot be held directly responsible, but which may adversely impact on the likelihood of patient compliance with anti-rejection treatment, may provide justification for the institution not to place an adolescent patient on the active transplant list or not to offer available donor kidneys. In pediatric patients with ESRD, a child's adaptive functioning skills may predict his or her adherence with prescribed medications and diet, and a family's behavioral response to the illness may be a clue to their ability to communicate with health professionals (Davis et al., 1996). Nonetheless, this type of information should not serve as the final word on providing or withholding a kidney transplant to a specific child. In these circumstances, the capacity to contribute to therapeutic decisions has been effectively taken away from the person who is being held accountable for the behavior that contraindicates renal transplantation.

The underage patient in fact does not have legal power to make decisions about treatment of life-threatening disease. However, pediatric nephrologists may undermine self-awareness that could ultimately facilitate long-term treatment success if surrogate decisions about an adolescent's worthiness to transplantation are made without full disclosure. Protocols for transplantation may require modification to overcome this unspoken bias against adolescent patients. For example, frank discussions about the importance of compliance with immunosuppressive medications despite side effects such as a Cushingoid facies, gingival hyperplasia, or hirsutism could be incorporated into the first encounter with an adolescent with ESRD. Open disclosure of the use of psychological assessment of the patient would ensure that all parties are aware of the importance of subjective factors in assessing fitness for renal transplantation. Direct communication of decisions made by the transplant team to the adolescent and delineation of alterations in behavior that would mandate reassessment of a decision not to offer renal transplantation would provide guidance to the adolescent as he or she seeks to improve his or her suitability for transplantation.

Kidney donation for transplantation

Pediatric donors

The technical aspects of performing a renal transplant in young children, especially those under the age of 6 years, are more demanding compared with the surgical requirements in adults with ESRD. Initially, it was felt that providing smaller kidneys to younger patients would be more appropriate for children because this might decrease the operative difficulties. However, this recommendation is controversial. A NAPRTCS report documented that in cadaveric renal transplantation, use of donors under the age of 6 years as associated with a significantly higher risk of early graft loss due to vascular thrombosis (Harmon et al., 1991). Small kidneys may compromise the nephron supply in the recipient and increase the risk of delayed allograft failure (Mackenzie et al., 1994). In contrast, the transplant team at the University of Minnesota has reported favorable outcomes in children given cadaveric kidneys, as a single kidney or as a two-kidney bloc, from donors as young as 4 years of age (Schneider et al., 1983; So et al., 1990). Conflict between the pressing need for organs and the optimal cadaveric donor from a technical perspective may create dilemmas for transplant teams as they allocate available organs to pediatric patients.

Cadaveric versus living-related transplantation

Many factors impact on the decision to proceed with renal transplantation. The assessment of the risk—benefit ratio for the donor and the pediatric recipient vary from family to family. The acceptance of the particular option for transplantation will also differ. For example, blacks are more reluctant to be living-related kidney donors (Meisler and Trachtman, 1989) and this accounts in large part for the lower rate of transplantation in non-white individuals (Kasiske et al., 1991). Surveys have indicated that people are more likely to donate organs from a relative who had just died than they are to donate their own organs (Manninen and Evans, 1985). Moreover, in 26 Finnish children under 5 years of age who received a kidney transplant, the outcome was similar regardless of whether they received a cadaveric or living-related allograft (Laine et al., 1994). Yet, there are transplant teams that have advocated living-related donation in children in an attempt to maximize the likelihood of long-term success following transplantation (Squifflet et al., 1981). Ethical practice mandates that this recommendation should be tempered in situations where there is a possibility of recurrent disease in the allograft, for example focal segmental glomerulosclerosis (Savin et al., 1996).

Anencephalic donors

One unique donor source has been explored for use in children in an effort to rectify the growing shortage of organs, the kidney removed from an anencephalic fetus. There are reports attesting to successful outcomes using these kidneys (Holzgreve et al., 1987). However, other experience indicated that outcomes in the recipient were poor because of abnormalities in renal function in the kidney removed from the anencephalic fetus (Harrison, 1986). Significant ethical problems arise if kidneys are procured from anencephalic infants. These include definition of personhood, quandaries related to the definition of brain death, and the reference to the proverbial 'slippery slope' if allowance is made to use kidneys from anencephalic donors (Botkin, 1988; Winslow, 1989). In point of fact, because of existing legal and administrative procedures, it is usually not feasible to procure solid organs that are suitable for transplantation from anencephalic infants (Peabody et al., 1989). An open dialogue must be maintained in which the pros and cons of this problem can be openly debated between bioethicists, nephrologists and transplant surgeons who care for young children with ESRD.

These are all concerns about kidney donation that are applicable primarily to children and not to adults with ESRD. Parents of these children must be made fully aware of all of the controversies surrounding the selection of a suitable cadaveric kidney in children. This information must be presented in a non-judgmental manner to parents who are probably considering the option of living-related donation. The efficacy of transplantation using kidneys donated altruistically by spouses or living non-related individuals has only been assessed in adult recipients (Terasaki et al., 1995). There is a single report describing 18 Arab patients, mean age of 13 years, who received commercially acquired kidneys (Frishberg et al., 1998). The allograft and patient survival in these children were comparable to standard cadaveric renal transplant recipients in Israel. However, the practice of procuring kidneys via commercial transactions has been, with rare exception (Radcliffe-Richards et al., 1998), opposed on ethical grounds in the United States and in Europe (World Health Organization, 1991).

Preference to pediatric recipients

According to the current criteria for allocating cadaveric kidneys that are utilized by the United Network of Organ Sharing (UNOS), extra points are given to children below the age of 18 years, especially those who are less than 11 years of age (Hauptman and O'connor, 1997). Although this systematic bias in favor of pediatric patients with ESRD may have an emotional appeal, it is important to explore the ethical justification for this stance. The primary argument in favor of giving priority to children is that providing them with a kidney transplant is likely to achieve a greater prolongation and improvement in the quality of life compared with adult recipients (Moskop, 1987). However, this approach minimizes the lasting impact on a family and community that can occur after the death of a parent and community member. A functioning adult represents actualized potential. The loss of such a person must be carefully weighed against the hope for the future that is invested in a child. There are analogous situations in which arguments are made in favor of one specific group of organ recipients, which is pitted against other patients awaiting a cadaveric organ. For example, in considering patients awaiting a first or a repeat solid organ transplant, some advocate giving priority to primary transplantation procedures because their mortality after the transplantation is lower (Ubel et al., 1993). In preparing this chapter, we have come to question the automatic preference that is currently given to children and we suggest alternative criteria such as tolerance of dialysis, the likelihood of reversing the primary disease, and prospects for full rehabilitation. Admittedly, these are subjective factors. However, they would mandate considering specific pediatric concerns such as the clinical burden of dialysis and the 'curability' of congenital renal anomalies. Ultimately, these problems reflect the moral dilemmas that arise when scarce medical resource must be rationed among competing groups of patients. Ideally, educational strategies to improve public awareness and to promote acceptance of transplantation among all segments of the population can be implemented that will foster a greater willingness to donate cadaver kidneys. This will increase the number of available solids organs and eliminate the tragic conflicts that arise among those who are on waiting lists for transplants throughout the country.

Screening for genetic renal diseases

General considerations

In discussing screening for genetic disease, there is no qualitative difference between renal problems and any other category of inherited disorders. There should be a clear benefit to the patient and or to the family in terms of available treatment options or prevention of disease (Allan, 1996). Medical indications for genetic screening include clarification of an uncertain diagnosis, definition of the prognosis if there is genetic heterogeneity, identification of disease prior to the onset of symptoms so that preventive measures can be adopted, carrier detection, and prenatal diagnosis. The only unique aspect of genetic testing in renal diseases may be for the purpose of identifying suitable living-related kidney donors (Marsick et al., 1998).

However, when considering genetic diseases in children, it is worthwhile to try to distinguish who is the primary beneficiary of the screening procedure. The extent of disease involvement during the pediatric years may influence the approach of clinicians to widespread application of screening tests. The benefits of testing to the child including savings in resources and anxiety must be weighed against the risks such as inappropriate assignment to a low-risk group or psychosocial harm caused by the awareness of carrying a disease gene (Harper and Clarke, 1990). Interestingly, the ethical predicament of screening one patient for genetic disease on behalf of another person has been vividly illustrated in our clinic by the occasional parent who balks at having their own urine tested during the evaluation of their child with hematuria.

When conducting genetic screening, there are currently no standard guidelines on how to balance the desires of parents *versus* their children, especially as their children mature and become more autonomous (Wertz et al., 1994).

The following two diseases illustrate some of these concerns in circumstances where the child already has readily detectable manifestations of disease, that is, Alport syndrome, and where the underlying disease is usually silent in children and adolescents, that is, autosomal dominant polycystic kidney disease (ADPKD).

Alport syndrome

Alport syndrome is an important genetic cause of kidney failure. In the most common variant, it is inherited as an X-linked dominant disorder and is the result of mutations in the COL4A5 gene. In the autosomal recessive forms, the disease arises because of mutations in the COL4A3 or COL4A4 gene on chromosome 2. Alport syndrome frequently presents in the first decade of life with microhematuria or gross hematuria after upper respiratory infections. As the patient grows older, proteinuria develops during the teenage years and other extra-renal manifestations of disease such as high-tone hearing loss will become evident (Kashtan, 1998).

At the present time, there is no reliable means of making this diagnosis except for a kidney biopsy. Genetic screening is not routine and this type of analysis is restricted to a handful of centers that perform the testing in select cases on an experimental basis (Pirson, 1999). Other tests such as skin biopsy to examine for the presence of COL4A5 or urinary measurements of collagen degradation products are not fully validated procedures. However, because the child has detectable abnormalities in the urinalysis and the occurrence of recurrent gross hematuria can be disturbing for parents, recommending a kidney biopsy in suspect cases is not considered ethically problematic. In fact, it may be fully justified in order to confirm a guarded prognosis when families are reluctant to rely on the clinical judgement of the pediatric nephrologist. Even though there is currently no specific therapy for Alport syndrome, the opportunity to implement non-specific treatments such as moderate protein restriction and administration of an angiotensin converting enzyme inhibitor lend further support to performing a kidney biopsy in a child suspected of having Alport syndrome.

Once the diagnosis of Alport syndrome is made in a child, this can have major repercussions within the family. Recently, 37 families who had a member with Alport syndrome were questioned about the impact of the diagnosis and its effect on future decisions to have children (Pajari *et al.*, 1999). Most respondents indicated that anxiety about ESRD was a major concern. They would support prenatal testing in an effort to predict health rather than for selective abortion and nearly all had a positive view towards genetic research. Nearly half of those surveyed felt that children should be told about their disease as soon as they start asking, preferably by the parent. This information tends to reinforce the notion that if a child has obvious manifestations of disease such as gross hematuria, then it is ethically justified to pursue the diagnosis and to inform the patient about his or her condition.

Autosomal dominant polycystic kidney disease (ADPKD)

In contrast to Alport syndrome, most children with ADPKD are completely asyptomatic during the pediatric period. There are some cases in which ADPKD can present during the neonatal period with an abdominal mass and/or hypertension (Cole *et al.*, 1987; Taitz *et al.*, 1987). However, most children do not have any clinical problems for which they are seeking explanation. In these circumstances, the pressure for screening is derived from the parents who want to know the status of their child. One cannot be as certain under these circumstances whether it is ethically justified to perform sonography or CT scanning to detect renal cysts in an otherwise healthy child.

A recent survey of 49 geneticists in the United Kingdom revealed that 61% would test a child for ADPKD (Wertz *et al.*, 1994). However, screening for ADPKD with renal sonography in children under 5 years of age has an unacceptably high 38% false negative rate (Gabow *et al.*, 1997). If the diagnosis of ADPKD is made in children older than 5 years, it is likely to have some adverse impact on the child's life such as closer surveillance by nephrologists and restriction of activities. The benefit of medical treatments such as the initiation of angiotensin-converting enzyme inhibitors or avoidance of over-the-counter cold remedies and caffeine-containing beverages to prevent hypertension is unproven. Thus, it seems reasonable to withhold screening until the risks and benefits are outlined to the child and the parent (Gabow, 1993). The child will have his or her own concerns while the parents may focus more on insurance issues and prospects for future marriage and children. Using the accepted standard of 9 years of age as the cut-off for obtaining assent in clinical research projects, we suggest that children above this age be involved in the decision-making process regarding screening for genetic renal disease. Obtaining permission from the child is even more imperative if detection of disease has an impact on day-to-day life-style.

The child in whom the diagnosis of ADPKD is made in the absence of a positive family history presents unique problems, that is, discriminating between a new mutation versus non-paternity. The identification of the most common form of the ADPKD gene has increased the accuracy of genetic testing (International Polycystic Kidney Disease Consortium, 1994). This only increases the pressure on nephrologists to be more vigilant and thoughtful in their approach to the asymptomatic child.

Conclusion

Ethical practices in medicine must be applied with equal enthusiasm in the most unusual and esoteric circumstances and in the most ordinary day-to-day situations. In reviewing this chapter, it is evident that much of it focuses on the rare instance of the child with ESRD. One could explain away the evident bias by claiming that 'real' problems are infrequent. However, this would avoid the need to learn lessons from these clinical scenarios that have broad utility for all children seen with nephrological disease. In writing this chapter, we have tried to provide a better understanding of the difficulties encountered when obtaining informed consent and delineating the risks and benefits of a treatment plan, the tendency to make substitute judgements for children instead of working with them to a shared decision, and the ethical dilemmas raised by genetic screening. The problems are rare but the approach crosses all disciplines and should be relevant for all children, their families, and their physicians.

References

Allan, D. (1996). Ethical boundaries in genetic testing. *Canadian Medical Association Journal*, 154, 241–4.
Ayanian, J. Z., Cleary, P. D., Weissman, J. S., and Epstein, A. M. (1999). The effect of patients' preferences on racial differences in access to renal transplantation. *New England Journal of Medicine*, 341, 1661–9.
Botkin, J. R. (1988). Anencephalic infants as organ donors. *Pediatrics*, 82, 250–6.
Bunchman, T. E. (1995). Chronic dialysis in the infant less than 1 year of age. *Pediatric Nephrology*, 9, S18–S22.
Cohen, C. (1987). Ethical and legal considerations in the care of the infant with end-stage renal disease whose parents elect conservative therapy: An American perspective. *Pediatric Nephrology*, 1, 166–71.
Cole, B. R., Conley, S. B., and Stapleton, F. B. (1987). Polycystic kidney disease in the first year of life. *Journal of Pediatrics*, 111, 693–9.
Committee on Bioethics (1995). Informed consent, parental permission, and assent in pediatric practice. *Pediatrics*, 95, 314–7.
Davis, I. D., Chang, P. N., and Nevins, T. E. (1990). Successful renal transplantation accelerates development in young uremic children. *Pediatrics*, 86, 594–600.
Davis, M. C., Tucker, C. M., and Fennell, R. S. (1996). Family behavior, adaptation, and treatment adherence of pediatric nephrology patients. *Pediatric Nephrology*, 10, 160–6.
Doyal, L. and Henning, P. (1994). Stopping treatment for end-stage renal failure: the rights of children and adolescents. *Pediatric Nephrology*, 8, 768–71.
Foulkes, L., Boggs, S., Fennell, R., and Sibinski, K. (1993). Social support, family variables, and compliance in renal transplant children. *Pediatric Nephrology*, 7, 185–8.
Frishberg, Y., Feinstein, S., and Drukker, A. (1998). Living unrelated (commercial) renal transplantation in children. *Journal of the American Society of Nephrology*, 9, 1100–103.
Furth, S. L., Hwang, W., Neu, A. M., Fivush, B. A., and Rowe, N. R. (1999). For-profit versus not-for-profit dialysis for children with end stage renal disease. *Pediatrics*, 104, 519–24.
Gabow, P. A. (1993). Autosomal dominant polycystic kidney disease. *New England Journal of Medicine*, 329, 332–42.
Gabow, P. A., Kimberling, W. J., Strain, J. D., Manco-Johnson, M. L., and Johnson, A. M. (1997). Utility of ultrasonography in the diagnosis of autosomal dominant polycystic kidney disease in children. *Journal of the American Society of Nephrology*, 8, 105–10.
Garg, P. P., Frick, K. D., Diener-West, M., and Powe, N. R. (1999). Effect of ownership of dialysis facilities on patients' survival and referral for transplantation. *New England Journal of Medicine*, 341, 1653–60.
Geary, D. F. (1998). Attitudes of pediatric nephrologists to management of end-stage renal disease in infants. *Journal of Pediatrics*, 133, 154–6.
Harmon, W. E., Stablein, D., Alexander, S. R., and Tejani, A. (1991). Graft thrombosis in pediatric renal transplant recipient: Report of the NAPRTCS. *Transplantation*, 51, 406–12.
Harper, P. S., and Clarke, A. (1990). Should we screen children for 'adult' genetic diseases? *Lancet*, 335, 1205–6.

Harrison, M. R. (1986). Organ procurement for children: The anencephalic fetus as donor. *Lancet*, **2**, 1383–5.
Hauptman, P. J., and O'Connor, K. J. (1997). Procurement and allocation of solid organs for transplantation. *New England Journal of Medicine*, **336**, 422–31.
Holzgreve, W., Beller, F. K., Bucholz, B., Hansmann, M., and Kohler, K. (1987). Kidney transplant from anencephalic donors. *New England Journal of Medicine*, **316**, 1069–70.
International Polycystic Kidney Disease Consortium (1994). Polycystic kidney disease: The complete structure of the PKD1 gene and its protein. *Cell*, **81**, 289–98.
Kashtan, C. E. (1998). Alport syndrome and thin glomerular basement membrane disease. *Journal of the American Society of Nephrology*, **9**, 1736–50.
Kasiske, B. L., Neylan, J. F. III, Riggio, R. R., Danovitch, G. M., Kahan, L., Alexander, S. R., and White, M. G. (1991). The effect of race on access and outcome in transplantation. *New England Journal of Medicine*, **324**, 302–7.
Laine, J., Holmberg, C., Salmela, K., Jalanko, H., Sairanen, H., Peltola, K., Ronnholm, K., Eklund, B., Wilkstrom, S., and Leijala, M. (1994). Renal transplantation in children with emphasis on young patients. *Pediatric Nephrology*, **8**, 313–9.
Mackenzie, H. S., Tullius, S. G., Heeman, U. W., Azuma, H., Rennke, H. G., and Brenner, B. M. (1994). Nephron supply is a major determinant of long-term renal allograft outcome in rats. *Journal of Clinical Investigation*, **94**, 2148–52.
Macklin, R. (1999). The ethical problems with sham surgery in clinical research. *New England Journal of Medicine*, **341**, 992–6.
Manninen, D. L., and Evans R. W. (1985). Public attitudes and behavior regarding organ donation. *Journal of the American Medical Association*, **253**, 3111–5.
Marsick, R., Limwongse, C., and Kodish, E. (1998). Genetic testing for renal diseases: Medical and ethical considerations. *American Journal of Kidney Disease*, **32**, 934–45.
Meisler, S. H., and Trachtman, H. (1989). Parental attitudes toward organ transplantation. *Pediatric Nephrology*, **3**, 86–8.
Merkus, M. P., Jager, K. J., Dekker, F. W., de Haan, R. J., Boeschoten, E. W., and Kredit, R. T., for the NECOSAD Study Group (1999). *Kidney International*, **56**, 720–8.
Morel, P., Almond, P. S., Matas, A. J., Gillingham, K. J., Chau, C., Brown, A., Kashtan, C. E., Mauer, S. M., Chavers, B., Nevins, T. E., Dunn, D. L., Sutherland, D. E. R., Payne, W. D., and Najarian, J. S. (1991). Long-term quality of life after kidney transplant in childhood. *Transplantation*, **52**, 47–53.
Moskop, J. C. (1987). Organ transplantation in children: Ethical issues. *Journal of Pediatrics*, **110**, 175–80.
National Commission for the Protection of Human Subjects of Biomedical Research and Behavioral Research (1978). The Belmont Report: ethical principles and guidelines for the protection of human subjects of research. Government Printing Office, Washington, DC.
Nevins, T. E. (1987). Transplantation in infants less than 1 year of age. *Pediatric Nephrology*, **1**, 154–6.
Pajari H., Koskimies, O., Muhonen, T., and Kaariainen, H. (1999). The burden of genetic disease and attitudes towards gene testing in Alport syndrome. Pediatric Nephrology, **13**, 471–6.
Peabody, J. L., Emery, J. R., and Ashwal, S. (1989). Experience with anencephalic infants as prospective organ donors. *New England Journal of Medicine*, **321**, 344–50.
Pirson, Y. (1999). Making the diagnosis of Alport's syndrome. *Kidney International*, **56**, 760–75.
Potter, D. E., Najarian, J. S., Belzer, F., Holliday, M. A., Horns, G., and Salvatierra, O. Jr. (1991). Long-term results of renal transplantation in children. *Kidney International*, **40**, 752–6.

Radcliffe-Richards, J., Daar, A. S., Guttmann, R. D., Hoffenberg, R., Kennedy, I., Lock, M., Sells, R. A., and Tilney N. (1998). The case for allowing kidney sales. *Lancet*, **351**, 1950–2.

Reinhart, J. B., and Kemph J. P. (1988). Renal transplantation in children: Another view. *Journal of the American Medical Association*, **260**, 3327–8.

Savin, V. J., Sharma, R., Sharma, M. and Trachtman, H. (1996). Circulating factor associated with increased glomerular permeability to albumin in recurrent focal segmental glomerulosclerosis. *New England Journal of Medicine*, **334**, 878–83.

Schneider, J. R., Sutherland, D. E. R., Simmons, R. L., Fryd, D. S., and Najarian, J. S. (1983). Long-term success with double pediatric cadaver donor renal transplants. *Annals of Surgery*, **201**, 439–42.

So, S. K. S., Gillingham, K., Cook, M., Mauer, S. M., Matas, A., Nevins, T. E., Chavers, B. M., and Najarian, J. S. (1990). The use of cadaver kidneys for transplantation in young children. *Transplantation*, **50**, 979–83.

Squifflet, J. P., Pirson, Y., Van Cangh, P., Otte, J. B., Van Ypersele de Strihou, C., and Alexandre, G. P. J. (1981). Renal transplantation in children: A comparative study between parental and well-matched cadaveric grafts. *Transplantation*, **32**, 278–81.

Taitz, L. S., Brown, C. B., Blank, C. E., and Steiner, G. M. (1987). Screening for polycystic kidney disease: Importance of clinical presentation in the newborn. *Archives of Diseases in Childhood*, **62**, 45–9.

Terasaki, P. I., Cecka, J. M., Gjertson, D. W., and Takemoto, S. (1995). High survival rates of kidney transplants from spousal and living related donors. *New England Journal of Medicine*, **333**, 333–6.

Truog, R. D., Robinson, W., Randolph A., and Morris A. (1999). Is informed consent always necessary for randomized, clinical trials? *New England Journal of Medicine*, **340**, 804–7.

Ubel, P. A., Arnold, R. M., and Caplan, A. L. (1993). Rationing failure: The ethical lessons of the retransplantation of scarce vital organs. *Journal of the American Medical Association*, **270**, 2469–74.

Warady, B. A., Hebert, D., Sullivan, E. K., Alexander, S. R., and Tejani, A. (1997). Renal transplantation, chronic dialysis, and chronic renal insufficiency in children and adolescents: The 1995 annual report of the North American Pediatric Renal Transplant Cooperative Study. *Pediatric Nephrology*, **11**, 49–64.

Wertz, D. C., Fanos, J. H., and Reilly, P. R. (1994). Genetic testing for children and adolescents: Who decides? *Journal of the American Medical Association*, **272**, 875–81.

Winslow, G. R. (1989). No–the law on anencephalic infants as organ sources should not be changed. *Journal of Pediatrics*, **115**, 829–32.

World Health Organization (1991). Guiding principles in human organ transplantation. *Lancet*, **337**, 1470–1.

PART III

Societal and economic issues

12
Societal allocation of resources for patients with ESRD

Daniel Callahan

I approach the topic of resource allocation for patients with end-stage renal disease with trepidation and chagrin. The trepidation comes from the difficulty of the topic, one that becomes harder, not easier, as time goes on. More people need dialysis, more can benefit from it, more seem inappropriate users, and more and more money is needed to pay for it. How are we supposed to deal with that? The chagrin comes from the fact that I have been saying for at least 20 years, in a voice reminiscent of Chicken Little, 'this can't go on, it just can't'. But it has gone on and, in the near term, will no doubt continue to go on.

I am relieved to note that I am not alone in my dire, so far unfulfilled, predictions. Richard Rettig, our most distinguished and perceptive American commentator on ESRD over the years, has said much the same thing: 'short-term cost containment pressures will be severe . . . and the longer-term issue of limiting access to care cannot be avoided forever' (Rettig, 1996, p. 1123). Moreover, when the much discussed 1984 book, *Painful Prescription: Rationing Hospital Care*, was published, detailing for an American audience the UK practice of setting a *de facto* covert age limit for dialysis, it was not hard to imagine something like that eventually happening in the United States as well (Aaron and Schwartz, 1984). Yet it has not happened, as least so far as can be seen. To add further confusion, more recent reports from the United Kingdom indicate that dialysis-rationing is not nearly so severe there any longer, even though the proportion of gross domestic product (GDP) spent on health care in the UK has not notably increased over the years—the money must be taken from somewhere else (Nicholson, 1998; Chandna *et al.*, 1999).

I mention these points to underscore what should by now be obvious: there is no rational way to predict how the United States (and maybe other countries as well) will respond to financial stress due to ESRD or to any other medical condition. The United States could conceivably muddle through for the indefinite future, wringing its collective hands now and then, introducing one cost-cutting scheme after another to save the day. Or there could be a future national financial crisis, forcing severe changes—even though some of us will take care not to predict just when that will happen. Another alternative would be to say that, even if we are experiencing no palpable crisis, we ought to be doing so, that it is wasteful and irresponsible to be spending so much money on ESRD when there are far more pressing medical and health care needs.

The future foreshadowed

However the country comes out on allocating resources to ESRD in the long run, two preliminary considerations are worth noting. One of them foreshadows the kind of problems that would become endemic if our country ever gets universal health care: every major disease would run the risk of incurring an ever-growing budget if it had cost controls no more effective then the present federal ESRD budget—up, up, and away. The other point is that, at least with dialysis, ESRD is the very model of a problem that is already endemic, that is, a severe, life-threatening disease for which, when dialysis is the only alternative, there is no cure, no inexpensive treatment, and no guarantee that those who receive the available treatment will have a decent quality of life. The AZT 'cocktail' for AIDS offers a similar example, as do many forms of desperate chemotherapy for advanced cancer, or efforts to forestall congestive heart failure, or recent drugs to keep Alzheimer's disease at bay for a year or so. The recent history of high-technology innovations is full of examples of expensive treatments producing only marginal benefits—but 'marginal' only from some social or financial perspective, but possibly benefiting those who receive them: better marginally treated than wholly dead (if not always).

I begin with these two considerations because it is important to situate the problem of resource allocation for ESRD in the right way. I confess I do not really know just what the 'right' way is, but I will offer some considered guesses about where policy might move. A wrong way of going should at once be put aside. That is to deal with it as an *ad hoc* problem, taking it out of the context of the health care system as a whole.

The characteristic way this is done is simply to ask 'How much should a country be spending on ESRD?' There is no reasonable way of answering that question without nesting it within a number of far broader questions. There is the economist's classic query about the opportunity costs of the program: are there some other ways of spending the money that would produce a better overall health outcome for the country? To which the answer is: possibly so. There is the egalitarian's question whether it is fair to single out—without any comparative policy analysis at all—one disease among many and make it, and it alone, the beneficiary of a seemingly limitless federal entitlement? To which the answer is simple: no.

Then there is the question that devotees of quality-adjusted life years (DALYs) and disability-adjusted life years (QALYs) can ask, whether there is a good return for the money (Harris, 1987; Barker and Green, 1996; Bleichrodt and Johannesson, 1997; Hyden, 1998; Murray and Acharya, 1997)? To which the answer is: well, it is a better investment than, say, bone marrow transplants for late-stage breast cancer, which is widely used despite the lack of any good evidence of its efficacy.

There is, finally, the question an advocate of formal priority setting for limited health care budgets can ask: after a lengthy public debate and a comparison with other health care needs, what priority would ESRD merit (Donaldson and Mooney, 1991; Ham, 1997)? Maybe not so high as at present, which is in effect at the very top of the list—but then it is the only disease as such on the entitlement list in the United States. In any event, most present trends indicate that the future of health care in the United States will be marked by a general increase in medical and economic circumstances similar to those characteristic of ESRD. It thus stands as an apt model of what will increasingly be a generic resource allocation issue.

My approach to the problem will begin with a number of assumptions, none of which I believe are particularly controversial (Levinsky and Rettig, 1991; Nissenson and Rettig, 1999; Rettig, 1996). For the foreseeable future it is reasonable to expect that dialysis will, in the absence of a sufficient supply of transplantable kidneys, be the main line of defense against ESRD; that the number of dialysis patients will continue to grow and that the majority of patients in the future will be over 65, with a potentially great (though not inevitable) increase of those over 75; that the future of the ESRD program will be affected by the future of Medicare's more general response to the costs of care for the elderly; that the cost per patient will continue to climb, fueled by improved technology and greater longevity on dialysis; that the quality of life on dialysis will remain poor, even if acceptable to most of those receiving it; and that, in general, the benefit of dialysis will remain marginal, offering a costly treatment with a comparatively short life expectancy. This last-mentioned feature places it in the growing category of other marginal treatments that do not cure, do not offer a restoration to normal functioning, but expensively prolong a life of chronic invalidism, all of which may be acceptable, if not prized, by patients.

My final assumption, tentatively at least for most of this paper, is the most stark: it will be necessary in the United States in the near future, as Medicare runs into more serious problems, to limit the ESRD program, and that will principally mean limiting dialysis. The sooner there is a national debate about how to do that, the better. The public will not then be surprised by what could appear a precipitate conclusion. Note that I do not assume a solution to the shortage of donated organs or that xenotransplantation will come along to save the day. Sobriety requires that an analysis of resource allocation problems does not assume a great technological breakthrough; that is just a way of evading the problem. If such a breakthrough should come, then well and good, that would be wonderful, but that possibility is no excuse not to use the knowledge and information at hand—and only that—as the foundation for any serious reflection on the allocation problem.

Tactics for the control of costs

There are probably no more than four possible ways of controlling—that is, of limiting—ESRD expenditures in the future, and in one way or another each is a form of rationing: (1) to establish publicly visible and known criteria of a medical kind for treatment eligibility as a federal entitlement; (2) to establish a publicly visible age limit on entitlement; (3) to establish some kind of budget cap on dialysis expenditures but leave the choice of eligible patients up to physician discretion; and (4) to use a means-testing approach.

That none of these approaches has passed muster in the past is no reason not to reconsider them. As long as money was, and still is, available to provide dialysis to all comers, and the day of reckoning always put off, there was no real incentive to ration—and plenty of political and other reasons to dodge the matter altogether. My discussion presupposes, *ex hypothesi*, that the problem *must* be solved, and that the available choices will each be unpleasant, probably painful. We will then be faced with a classical moral and political problem, that of choosing the least bad solution.

Explicit, publicly known medical criteria for eligibility

At first glance, the idea of specifying medical criteria as the basis for an entitlement seems obvious and fair. It is obvious in the sense that it appears compatible with recent efforts to establish evidence-based medicine as a key component of efficient, cost-effective health care: provide treatment when the evidence for its efficacy is, on balance, strong. It seems fair because it does not use any criteria other than impersonal medical benefits as a means of distributing scarce resources. The use of QALYs has been one frequently proposed method for making such determinations, with DALYs as an alternative approach. In both cases, the specific aim of these techniques has not been to determine if a particular patient should receive a treatment but whether a class of treatments (e.g., dialysis) offers a better use of resources than some alternative uses of the same resources (e.g., prenatal screening programs). These techniques could be adapted to screen individual patients.

For all of its apparent moral congeniality (if I may so put it), efforts to specify medical criteria for the treatment of life-threatening conditions have never fared well (save for cardio-pulmonary resuscitation with terminally ill patients). The main objection has focused on the discrepancy between what outside observers take to be a life of acceptable quality and functioning and what patients themselves consider tolerable (Evans *et al.*, 1985). It is a common phenomenon (and not just with dialysis) that people adapt to a loss of function and an increase in pain and discomfort much better than they themselves expect in advance. The fashioning of a new self-identify is probably the necessary price to be paid for such adaptation, but it can be and is commonly achieved. The elderly seem more able to change in that respect than the young. If they are no longer working, and no longer have the responsibility for child care, they have the time and possibility of living with conditions that might undo younger people.

Now it might well be argued that, even if patients are prepared to put up with a low quality of life for a short period of time, dialysis is simply not a good investment of societal resources. Surely better ways of spending the money to improve health could be found. With that kind of judgment in mind, it might be perfectly possible to fashion some strict treatment standards. But the almost immediate retort to such a proposal is to ask: but whose standard of the quality of life is to be used? That of some expert body or commission, or the patient's physician, or the consensus of nephrologists? But who can claim to be an 'expert' on what kind of life if worth living? Recall the title of a play from the 1970s: *Whose Life Is It Anyway?* If it is the length of life after a treatment that is at stake, a seemingly objective enough criterion, little imagination is required to think of people who, for family or other reasons, would be happy to have a few more years, just a few; and, in any case, much money is spent in other health domains where the prospects are no better.

Surely it might be possible to fashion some ostensibly 'objective' medical standards for eligibility. But it would be hard to demonstrate to almost one and all that they were not arbitrary and that they did not seem to impose some stranger's notion of what would count as a life worth living, or a life worth saving. Anything less than meeting that stringent test would have a poor chance of gaining political acceptance.

Age-based eligibility limits

Since the greatest increase in dialysis patients in recent years has been among those over age 65, with even greater increases expected in the future, it is only reasonable to consider the use of age itself as a standard for the setting of limits (Callahan, 1987). An age limit of, say, 70 or 75 for dialysis eligibility could make an enormous financial difference (and, for the record, I write this as someone who is now 70; hence, it is 'us' I am talking about, not 'them').

Apart from simply saving money, an age limit would have three advantages. First, it would use an objective standard, chronological age, that could be equitably applied to everyone, much as a driving age of 16, or a drinking age of 21, is applied to the young in the United States—and of course it is a standard, with 65 as the starting point, for the US Medicare program itself. Few have ever claimed that the use of 65, a specific age, as a requirement for Medicare eligibility is itself unfair or ageist, even though many have sought to lower that age to take care of those in need below that line. Second, unless one holds that it is the purpose of medicine, and the goal of federal entitlement programs, to carry out an unrelenting war against death, whatever a person's age and whatever the cost, then there is nothing inherently wrong in allowing someone to die from disease in old age. Few previous cultures have considered such deaths evil (even though they often did consider them sad) (Reynolds, 1991). A reasonable goal for a health-care system is to help the young become old, not to help old people become indefinitely older.

Third, since it is the working young who pay for most health-care costs of the elderly, it can be an unfair burden on them to demand that they support an unrelenting battle against mortality in old age, and at that time of life when they have their own families and lives to support. Money taken from the young to pay for the old, particularly if too much money, can also be seen as money that might better be used to improve the health of the young—to help them become old. Nor can it plausibly be argued that, because they will when they become old be the beneficiaries of the next younger generation, there is no problem in their now paying for the present health-care costs of the elderly. Those costs could, if significantly increased, still be an enormous burden, crippling their ability to meet the present needs of their families. It may be a consolation that they will have a better future when old—but that does not help pay their present bills.

Despite what have always seemed to me some compelling arguments in favor of age-based rationing, I soon discovered it is an idea that just about everyone loves to hate (Barry and Bradley, 1991; Binstock and Post, 1991; Vape Kamp, 1998). For many it reeks of ageism, that of using chronological age to stigmatize the old, putting them in a category they have no choice about and then using that to deny them life-saving or life-improving treatments. The campaign against ageism, inspired in great part by the work of Robert Butler in the 1970s, has worked relentlessly to demolish stereotypes about the old and to give them a full share of life unburdened by fixed and often mythical ideas about old age (Butler, 1975). It is then a bucket of harshly cold water to reintroduce age as a standard for discriminatory use, to in effect blame the elderly—so the charge goes—for being a social and economic burden.

A no less common objection is that the aged are an exceedingly heterogeneous group, more so than other age groups, and that a person's chronological age is a meaningless predictor of a person's health or life prospects. An age-based rationing standard would be grossly unjust, treating every elderly person alike, though they are not, and ignoring massive evidence of the gap between chronological age, on the one hand, and health and quality of life, on the other. It could also produce the perverse result of allowing younger people with poor health prospects to receive care that would be denied an older person with otherwise good, even better, health prospects.

Fixed budgets and physician discretion

The essence of the UK way of controlling the cost of dialysis is by forcing doctors to live with fixed budgets but at the same time allowing them considerable freedom in deciding how to spend the money they are allotted. The high cost of dialysis and its obviously heavy burden on any fixed budget makes it a natural target for rationing, particularly for the elderly. (Wing, 1990). The rationing in the UK is accomplished not by any formal, explicit rules against dialysis for the old, but by informally limiting referrals to specialist consultants who treat ESRD. The rationale given to patients is typically not an economic rationale at all, but instead a medical excuse; that is, that a patient is just not a good candidate for dialysis. A medical myth is thus maintained, seemingly having nothing to do with health-care budgets.

While the average age of referrals to dialysis has gone up significantly in recent years, well above the age 55 first reported in *The Painful Prescription*, the dialysis rate in the United Kingdom is still below that of the United States. There is also a great variation in those rates and the informal age standards from region to region. Better informed and more aggressive patients, moreover, know how to use pressure and knowledge to gain dialysis that might otherwise be denied.

In their much praised book *Tragic Choices*, Guido Calabresi and Philip Bobbit (1978) argued that when societies are faced with unpalatable tragic choices they will frequently hide those choices. That is what the British have traditionally done with dialysis, right up to the present, and there is some evidence this happens in Canada as well (Levine, 1998; McKenzie, 1998). The advantages of this strategy are many: it avoids the nasty politics of open rationing, it allows physicians considerable freedom to do as they choose, and it offers patients a plausible reason for the care denied to them. The disadvantages are no less apparent: the public is deceived about what is going on, physicians are given discretionary power but with no formal accountability for its use, and there is no open debate about where, if rationing is needed, it should at best be focused. Dialysis is picked on principally because of its cost.

At the same time, I should note, I have heard many American nephrologists say that they feel their hands are tied by the present system. Since the treatment is provided free by Medicare, there are no economic reasons to say no to patients, and because the patient is left to be the final judge of what constitutes an acceptable reason for going on dialysis, the physician's judgment is bypassed. If UK physicians are effectively forced by budget restraints to say no to some patients, they are also left with the freedom to use their clinical judgment to say yes. In that sense, they have the best of both worlds: they can provide dialysis if they choose to do so on clinical grounds, and they can use clinical grounds as a cover for an economic decision if they choose not to do so.

But it is precisely this combination of discretion and disingenuousness that can be the source of injustice and an arbitrary use of physician power. It is hard to imagine that this kind of system would be acceptable in the United States, though not hard to imagine that something like it might be tried. If dialysis was ever put in the hands of Health Maintenance Organization (HMO) managers who had to live with tight budgets, subterfuge of this kind might well be tempting (though I would hope that the temptation would be rejected and more open, fairer methods of rationing chosen).

Means-testing

As has been much discussed in the debate about the future of Medicare, the idea of some form of means-testing offers one seemingly attractive option. The argument is simple and straightforward: why should patients receive free what they could afford to pay for, in whole or part? This argument applies, for example, in the United States where the Medicare program as a whole is projected to run into devastating financial problems in the years ahead (Bipartisan Commission, 1994). Even if some strict means-testing plan seems unfeasible—cutting the highly affluent off from the entitlement altogether—would it not at least make sense to institute some kind of co-payment plan, scaling it according to ability to pay? To add strength to such arguments, public opinion surveys in the United States have shown that some form of means-testing is, at this point, about the only acceptable way of controlling Medicare costs (Kaiser Family Foundation, 1994).

Yet neither the commonsensical quality of the arguments nor the findings of public opinion polls will necessarily carry the day. In the United States, a large number of people believe that Medicare is an entitlement program that is not an act of charity by Congress, but something that people are owed by virtue of money taken from them by payroll taxes over the years. It is an entitlement based on a congressional promise to return benefits based on worker's contributions over the years. Many liberals look with horror at the idea of means-testing, not so much because the affluent would have to pay for what is now free, but because Medicare has always been seen as a forerunner of universal health care and a model of the way the health care system as a whole should be run.

There are some even more severe economic concerns about means-testing, at least if it is seen as a cost-saving panacea. The high average cost of dialysis, now over $50000 a year, would put it either totally out of the range of most elderly people or force many of them to beggar themselves to find the money (as is often now the case with long-term care). Some people could surely pay for it, but probably not enough—and especially those over 75—to realize significant savings. The fact that minorities, and African-Americans in particular, are far more likely than whites to suffer from

ESRD and are also poorer in old age, would almost surely raise the specter of racism if means-testing was required; and that would be true, I suspect, even if few blacks would be kept from dialysis because of such tests.

As for younger people, now covered by Medicare for ESRD, if they ended in the marginal category of those too well-off to qualify for full coverage but not well off enough to comfortably afford the costs of a frugal means-testing program, many would be faced with giving up a large portion of their income needed for their own families. The history of Medicare offers many cautionary tales about means-testing, from fraud in gaining coverage, through the indignity of financial screening, to the point of just missing the eligibility cut-off point. The fact that the large majority of the 44 million or so uninsured in the United States have too high an income to qualify for Medicaid, but not enough money to afford health insurance, is not a history encouraging to the idea of means-testing.

No exit?

A review of the history of arguments about controlling the escalating costs of the ESRD program, and of US Medicare more generally, is not one to encourage optimism about setting limits for that program. Just about every possible policy direction has its critics lined up and ready to leap out with their knives sharpened. But haven't I forgotten one possible policy solution? What about having a fixed or otherwise limited budget and then organizing local or regional committees to make patient-by-patient allocation decisions? If that idea sounds familiar, it is because that is where the dialysis struggle first began in the early 1970s when dialysis machines were in short supply.

As is well known and often recalled, a committee in Seattle was formed to choose patients for the limited number of machines. It turned out to be terrible to make such decisions, to pit one life against another, and it was the failure of that committee to find a satisfactory way of making its decisions that was responsible in part for the 1972 ESRD legislation. One might speculate, moreover, whether it would not now be even more difficult to cut back on a long-standing entitlement, forged out of distress at the prospect of nasty rationing, then it was to put it into place at the outset. My guess is that it would be, but much will depend on available resources.

Another reflection suggests itself when the history of ESRD legislation in the United States is considered. The failure of Congress to create comparable entitlement programs for other diseases—or the universal health care necessary to cover all diseases—suggests that it learned a kind of lingering, hard-to-forget lesson: once open-ended entitlement programs are in place, it will be exceedingly difficult to reduce their coverage if life itself is at stake. The mid-1970s was one of those periods when talk of universal health care was once again in the air in the United States, and a bipartisan bill toward that end was introduced—unsuccessfully—in the US Senate by Senators Edward M. Kennedy and Jacob Javits in 1975. At least one reason it failed was precisely an anxiety about the control of costs once such a program was underway. The Medicare program, and the ESRD program, both of which saw costs quickly escalating beyond early predictions, were object lessons hard to ignore.

Is there no exit here? The picture I have drawn is one in which every way out seems blocked by ethical and political objections, and they have been sufficient to keep the ESRD program going. I say 'sufficient' because it is likely also the case that there has always been enough money available from the US federal government to pay for the program, and that has been the 'necessary' condition for its continuance.

There are three plausible future possibilities, each of them stemming from quite different situations but all pointing to the same policy outcome. One of them is a severe national economic crisis at some point in the future, an epic depression, forcing cutbacks in even the most well-established and popular entitlement programs. Another is the prospect of severe rationing in the next 20 years or so as the Medicare program (and perhaps other national health programs) is forced to reduce its pace of program growth needed to keep up with the retiring baby boom generation. Still another prospect is that, finally, a universal health care bill will be passed. If that is the case, and if the cost of such a bill is to be sustainable, then there will have to be some rationing (as is the case in every other country with such legislation).

Which ever of these possibilities presents itself, something would have to be done about the program. And at that point, the strategies I discussed above—all of which have hitherto been found wanting—would have to be reconsidered. I have long felt that, for the reasons outlined above, a formal age limit on expensive, high-technology medicine (though coupled with good primary care as well as decent long-term care) would be the fairest solution—if democratically implemented, and with the agreement of the elderly themselves. But no country has ever put in place such a formal policy and I have come to doubt that any country, and particularly the United States, ever will. Politically, it would be much too blunt and much to easy to identify those who would be the losers under such a policy.

Indeed, if the past history of efforts to ration health care is any guide, no policy that is too open in its tactics and whose victims would be too easily identifiable is likely to succeed politically. The rationing would have to be obscured by ambiguous policies and its victims be 'statistical' not identifiable victims. That would also mean that the use of specific medical criteria for denying treatment would have to be ruled out as well. For it too would have identifiable victims. I say this not out of cynicism but because it is probably true, as Calabresi and Bobbit (1978) argued in *Tragic Choices*, that it is too hard to openly face truly nasty decisions. An official pretense of ignorance at what is happening will most likely prevail.

If that last speculation is correct, that leaves two realistic possibilities. Means-testing is one of them, almost certain in any case for the future of Medicare in the United States, and likely to gain public support. But, as suggested earlier, that policy would probably not realize a significant saving, given the high annual cost of dialysis and the likelihood that the majority of patients could not afford it.

We are left then with the plausible possibility of forcing physicians to work with set budgets, leaving it to them to make the hard decisions behind a veil of discretion if not secrecy—but sparing them, in return, from invasive oversight and the threat of law suits and criminal prosecution. That is the way the UK system has been run, and not unsatisfactorily even though there are from time to time complaints about the denial of life-saving treatments to patients. But these complaints have not been effective in increasing the budget of the National Health Service. There are, as noted, great possibilities for injustice to individuals in that kind of system, but also tacit respect for the needs of different age groups. An open-ended spending of money to extend the life of the elderly, who have already run the race of life, is not considered a 'need' of the elderly as a group.

There is one option I have not explored here, and to me it would be the ideal. It would be a priority-setting scheme along the lines of that now used by the US state of Oregon in its Medicaid program for the poor. That scheme blends public contributions and professional judgment to develop a rank-ordering of treatments, to be funded according to the available budget allocated by legislatures. But no other state has chosen to emulate Oregon, and it is even less likely it could be achieved at a national level. In the Oregon plan, moreover, life-saving therapies have a high ranking and it is easily imaginable that they would continue to do so in any other state or national plan (because of the identifiable victim stigma).

There is one final plausible possibility, flying in the face of my initial assumption that something decisive must be done about the ESRD program: that the US will remain prosperous enough, and the critics of rationing strong enough, that muddling through as is now done will continue to prevail. There would surely be much nibbling around the edge of the program, shaving costs, cutting moral corners—continuing to refuse, for instance, to build inflation into dialysis reimbursement as is now the case—and maybe some discreet *ad hoc* rationing at the bedside by physicians, but leaving an intact if increasingly starved program.

The United States has proven itself exceedingly adept at not solving, or even directly confronting, long-standing problems. That one generation of reformers after another ever since the Second World War has predicted, wrongly so far, the creation of a universal health plan tells a sad but persistent story of hopes dashed and irrationality continued. The ESRD story may, for some at any rate, have a somewhat different and happier moral. That is the capacity of the country to continue financing a program that has so much going against it financially, and yet has saved so many lives over the years. For those who hold this view, it will be the capacity of the ESRD program to *resist* radical reform that will be the great victory.

References

Aaron, H. J., and Schwartz, W. B. (1984). *Painful prescription: Rationing hospital care*. The Brookings Institution, Washington.

Barker, C., and Green, A. (1996). Opening the debate on QALYs. *Health Policy and Planning*, 11, 179–83.

Barry, R. L., and Bradley, G. V. (1991). *Set no limits: A rebuttal to Daniel Callahan's proposal to limit health care for the elderly*. University of Illinois Press, Urbana, IL.

Binstock, R. H., and Post, S. G. (1991). *Too old for health care?* The Johns Hopkins University Press, Baltimore, MD.

Bipartisan Commission on Entitlement and Tax Reform (1994). *Final Report*. Superintendent of Documents, Washington.

Bleichrodt, H., and Johannesson, M. (1997). The Validity of QALYs. *Medical Decision Making*, 17, 21–32.

Butler, R. N. (1975). *Why survive? Being old in America*. Harper & Row, New York.

Calabresi, G., and Bobbit, P. (1978). *Tragic choices*. W. W. Norton, New York.

Callahan, D. (1987). *Setting limits: Medical goals in an aging society*. Simon & Schuster, New York.

Chandra, J. M., Schulz, J., Lawrence, C., Greenwood, R. N., and Farrington, K., (1999). Is there a rationale for rationing chronic dialysis? *British Medical Journal*, **318**, 217–23.

Donaldson, C., and Mooney, M. (1991). Needs assessment, priority setting, and contracts for health care: An economic view. *British Medical Journal*, **303**, 1529–30.

Evans, R. W., *et al.* (1985) The quality of life of patients with end-stage renal disease. *The New England Journal of Medicine*, **312**, 553–9.

Ham, C. (1997). Priority setting in health care: Learning from international experience. *Health Policy*, **42**, 49–66.

Harris, J. (1987). QALYfying the value of life. *Journal of Medical Ethics*, **13**, 117–23.

Hyder, A. A., Rotllant, G., and Morrow, R. H. (1998). Measuring the Burden of Disease: Healthy Life Years. *American Journal of Public Health*, **88**, 196–202.

Kaiser Family Foundation/Harvard School of Public Health (1998). *National survey on Medicare: The next big health policy debate?* The Kaiser Family Foundation, Menlo Park, California.

Levine, D. Z. (1998) Would you Deny this patient dialysis? *American Journal of Diseases*, **31**, 131–2.

Levinsky, N. G., and Rettig, R. A. (1991). The Medicare end-stage renal disease program. *The New England Journal of Medicine*, **324**, 1143–8.

McKenzie, J. K. (1998) Dialysis decision making in Canada, the United Kingdom, and the United States. *American Journal of Kidney Diseases*, **31**, 12–18.

Murray, C. J. L., and Acharya, A. K. (1997). Understanding DALYs. *Journal of Health Economics*, **16**, 703–30.

Nicholson, R. H. (1998). Truth lies somewhere if we knew but where. *Hastings Center Report*, **22**, 1999.

Nissenson, A. R., and Rettig, R. A. (1999). *Health Affairs*, **18**, 161–79.

Rettig, R. A. (1996). The social contract and the treatment of permanent kidney failure. *Journal of the American Medical Association*, **275**, 1123–6.

Reynolds, R. (1991). Natural death: A history of religious perspectives. In *Life span: Values and life-extending technologies* (ed. Veatch, R. M.). Harper & Row, New York.

Varekamp, L. J. (1998). Age rationing for renal transplantation? The role of age in decisions regarding scarce life extending medical resources. *Social Science and Medicine*, **47**, 113–20.

Wing, A. J. (1990). Can we meet the real need for dialysis and transplantation? *British Medical Journal*, **301**, 897–90.

13
Economic issues in nephrology practice: Ethical dilemmas

William M. Bennett

On some positions, cowardice asks the question, is it expedient? And then expedience comes along and asks the question—is it politic? Vanity asks the question—is it popular? Conscience asks the question is it right? There comes a time when one must take a position that is neither safe nor politic nor popular—but he must do it because conscience tells him it is right. (Martin Luther King, Jr. 1968)

Introduction

It is clear that since the 1970s health care has become a tremendous economic force in the United States. Nearly 15% of the nation's gross national product is spent on health care-related programs and there are increasing numbers of professionals and non-professionals whose livelihoods are involved in the health care enterprise. For practising physicians in the United States, both academic and private, this has presented a challenge to the traditional doctor–patient relationship that placed the physician in the major advocacy position for patients and their health care needs. Health maintenance organizations and managed care in general are based on the assumption that the financial risk of care can be shared among populations of people. These movements are largely driven by economic considerations, with the serious consequences of erosion of the traditional doctor–patient relationship.

The basic major ethical principle underlying the practice of medicine demands that the physician who assumes responsibility for the care of a patient has an implied contract with that patient to provide his best judgment as to the most appropriate medical care for that individual. The physician's relationship to the whole of society, hospital administrators, economic bottom lines, and other important factors in the entire health care picture should be subservient to the doctor–patient relationship. This principle was articulated by the scholar Moses Maimonides in the twelfth century, 'Do not allow thirst for profit and vision of renown and admiration to interfere with my profession for they are the enemies of truth and of love for mankind and they can lead astray in the great task of attending to the welfare of thy creatures' (Maimonides, 1128–1204). The Oath of Hippocrates, which is the foundation of modern medical ethics, states that 'I will follow that system or regimen which according to my ability and judgment I consider for the benefit of my patients and abstain from whatever is deleterious and mischievous' (Hippocrates, 460–377 BC). These historic statements and principles are under constant attack from policy makers within government and market-driven economic forces. For nephrologists who largely care for complex, seriously ill patients, the imposition of other forces affecting clinical behavior and the implied doctor–patient contract is eroding the basic core values of the profession. Pellegrino and Relman (1999) have recently argued that professional societies must subscribe to ethical principles similar to those of their individual member physicians. In their view, nephrologists should be members of a moral community dedicated to improving the lot of the patients they serve.

Generalist and specialist physicians

Many health care managers believe that general physicians, including family practitioners, general internists, and even obstetricians and gynecologists, can care for most clinical problems competently. By their calculations, this is also the least expensive way to provide care since in general less specialized physicians are paid less than more specialized physicians and use less medical resources. Medicine seems to be the only field of endeavor where knowing less and having less training and experience is thought to be better than knowing more (Culliton, 1994). Easy access to specialists for patients with complex problems such as chronic renal failure is explicitly discouraged by many managed care plans in the United States and by a number of governmental health plans in other countries. The politically popular concept of the generalist physician functioning as a barrier to specialist referral also has been embraced widely in academic centers in the United States. This concept is largely driven by economic forces; many believe that specialty care must be limited in its scope if society is to afford comprehensive medical care for the population. This concept has never been studied adequately and has in effect been imposed by managers as a fait accompli without the informed consent of the people. In fact, the few studies that have been performed show that superior diagnostic and clinical skills in caring for complex medical problems permit the specialist get to a correct answer more quickly and less expensively than less well trained providers. The latter usually have not seen adequate numbers of patients with such problems to be able to provide comparably efficient and effective diagnosis and treatment (Jaspen 1997; Nash *et al.*, 1997).

For patients burdened with chronic renal disease, it is clear that dual medical care by general physicians and subspecialists is inefficient and burdensome. Since all nephrologists are by training general internists first and nephrologists second, there seems to be no a priori reason to presume practicing nephrologists who see patients frequently have lost their general medical knowledge and skills (Bennett and Langdon, 1997). In many US managed-care plans, both for-profit and not-for-profit, the determination of medical necessity by untrained people compounds the problem (Rosenbaum *et al.*, 1999). Specialists such as nephrologists are sometimes accused of excessively aggressive medical care, for example, the use of dialysis in the very elderly. There is no evidence that subspecialists provide futile care more often than generalist physicians. However, it is important to define futility narrowly as medical care that has no more than a remote chance of maintaining or restoring a quality of life acceptable to the patient. It must be separated sharply from complex, expensive care *per se* or from care of the elderly who are presumed to be 'at the end of life'. Futility should not be used as a justification for implicit rationing. Implicit rationing of complex healthcare by private managed-care organizations or national health plans may be financially desirable but it risks discrimination against older patients, patients likely to have poor outcomes because of comorbid disease, and more generally all those who are seriously ill. While this may be good economic and public policy on a societal level, it leaves the physician with the ethical dilemma of fulfilling the implied contract with patients in a hostile environment with artificial barriers interposed (Rosenbaum et al., 1999). By submitting to such non-patient factors in clinical decision making, the individual physician will erode the trust of patients in the fundamental ethical contract. They will no longer believe that their doctors are fiduciaries for the welfare of their patients.

Explicit rationing, in which society decides to set limits on available medical care by a public process, is ethically more acceptable than hidden or implicit rationing. However, it is far more difficult to impose. An illustrative case was the program in the US State of Oregon. The Governor, in proposing an explicit rationing program for poor people whose health care is supported by the governmental Medicaid program, stated that 'the Hippocratic Oath is outdated for the 20th century' (Greenberg, 1991; Crawshaw, 1992). Fortunately for poor, sick patients, his controversial program has never been fully implemented, since the political will to carry it out was lacking.

In reaching their conclusions about these matters, physicians need to ask themselves what care they would want for their own families. Would they want a family practitioner to provide the gynecologic and obstetric care for their family? Would they want a generalist physician deciding on diagnosis and treatment of nephrologic disorders? I do not think so. However, when this issue is impersonal and framed in the context of the general debate about the cost of healthcare it becomes easy to disenfranchise those who are poor and seriously ill (Burck et al., 1992). Nephrologists need to be accountable according to the professional model rather than economic or political models, as defined by Emanuel and Emanuel (1996). In my view, specialists need to stand up for excellent medical care in this new millennium of dazzling science. We must insist that the care of patients with serious problems be determined by good medical practice. This is not to say that cost and access are irrelevant. However, physicians ultimately have a moral and ethical obligation to patients, not to health care systems.

Access to health care

The passage in 1972 of the US law that funded treatment of end-stage renal disease with dialysis or transplantation by Medicare was unique; no other entitlements for care of a specific disorder have been enacted to this date in the United States. In part this is because Medicare expenditures for end-stage renal disease have increased far beyond original projections. The advent of this program was a blessing to physicians and others who were trying to allocate limited resources to very ill people (Rettig and Levinsky, 1991). This program serves as a model for any complex chronic disease and should be highlighted in the debate about health care delivery systems and access to care. The growth of expenditures is due to the increasing ability of nephrologists to care for older patients and those with co-morbidities such as diabetes, in addition to the younger patients without major co-morbidities originally expected to be the beneficiaries of the program. The cost per dialysis treatment has actually been reduced by about two-thirds since 1972, due to technological advances and economies of scale. The expanded numbers of people who are being treated in 1999 compared with 1970 and the favorable outcomes of those patients—restored to a quality of life acceptable to them albeit not normal—seem to me to be a success rather than an expensive aberration, as some have argued.

A current problem is late referral of patients to end-stage renal disease programs, which is an important determinant of inferior outcomes (Kliger, 1998). Emergency placement of vascular access less than 30 days prior to start of dialysis is a good example. Why are these patients subject to late referral? The most logical explanation is they have little access to health care prior to their presentation as end-stage renal disease patients. The burden of end-stage renal disease is disproportionately large in African-Americans and Hispanics. These are the people, particularly in areas where large minority populations exist, who have the least access to medical care and are the most underserved. Furthermore, the increasing focus on the 'bottom line' even of institutions formerly devoted to the care of the poor and underinsured, such as academic health centers, also has undermined the effort to provide care to the indigent. The public hospital mission has been changing to mimic private, for-profit hospitals even at prestigious institutions that were previously committed to community service. The 'cherry picking' of high-paying patients and insured patients by some health care providers leaves those who are less well endowed to use delivery systems that do not welcome them. This is the case for many nephrologic patients and is a source of discouragement and frustration for many physicians. Providing medical care only to the population that can most afford it violates the basic ethical precepts of medicine, be it academic or private.

Industrialization of nephrology

Industrialization and consolidation of the end-stage renal disease industry has been dramatic during the 1990s. This is shown on page 216 in Figure 13.1. Five to six large companies now provide the dialysis care for the majority of patients in the United States (and in several European countries). There has been a transfer of proprietorship of dialysis units from individual physicians or not-for-profit hospitals to these for-profit companies. Shares in these companies are traded on Wall Street and other equity markets. Some companies are vertically integrated and sell not only dialysis treatments but also dialysis machines and other equipment and laboratory tests. Putative advantages of corporate ownership are efficiencies due to standardized protocols, advanced information systems and purchase of drugs and supplies in bulk. The latter gives the large corporations the power to negotiate favorable rates. One of the major variable costs in dialysis care is the lack of predictability of physicians' clinical behavior. The control of physicians looms as an impending threat if these companies start to lose profit margin and/or their share prices fall. Health care stocks have declined in value while pharmaceutical and biotechnology companies flourish.

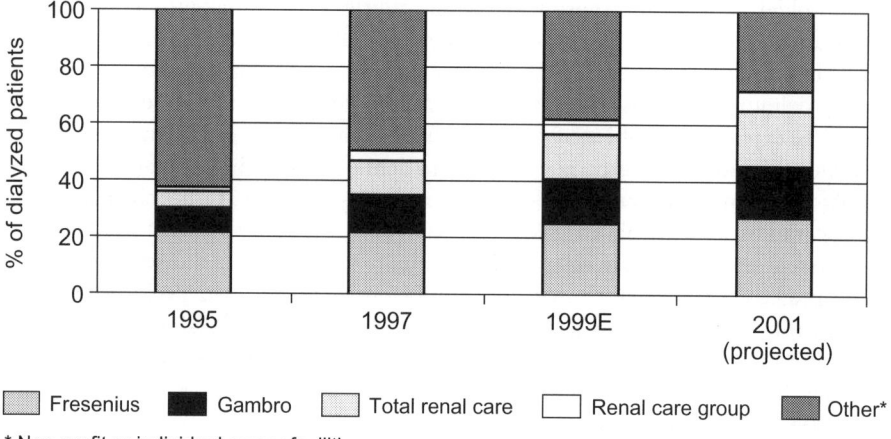

Fig. 13.1 Changes in ownership of U.S. dialysis facilities since 1995.

According to Kuttner (1999) and Massey (1997), pressure to protect profit margins has led to avoidance of cost manifested by denial of care, shunning of sick patients and micromanagement of physicians. Although there is no evidence that the nature of the dialysis procedure itself is altered by unit ownership, there are certainly corporate pressures to increase efficiency and to save money. It should be obvious that better management could present a 'win-win' situation for patient and owner. However, the physician should realize the fine line between efficiency and decreased quality of care. The ethical responsibility of a for-profit chain and a not-for-profit proprietor are not different in terms of patient responsibility. Financial incentives for physicians to control costs are not evidence of misconduct but doctors should be aware of the appearance of conflict of interest. A good rule of thumb for any physician–industry financial relationship is the comfort of the physician with public disclosure.

The industrialization of dialysis ownership can pose many potential ethical conflicts. The complex arrangements for payment of physicians by companies and by Medicare in the United States provide any number of examples, some of which are relevant in other countries. In the United States, nephrologists are compensated for dialysis patients by a capitated fee based on a bundle of services provided monthly. If the patient is hospitalized, in-patient fee for service payment predominates. Compensation of nephrologists by these two mechanisms is generous, in that few nephrologists see their out-patients more often than once or twice per month (Hull, 1999). This is distinctly different from other parts of the world, where patients are seen more frequently, often at each session. It is possible that the higher mortality in US dialysis units versus those in Europe is related in part to the intensity of physician involvement.

Many nephrologists serve as medical directors of dialysis units. They receive compensation for administrative services that are often incompletely defined. In addition to their monthly capitated fees for direct patient care, physician medical directors usually receive $1000–2000 (US) per year per patient for the administrative job. In some units, the medical director designation is dependent on the number of patients that any individual physician has in a dialysis unit. In other words, the nephrologist who refers the most patients is appointed director. This arrangement comes perilously close to breaking laws that prohibit referral to a health care entity in which the owner has a financial interest (Health Care Financing Administration, 1998). Although dialysis is a specific exemption under these regulations, to the extent that companies that provide dialysis services compensate medical directors based on referrals or patient volume, this verges on a violation and probably would not stand outside investigation and scrutiny (Caeser, 1998).

The medical directors in a unit run by a dialysis provider may have subtle pressures or incentives to use the products made by, and laboratory services provided by, that company exclusively even if there are better alternatives. There is no evidence as to how often this occurs but the potential conflict and ethical dilemma for the physician are evident. An example of the conflict between best practice and company economics is whether to prescribe erythropoietin by the intravenous or the subcutaneous route. There is general agreement that the latter has equivalent efficacy and safety with considerably lower doses. Intravenous medications are responsible for much of the profit margin of dialysis units; intravenous administration of drugs such as erythropoietin, iron and to a lesser extent, vitamin D is reimbursed by the federal government at prices negotiated with the drug manufacturer that are high enough to leave a profit margin. The ethical dilemma for the physician is that judgments about best medical practice may be in conflict with the economics of the owner of the dialysis unit. Patient advocacy should be the first consideration of the nephrologist.

Medicine has moved towards practice guidelines to standardize therapy and to improve quality of care. In nephrology, practice guidelines might affect the use of particular products or services. It is apparent that practice guidelines should be free of commercial influence or even the appearance of such. Since each guideline costs at least $100000 (US) to develop, industry support is often sought for developing guidelines. The accumulation of evidence, content of the guideline and application in practice need to be completely independent of the sponsor. Experts from the sponsoring organization should not participate at any level in practice guideline development to avoid conflicts of interest, although the appearance of influence may be hard to avoid completely.

Does ownership influence patient outcomes?

The key issue in evaluating whether the industrialization of dialysis is beneficial or harmful is whether it influences patient outcomes, such as morbidity and mortality. A sparse but growing literature has begun to address this issue. For-profit dialysis facilities in the United States administered lower doses of erythropoietin than not-for-profit facilities at a time when reimbursement policy made this practice more profitable (deLissovoy *et al.*, 1994). Held *et al.* (1991) reported that patients in for-profit facilities underwent fewer hours of dialysis than patients in not-for-profit facilities. Recently, Garg *et al.* (1999) investigated the effect of dialysis facility ownership on patient outcomes. Using the United States Renal Data System database, they found that crude mortality rate per 100 person years was 21.2 for patients treated by for-profit facilities and only 17.1 for patients treated in not-for-profit facilities. This difference of 20% was statistically significant. In addition, the study by Garg *et al.* showed that the likelihood of being placed on a waiting list for a kidney transplant was 26% lower for patients at for-profit centers. However, Ayanian *et al.* (1999) did not find that the profit or non-profit status of the dialysis facility made any difference in access to transplantation. Firm conclusions about these outcome measures are difficult to draw. However, the specter that financial incentives drive reduction in key components of dialysis that in turn compromise quality of care must be considered. My conclusion thus far is that these data demand further study of the influence of ownership on the quality of care of patients with end-stage renal disease.

Academic medicine and nephrology

Institutions that engage in training, teaching, and research as well as patient care also have ethical dilemmas with respect to modern nephrology practice. Some of these issues are relatively subtle. There are major motivations for academic medical centers to be associated with the dialysis industry, providers of health care products and companies that make pharmaceutical preparations useful for patient care. They may include notoriety, support for research infrastructure and opportunities for the academic nephrologist to earn income and other benefits that potentially could compromise a primary mission of patient advocacy and service. Sometimes the incentives that are provided are not necessarily financial (Dieppe *et al.*, 1999).

Much of the research that is directly sponsored by industry is done for the regulatory purposes only and is not of high quality, inasmuch as major research questions are subservient to the FDA drug approval process. Publications are often in journal supplements and are not submitted to critical peer review. Ghost writing of articles by hired writers supported by grants from pharmaceutical companies is common. As opposed to traditional research, industry usually approaches the academic physician rather than the reverse and most of the ideas and protocols are devised by the industry. An interesting study by Shah *et al.* (1999) showed the results in terms of immunosuppressive drugs and transplantation when studies were double blind as opposed to open label, for the same immunosuppressive compounds. Results in terms of efficacy were greater in the open label studies and while adverse effects were fewer. This is perhaps not surprising nor peculiar to nephrology but in these very competitive areas the physician using his academic title has implied authority and impartiality. The doctor serving as a consultant, a member of a speaker's bureau or even owning stock may be compromised in his choice of medications by incentives that are not directly related to patient care.

The educational activities of academic health centers are heavily subsidized by the pharmaceutical industry. While there are established guidelines for such relationships mandating that responsibility for content must rest with the educator, these principles are often eroded. At times pharmaceutical companies and dialysis companies organize and direct educational programs. There is evidence that physician–pharmaceutical company and for-profit company interactions misinform physicians, leading to inappropriate prescribing (Chren, 1999). Waxman and Kimball (1999) point out that continuing medical education is a multibillion dollar industry designed to market products. They call for educational programs in the future that are accountable for the use of clear outcome measures. Industry motivations are usually couched in terms of educating physicians, particularly nephrologists, in high-quality patient care and improved outcomes. However, in a vertically integrated company, this can be self-serving (Chren, 1999). In my view, the profession should resist such incursions by industry into the educational arena and stick closely to guidelines for educational programs that mandate independent professional control.

Conclusion

Modern nephrologic practice is subject to a variety of influences that compromise the traditional doctor–patient relationship. The profession is in danger of abandoning its primary mission and responsibility, which is to speak and act as an advocate for patients. To the extent that this happens it will be a lesser profession. The ethical issues are not particularly difficult to understand but they are very difficult to apply. As in all ethical matters, we should strive to do the right thing as outlined in the quote by Martin Luther King, Jr at the beginning of this chapter.

References

Ayanian, J. Z., Cleary, P. D., Weissman, J. S., and Epstein, A. M. (1999). The effect of patients' preferences on racial differences in access to renal transplantation. *New England Journal of Medicine*, **341**, 1661–9.

Bennett, W. M., and Langdon, L. O. (1997). The nephrologist as the principal care provider for patients with chronic renal disease: The perspective of the American Board of Internal Medicine. *Seminars in Dialysis*, **10**, 324–5.

Burck, R., Sheldon, M., Burton, L. A., Williams, J., Foster, P., Bone, R., Jensen, D., Sankary, H., and Rosenblate, H. (1992). Limiting access and patient selection in liver transplantation. *New England Journal of Medicine*, **326**, 413.

Caeser, N. (1998). Remuneration arrangements important part of Stark II Regulations. *Managed Care*, **7**, 65–6.

Chren, M. (1999). Interactions between physicians and drug company representatives. *American Journal of Medicine*, **107**, 182–3.

Crawshaw, R. (1992). The Oregon Medicaid controversy. *New England Journal of Medicine*, **326**, 642.

Culliton, B. J. (1994). Primary care is not the answer. *Nature*, **370**, 501.

deLissovoy, G., Powe, N. R., Griffiths, R. I., *et al.* (1994). The relationship of provider organizational status and erythropoietin dosing in end-stage renal disease patients. *Medical Care*, **32**, 130–40.

Dieppe, P., Chard, J., Tallon, D., and Egger, M. (1999). Funding clinical research. *Lancet*, **353**, 1626.

Emanuel, E. J., and Emanuel, L. L. (1996). What is accountability in health care? *Archives of Internal Medicine*, **124**, 229–39.

Garg, P. P., Frick, K. D., Diener-West, M., and Powe, N. R. (1999). Effect of the ownership of dialysis facilities on patients' survival and referral for transplantation. *New England Journal of Medicine*, **341**, 1653–60.

Greenberg, D. S. (1991). The Oregon plan on Capitol Hill. *Lancet*, **338**, 808–9.

Health Care Financing Administration (1998). Medicare and Medicaid Programs; Physician referrals to healthcare entities with which they have financial relationships. *63 Federal Register 1659*, **January 9**.

Held, P. J., Levin, N. W., Bovbjerg, R. D., Pauly, M. V., and Diamond, L. H. (1991). Mortality and duration of hemodialysis treatment. *Journal of the American Medical Association*, **265**, 871–5.

Hippocrates of Cos (460–377 BC). Oath of Hippocrates.

Hull, A. R. (1999). Slipping away: Nephrologists are losing control of managing their renal patients. *Nephrology News and Issues*, **September**, 12–4.

Jaspen, B. (1997). Cost effectiveness of cardiology cases handled by generalists studied. *Modern Healthcare*, **March 17**, 23.

King, Jr., M. L. (1968). Sermon entitled 'Remaining Awake Through a Great Revolution' given on 31 March 1968. In, A Knock at midnight: Inspiration from The Great Sermons of Reverend Martin Luther Ling, Jr. Eds. Carson, C., Holloran, P. Warner Books, New York, 1998.

Kliger, A. S. (1998). Clinical practice guidelines and performance measures in ESRD. *American Journal of Kidney Diseases*, **32**, S173–6.

Kuttner, R. (1999). The American health care system: Wall Street and health care. *New England Journal of Medicine*, **340**, 664–8.

Maimon, Rabbi Moshe Ben (AD 1138–1204). Oath of Maimonides.

Massey, R. U. (1997). The industrialization of medicine. *Medicine and Health, Rhode Island*, **80**, 107–8.

Nash, I. S., Nash, D. B., and Fuster, V. (1997). Do cardiologists do it better? *Journal of the American College of Cardiology*, **29**, 475–8.

Pellegrino, E. D., and Relman, A. S. (1999). Professional medical associations: ethical and practical guidelines. *Journal of the American Medical Association*, **282**, 984–6.

Rettig, R. A., and Levinsky, N. G. (eds) (1991). *Kidney failure and the federal government*. Committee for the Study of the Medicare ESRD Program, Institute of Medicine, Washington, DC, National Academy Press.

Rosenbaum, S., Frankford, D. M., Moore, B., and Borzi, P. (1999). Who should determine when health care is medically necessary. *New England Journal of Medicine*, **340**, 229–32.

Shah, M. B., Martin, J. E., Schroeder, T. J., and First, M. R. (1999). The evaluation of the safety and tolerability of two formulations of cyclosporine: Neoral and Sandimmune. *Transplantation*, **67**, 1411–7.

Waxman, H. S., and Kimball, H. R. (1999). Assessing continuing medical education. *American Journal of Medicine*, **107**, 1–4.

PART IV

Ethical issues in non-Western cultures

14
Japan

Atsushi Asai, Yasuhiko Miura, Shizuko Nagata, Shunichi Fukurhara, and Kiyoshi Kurokawa

Introduction

In Japan as in many other countries, health care professionals and society as a whole have become increasingly aware of a growing number of ethical issues in health care since the 1980s. Many issues remain controversial even today; they include to what extent respect for patient autonomy is relevant in decision making; whether or not brain death is the death of the individual; and how decisions about life-prolonging treatments and end-of-life issues should be determined, to name only a few. Under these circumstances, it was not until the end of the 1990s that ethical problems in nephrology began to attract physicians' attention. The available descriptive data on actual practices in nephrology are scant. For instance, discussion about advance directives and termination of dialysis began only in the mid-1990s. The purpose of this chapter is to address the ethical issues involved in Japanese health care in general and to examine those in nephrology in particular. First, as background information, how the Japanese health care system and major religions influence Japanese moral values will be mentioned briefly. Second, the ethical issues affected by the physician–patient relationship, patient autonomy, brain death, and end-of-life decisions will be summarized. Third, the ethical issues in clinical practice in nephrology and kidney transplantation will be discussed.

The health care system, religions, death, and ethics in Japan

The health care system

Japan has a national health care insurance system, and universal coverage has been achieved at relatively low cost. Such health indices as infant mortality and life expectancy at birth are among the best in the world (Ikegami and Campbell, 1995). There are three types of health insurance plans available, including community-based (mainly for the self-employed and pensioners who are aged less than 70), employer-based (employees of most businesses and of national and local government), and health insurance for the elderly aged 70 or above (including bed-ridden elderly aged 65 or above). Every single Japanese is required to be enrolled in one of the three insurance plans, and in principle all patients are free to select the physician or medical institution that gives them care. Few people fail to seek health care because of the possible financial consequences (Tierney, 1994). The majority of medical care providers in Japan are private, but most large hospitals are owned by the national or local governments, voluntary organizations, or universities. The reimbursement is based on a fee-for-service schedule. National fee schedules apply to all Japanese regardless of their health plans and regardless of where they receive care. All physicians can decide by themselves, which medical interventions are appropriate for their patients, provided the recommended procedure or therapy is covered by their insurance (Tierney, 1994; Ikegami and Campbell, 1995). The average duration of hospitalization in Japan is about 35 days, which is much longer than in most Western nations. It is argued that the over-treatment of the elderly, particularly in long-term care, is one of the major problems in the Japanese health-care system (Ikegami and Campbell, 1995). For the elderly, hospitals often function as nursing homes. Hospitalizations for social rather than medical reasons are common: the social reasons include the family's inability to care for their elderly patient in their own home, lack of an available nursing facility, and absence of a family member able to take care of the elderly patient. It is frequently said that the Japanese health-care system's main problem is its low quality. Observers have also criticized the lengthy waiting times and very short patient contact with physicians, insufficient physician explanations to patients about their diagnosis, prognosis, treatment, poor physical facilities, and inadequate medical education and clinical research (Ikegami and Campbell, 1996).

The influence of religion and definitions of death

Ancient religions such as Buddhism and Shintoism (the Japanese traditional belief system arising from a long history of ancestor worship) remain widely influential in Japan (Tierney, 1994). Confucianism has also taken root in the Japanese psyche and influenced behavior for centuries. In combination with the influence of Buddhism and Confucianism, Shintoism, which has governed Japanese spirituality, long ago established a view of death as a curse, of corpses as polluting, and of the spirit of the deceased as something frightening (Young, 1995). Life and this world are valued highly; death is denied and abhorred. The Japanese seldom consider death as an invitation by the Creator (Kodera, 1989). In Confucianism and Shintoism, the body and the soul are viewed as being one in the 'next life' as well as this life, and the dichotomy of body and soul is apparently rejected by a considerable number of Japanese (Kaji, 1990; Tierney, 1994). It is argued that the traditional Japanese image of the human being is one of a completely integrated mind–body unit, rather than distinct and separate units of mind, body, and spirit (Fujita, 1980). This is why some Japanese are extremely reluctant to accept autopsy and brain death. It is also said that some Buddhists regard the extension of life by accepting organs from another individual's body as unnatural, and something unnatural is often regarded as unethical in traditional Japanese culture. In addition, according to Buddhist notions, consciousness is not located solely in the brain, and therefore the cessation of functioning by any one part or organ of the individual is not regarded as the death of the individual (Fujii, 1991; Tamaki, 1993).

Under these circumstances, after an almost 30-year history of debate, a law legally authorizing organ transplantation from a brain-dead individual was enacted by the Japanese government in October 1997 (Akabayashi, 1997). The law provides that brain death may be clinically determined only when a patient has a donor card proving that the patient accepts brain death as his or her death and when the patient's family consents to accept the patient's will. At the time of writing (December 1999), four cases of organ transplantation from brain-dead patients have been reported.

Ethics in Japanese clinical practice: An overview

It is argued that interdependence and harmony have great significance as social values in Japan and that the family or close community has been fostered as the most fundamental social unit in Japanese culture (Tierney, 1994; Fetters, 1998). It is even asserted that a person does not exist as an individual, that is, as an autonomous unit, but only as a member of the family, the community, or society (Tanida, 1996). Under the persistent influence of Confucianism, the Japanese tend to think that ethical obligations are determined by an individual's social position and that his or her duties towards others are those of the person's social roles. Moral duties derived from social roles are often perceived to be more important than those based on simple humanity or personal relations. The Japanese also tend to accept hierarchical human relations and are sometimes willing to follow decisions or recommendations given by authorities such as physicians or bureaucrats without being informed on all the relevant facts.

Ethical decisions in Japanese clinical practice have naturally reflected the aforementioned traditional ethics and morality of Japanese society and culture to a great extent. For example, the physician–patient relationship can be called paternalistic in many cases, and the autonomy of patients' decisions is not regarded as important by physicians, their families, or even the patients themselves (Ishiawata and Sakai, 1994; Asai, 1996). Despite recognition in the press and the literature written in Japanese, informed consent has not yet become well established in actual clinical settings. Medical information of grave importance is not always fully disclosed and the patient is not always told the truth in every instance of patient care, because a considerable number of patients and their family members do not want their caregivers to divulge the complete truth about their conditions (Asai, 1996). It might be argued that, in the medical culture of Japan, no pure bilateral relationship has ever existed between a physician and patient; instead, rather complicated trilateral relations among the physician, the patient's family, and the patient have played significant roles in medical decision making. With regard to end-of-life decisions, which are undoubtedly among the most crucial ethical issues confronted in any clinical setting, much remains inconclusively addressed or controversial in Japan.

Several medical associations and committees consisting of academics and intellectuals have stated their positions on the ethicality of judgments at the end of life. However, these statements and decisions have yet to be legally sanctioned. Legally binding advance directives and do-not-resuscitate orders, for example, do not yet exist in Japan. Even informed consent is not legally regulated in clinical settings. Recent data suggest that Japanese physicians tend to treat terminally ill patients and those in persistent vegetative states aggressively, even when the patients wish or would want otherwise (Asai *et al.*, 1995, 1999). Patients' wishes or advance directives about death with dignity or about peaceful death may frequently be disregarded. The withholding or withdrawal of life support is sometimes perceived as abandonment of the dying patient by the family or the physician in charge (Asai *et al.*, 1997, 1998). Lack of practical and generally accepted guidelines about health-care ethics may lead to inconsistent and idiosyncratic judgments by individual physicians or other health-care professionals. On the other hand, surveys of the general public and patients show that the majority of Japanese want to have their advance directives respected and followed (Akabayashi *et al.*, 1997; Vpltz, 1998).

As for physician-assisted death, two published 'euthanasia' cases in the 1990s triggered a hot debate about the ethicality of mercy killing and the significance of informed consent. In 1995, a Yokohama court defined four essential prerequisites for active euthanasia: (1) that the patient is experiencing intractable physical suffering; (2) that the terminal patient's death is unavoidable; (3) that every method to alleviate the patient's physical suffering has already been exhausted and no alternative is available; and (4) that the patient explicitly expresses the desire to terminate his or her life (Sakamoto and Kitazawa, 1996). A survey on Japanese physicians' attitudes toward voluntary active euthanasia showed that only one of 10 thought it acceptable, even if all of the four prerequisites were met. Another study suggests that more than 60% of Japanese physicians who often care for dying patients regard as ethically acceptable neither voluntary active euthanasia nor assisted suicide and do not apparently make an ethical distinction between voluntary active euthanasia and assisted suicide (Asai *et al.*, 1998). The lack of data makes it impossible to know whether and to what extent physician-assisted deaths are actually occurring in Japan at this moment. Finally, it should be noted that ethical attitudes in clinical practice and the moral values of the Japanese may be in the course of drastic change because of modern means of global communication and the resulting exposure to the strong and rapidly growing influence of Western, especially American, culture. Although Japan is currently Westernizing its medical system, no one can predict what changes in ethical values will occur in Japan in the future.

Ethical issues in nephrology

Current practice in dialysis and organ transplantation: An overview

The Japanese Medical Association of Dialysis reported in 1998 that more than 175 000 patients are currently undergoing chronic dialysis in Japan. The average age of patients undergoing dialysis is 62 years; of all patients undergoing dialysis, approximately 37% are over 65 years old and 23% are 70 or older (Nihon Tokei Igakukai, 1998). It is also reported that the total number of patients undergoing dialysis in Japan comprises about one-fourth the total of all such patients in the world (Miura, 1998). More than 15% of Japanese patients undergoing dialysis require special supportive care because of their disability, and about 5% of inpatients are hospitalized for 'social' reasons (Zenkoku Jinzoubyou Kanja Renrakukaigi, 1997). A 1994 survey shows that 11% of all patients undergoing dialysis are hospitalized, of whom 63% have been in the hospital for more than one year, and about one-fifth have been in the hospital for more than 5 years (Nihon Tokei Igakukai, 1995). Hemodialysis costs from 300000 to 350000 yen on average a month and the cost of continuous ambulatory peritoneal dialysis is about the same. Because of the increase in the number of patients undergoing chronic dialysis, the cost of dialysis accounts for 3.4% of Japan's total health-care expenditure. The Japanese national health-care insurance system has covered the cost of dialysis since 1967. Currently, because of subsidies provided by local communities and government, the amount that a patient undergoing chronic dialysis must pay is no more than 10000 yen a month, and the full cost is covered in many cases (Miura, 1998; Nihon Tokei Igakukai, 1998).

On the other hand, kidney transplantation has been infrequent, and the number of kidneys transplanted annually has gradually decreased. For example, 867 kidney transplants were performed in 1989, 707 in 1991, 662 in 1993, and only 638 in 1996. Data are not available on the relative frequency of organ transplants from cadaver donors and live donors since organ transplantation from brain-dead patients was first legally authorized in Japan, but on average, between approximately 400 and 500 kidneys have been transplanted from live donors and the rest, a few hundred, from cadavers. Even taking the difference in population between Japan and the US into consideration, only one-third as many live donor kidney transplants and one-twentieth as many cadaver donor kidney transplants occur in Japan as in the US (Ohshima and Ono, 1998). There is a very great potential demand for kidneys: in 1997, 84000 patients under the age of 60 were on dialysis and 15000 registered as potential kidney transplant recipients (Amemiya, 1999).

Ethical issues in dialysis and kidney transplantation

Termination of dialysis and advance directives

The exact number of deaths due to termination of dialysis is not known, because the format of medical statistics employed in Japan does not specify this cause of death. In 1995, the total number of deaths of patients who had been undergoing chronic dialysis was 14 200, and 122 deaths were classified as suicide or refusal to undergo dialysis (0.9%) (Maeda, 1997). The available relevant data focusing exclusively on the termination of dialysis have been reported by Seiji Ohira and Sehgal et. al. (Sehgal *et al.*, 1996; Ohira, 1995, 1998); a survey of Japanese nephrologists in 127 medical institutions was conducted by Ohira in 1996 in Hokkaido. About one-third of the responding institutions reported cases where dialysis was discontinued; they reported a total of 105 cases of termination of dialysis. Of these, only 1.9% of the patients left written advance directives, and about one-third reportedly had left an advance directive orally. Approximately one-fourth of the patients were competent and made informed decisions with regard to withdrawal of dialysis. Patients' families and the physicians in charge of these cases made relevant decisions in the remaining cases (72%). When the decision is made to terminate dialysis, one-third of the patients were on ventilators and two-thirds required total parenteral nutrition. In none of the cases was the decision to discontinue dialysis overturned by the patients' families. An international survey of nephrologists in the US, Germany, and Japan conducted by Sehgal et al. in 1995 revealed that Japanese nephrologists withdrew dialysis from 0.7% of their patients in the last year (Sehgal et al., 1996). Only 0.3% of Japanese patients had completed advance directives and such directives were used in decision making for 0.09% of patients. Another survey on Japanese patients conducted by Miura et al. reported that only 16 of 520 patients (3%) answered that they had completed an advance directive or mentioned their wishes directly to their physician in charge (Miura et al. 1997). Thus, discontinuation of dialysis seems to have occurred infrequently and patients presenting advance directives are even more rare in Japan than elsewhere.

Attitudes of patients and physicians towards advance directives affecting dialysis

As shown in the previous section, the use of advance directives is not established in Japan, and the percentage of patients who have completed written advance directives is very low. The findings on Japanese attitudes toward the use and significance of advance directives is summarized in the following. Miura et. al. conducted a nationwide cross-sectional survey of 630 patients undergoing dialysis in 1997 (Miura et al., 1997). Of those who responded (the response rate was 83%), more than four-fifths of the patients desired to leave advance directives expressing their wish not to undergo unwanted life-sustaining treatments, including dialysis. As for the format of advance directives, most patients wanted to talk to their family about their wishes (oral advance directive) and less than one-fifth wanted to complete a written advance directive. The patients varied greatly in how much leeway they would give surrogates or physicians to override their advance directives: 'no leeway' (12%), 'a little leeway' (35%), 'a lot of leeway' (37%), and 'complete leeway' (9%).

Miura et al. (1998a) also conducted a group interview with Japanese nephrologists to reveal their attitudes toward advance directives and death with dignity. It revealed that Japanese nephrologists, like Japanese physicians in general, thought that advance directives were useful in decision making and wished to respect them. On the other hand, the participating physicians expressed certain worries about advance directives, including, for example, the possibility that patients might change their minds, that patients' families might file law suits for murder, and that differences in the health-care and legal systems and culturally distinctive attitudes towards individual dignity in Japan might impair the functioning of advance directives in Japan. The aforementioned study by Sehgal et al. (1996) of nephrologists in three nations and the frequency with which they terminate dialysis also suggested that the family has a major influence upon Japanese physicians' decisions. It showed that 88% of physicians responding to a hypothetical vignette would withdraw hemodialysis from an incompetent patient if a patient left an advance directive expressing his or her wishes to do so and family members agreed with his or her advance directive, while less than one-fifth would withdraw dialysis from such a patient if a family member insisted on continuing dialysis despite the patient's advance directive not to do so. Another small-scale study conducted in one Japanese hospital showed the same tendency (Maeda, 1998). The results suggest that the majority of physicians and nurses questioned would terminate dialysis if both a patient and his or her family wanted to discontinue it, while considerably less than half would do so if only the patient desired dialysis to be withdrawn. Thus, in Japanese clinical settings, the patient's family plays a significant role in decision making. These studies suggest that the wishes of the patient's family have serious impacts on physician's medical decisions, especially end-of-life decision making.

Predictions of patients' wishes about advance directives regarding withdrawal of dialysis

Surrogate judgment by the patient's family, or sometimes by the patient's physician, has been proposed as a method of respecting the autonomy of the incompetent patient. In Japan, where informed consent is not yet well established and patients are not always told the truth about their condition, surrogate decisions are frequently used for the conscious and competent patient. It is argued—in fact, it is a die-hard belief—in Japan that people can communicate their thoughts or wishes to one another without explicit oral communication, a process called 'ishin-denshin' in Japanese. Being thoughtful for others, especially close relatives or friends, through this indirect communication has long been regarded in Japanese society as virtuous behavior. Little is known, however, about the accuracy of the predictions of patients' preferences made by the patients' family or physician in clinical settings. Miura and his colleagues conducted a survey to clarify to what extent the family and physicians can predict patients' wishes regarding their dialysis and end-of-life decision-making (Miura *et al.*, 1998b). The survey in 11 prefectures in Japan studied about 400 patients undergoing chronic dialysis, as well as one of the family members playing a key part in each patient's treatment decisions and the patient's nephrologist. The results show that neither the patient's family nor the physician can predict better than chance alone a patient's preferences regarding cardiopulmonary resuscitation (CPR), either in the patient's current medical situation, or in cases where the patient is affected by severe dementia, or in cases of terminal cancer. This is also the case for the patient's wishes regarding discontinuance of dialysis. For instance, the patient's family correctly predicted the patient's preferences regarding CPR while the patient is in the current medical condition in 65% of all cases; the Kappa coefficient in this case is just 0.24; physicians accurately predicted their patient's wishes regarding continuance of dialysis if the patient should suffer from severe dementia in 57% of all cases; the Kappa coefficient in this case is only 0.18.

Informed consent in dialysis and refusal of treatment

The significance and importance of informed consent in the initiation and maintenance of dialysis is being increasingly recognized, although it has been pointed out that obtaining valid and reliable informed consent is difficult. Patients who require dialysis often do not understand what dialysis is like, and some refuse it because they overestimate its discomfort. The fact that a patient requires dialysis to survive sometimes triggers desperation in the patient and refusal to allow treatment (Harada, 1997). Some nephrologists have reported specific cases of refusal of dialysis: for example, a

Buddhist monk with end-stage renal disease initially refused to undergo dialysis, maintaining that he would rather die, because living dependent on a dialysis machine would be inconsistent with his values. After several months of persuasion, however, he accepted dialysis and declared in the end that he had not imagined how simple the procedure was and that undergoing dialysis and surviving was the right choice (Miura et al., 1998a). Thus, it can be argued that a patient's difficulty in understanding the real nature of dialysis sometimes invalidates informed consent. Japanese physicians' inability to give adequate medical explanations to patients has also been noted: a survey on 1000 patients who have undergone dialysis for one or two years revealed that less than two-fifths of the patients were satisfied with their physician's explanation (Ohira, 1997). Due to the lack of data on the non-initiation of dialysis for severely ill patients with irreversible organ failure, it is not known what kind of disclosure is being given, what decisions are being made, and by whom they are being made.

One landmark decision by the courts in Japan, however, did rule on a physician's refusal to provide dialysis to a mentally ill patient (Nakatani, 1998). A 42-year-old woman with schizophrenia was brought into a prefectural hospital twice with severe diabetic renal failure requiring dialysis. A physician at the hospital refused to provide her with dialysis because of her psychiatric illness. The patient died three days after the refusal. Her parents sued the physician and the hospital. The court of appeals made the final decision that physicians have the legal duty to treat unless the provision of treatment is physically impossible. The defendant argued that the patient's medical condition made it impossible for her to continue long-term dialysis and that the patient's ability to understand the medical situation, self-management, and family support were necessary, but the court rejected this argument. This court decision has had a tremendous impact on decisions regarding initiation of dialysis made by nephrologists in Japan.

Ethical issues in kidney transplantation

As mentioned previously, the total number of kidney transplantations is lower in Japan than in other countries, the number performed annually has been decreasing for unknown reasons, and twice as many kidney transplants are performed from live donors as from cadaver donors. Thus far, Japanese attitudes toward life and death that make patients unwilling to undergo an organ transplantation and the lack of the spirit of mutual aid for others beyond close relatives have often been discussed as the main ethical issues (Ohkubo, 1995). A recent nationwide study on renal transplant recipients suggests that such patients tend to rate their own health status very low compared with patients in other countries. This, the authors argue, is because renal transplantation is a very unusual procedure and this realization itself can lower patients' perceptions of their own health status. Because they know that their lives depend on an extremely unusual form of treatment, it is reasonable for these patients to see themselves as being in very poor health (Tsujihayashi et al., 1999). Since October 1997, brain death has been accepted in Japan as the death of the individual; it is expected that this will lead to an increase in the number of kidney transplants and that new ethical issues, including fair resource allocation and transparency of transplantation medicine, may arise from these changes and confront Japanese society.

Conclusion

The care of patients with end-stage renal disease involves a variety of ethical problems, many of which remain unresolved. It is likely that new legislation permitting the retrieval of organs from brain-dead patients and increased recognition of the significance of patient self-determination through informed consent and advance directives will add more complicated moral dilemmas to clinical practice. Japanese society as a whole will confront the need to establish consistent ethical norms and a fair decision-making process in order to solve these problems and to satisfy patients' health-related preferences.

Authors thank Mr Christopher Holmes for his kind work in editing this chapter.

References

Akabayashi, A. (1997). Finally done–Japan's decision on organ transplantation. *Hasting Center Report*, 27, 47.

Akabayashi, A., Kai, I., Ito, K., and Tukui, M. (1997). The acceptability of advance directives in Japanese society. *Journal of the Japan Bioethics Association*, 7, 31–40.

Amemiya, H. (1999). Current status of organ transplantation in Japan. *Transplantation Proceedings*, 31, 1990–1.

Asai, A. (1996). Barriers to informed consent in Japan. *Eubios Journal of Asian and International Bioethics*, 6, 91–3.

Asai, A., Fukuhara, S., and Lo, B. (1995). Attitudes of Japanese and Japanese-American Physicians towards life-sustaining treatment. *Lancet*, 346, 356–9.

Asai, A., Inoue, S., Miura, Y., Tanabe, N., and Fukuhara, S. (1997). Medical decisions concerning the end of life: A discussion with Japanese physicians. *Journal of Medical Ethics*, 23, 323–7.

Asai, A., Miura, Y., Tanabe, N., Kurihara, M., and Fukuhara, S. (1998). Advance directives and other medical decisions concerning the end of life in cancer patients in Japan. *European Journal of Cancer*, 34, 1582–6.

Asai, A., Maekawa, M., Akiguchi, I., Fukui, T., Miura, Y., Tanabe, N., *et al.* (1999). Survey of Japanese vegetative states. *Journal of Medical Ethics*, 25, 302–8.

Fetters, M. M. (1998). The family in medical decision making: Japanese perspectives. *Journal of Clinical Ethics*, 9, 132–46.

Fujita, S. (1980). *Sei to shi no mirai* (Ethics of life and death). Asahi Shimbunsha, Tokyo.

Fujii, S. (1991). 'Buddhism and Bioethics' Theological Developments in Bioethics; 1988–1990. In (ed. B. Andrew Lustig) *Bioethics yearbook*, vol 1, pp. 61–8. Kluwer, Dordrecht.

Harada, T. (1997). Koreisha niokeru infomudo konnsennto (Informed consent for elderly patients). *Toseki Fronteer*, 7, 6–9.

Ikegami, N., and Campbell, J. C. (1995). Medical care in Japan. *New England Journal of Medicine*, 333, 1295–9.

Ikegami, N., and Campbell, J. C. (1996). *Nippon no Iryo* (Medical Care in Japan). Chuko Shinsho, Tokyo.

Ishiwata, R., and Sakai, A. (1994). The physician–patient relationship and medical ethics in Japan. *Cambridge Quarterly of Healthcare Ethics*, 3, 60–6.

Kaji, N. (1990). *Jukyo towa?* (What is Confucianism?). Nanika Kyuko Shinsho, Tokyo.

Kodera, S. (1989). Nippon-jin no seimei-kan. In (eds Tomoshi Tsukazaki and Naoki Kamo) *Seimei-rinri no genzai* (Japanese concept of life), pp. 51–69. Sekaishiso-Sha, Kyoto.

Maeda, K. (1997). *Wagakuni no touseki ryouhou no genjo as of December 31, 1996* (Current situation of dialysis treatment in Japan as of December 31, 1996). Nihon Toseki Igakukai, Tokyo.

Maeda, T. (1998). Japanese religious values, the philosophy of life and death of aged person, the dignity death, and the withdrawal of dialysis. *Rinshotoseki*, 14, 1315–24.

Miura, Y. (1998). Toseki chiryou no dounyu to kanja no rieki, (Introduction of dialysis and benefits of patients). *The Japanese Journal of Nursing*, 62, 26–34.

Miura, Y., Asai, A., Fukuhara, S., and Tanabe, N. (1997). Advance directives nikansura kenkyu (A study of advance directives). Kenkyu Hokokusho of a Grant for Scientific Research Expenses of the Ministry of Health and Welfare of Japan; Funds for Comprehensive Research on Long Term Chronic Disease (Renal Failure) 7–11.

Miura, Y., Asai, A., Fukuhara, S., Matsumura, S., Tanabe, N., Masakane, I, et. al. (1998a). Japanese physicians: Views of ethical problems in dialysis therapy and advance directives. *Tosekikaishi*, 31, 1221–5.

Miura, Y., Asai, A., Fukuhara, S., and Tanabe, N. (1998b). Advance directives nikansura kenkyu (A study of advance directives). Kenkyu Hokokusho of a Grant for Scientific Research Expenses of the Ministry of Health and Welfare of Japan; Funds for Comprehensive Research on Long Term Chronic Disease (Renal Failure) 10–15.

Nakatani, K. (1998). Discretion of medical doctors and law. *Rinshotoseki*, 14, 1315–24.

Nihon Toseki Igakukai Tokeichosa Iinkai. (1995). *Wagakuni no touseki iryouhou no genjo as of December 31, 1994* (Current situation of dialysis treatment in Japan as of December 31, 1994). Nihon Toseki Igakukai, Tokyo.

Nihon Toseki Igakukai Tokeichosa Iinkai. (1998). *Wagakuni no touseki iryouhou no genjo as of December 31, 1997* (Current situation of dialysis treatment in Japan as of December 31, 1997). Nihon Toseki Igakukai, Tokyo.

Ohira, S. (1995). Toseki no kyohi, keizoku, chushi. In (eds Ohhira, S., Miki, T., and Maeda, T.) Koreisha no toseki–Dounyu kara follow-up made (Treatment refusal, continuation, and termination of dialysis treatment: From introduction through follow-up), pp. 212–21. Nippon Medical Center, Tokyo.

Ohira, S. (1997). Toseki iryo kakudankai niokeru informed consent (Informed consent in the process of dialysis). *Tokeikaishi*, 30, 1347–62.

Ohira, S. (1998). Toseki no chushi (Termination of dialysis). *Rinsho Toseki*, 14, 1341–7.

Ohkubo, M. (1995). The quality of life after kidney transplantation in Japan: Results from a nationwide questionnaire. *Transplantation Proceedings*, 27, 1452–7.

Ohshima, S., and Ono, Y. (1998). Renal transplantation. *Nichigekaishi*, 99, 765–9.

Sakamoto, T., and Kitazawa, K. (1996). Confronted with 'death'. *Nikkei Medical*, 10, 46–60.

Sehgal, A. R., Weisheit, C., Miura, Y., Butzlaff, M., Kielstein, R., and Taguchi, Y. (1996). Advance directives and withdrawal of dialysis in the United States, Germany, and Japan. *Journal of the American Medical Association*, 276, 1652–6.

Tamaki, K. (1993). *Seimei towa nanika?* (What is life?). Hozokan, Kyoto.

Tanida, N. (1996). 'Bioethics' is subordinate to morality in Japan. *Bioethics*, 10, 201–11.

Tierney, L. M. (1994). An experience in Japanese academic medicine. *Western Journal of Medicine*, 160, 139–45.

Tsujihayashi, Y., Fukuhara, S., Green, J., Takai, I., Shinazato, T., Uchida, K., et al. (1999). Health-related quality of life among renal-transplant recipients in Japan. *Transplantation*, 68, 1331–5.

Vpltz, R., Akabayashi, A., Reese, C., Ohi, G., and Sara, H. M. (1998). End-of-life decisions and advance directives in palliative care: A cross-cultural survey of patients and health-care professionals. *Journal of Pain and Symptom Management*, **16**, 153–62.

Young, K. K. (1995). Death: Eastern thought. In (ed. Reich WT). *Encyclopedia of bioethics* (revised edn), pp. 487–97. Macmillan Library Reference USA, New York.

Zenkoku jinzoubyou kanja renrakukaigi. (1997). Youkaigo tokeikanja mondai (Problems with dialysis patients who require nursing care). *Zenjinkyou SSKA*, **160**, 3–8.

15
China
Lei-Shi Li and Xiao-Dan Yao

Introduction

China has a long cultural history of more than 5000 years, and traditional medicine has been an important part of this ancient civilization. In the long run of medical practice, traditional Chinese medicine has developed a classic system of its own ('*YIN-YANG WU-XING*' theory), which is still widely accepted and practised among the vast population of China. In the practice of traditional medicine, ethical disciplines have been established and generally accepted. Confucianism and Buddhism exert prominent influence on medical practice as well as medical ethics. All these combine to form the unique aspect of Chinese medical ethics, which is distinctly different from that of the Western world.

Ethical issues were discussed in both philosophical works of literature and classics of traditional Chinese medicine. The ethical essence of compassion and saving lives is found in the earliest record of '*DIWANG SHIJI*', a classic of traditional Chinese medicine more than 4000 years old. About a hundred years ago when Western medicine (now the dominant mode of medical practice over this country) was introduced into China, medical ethics in China adopted many new characteristics. The key ethical principle of saving lives remain the same while conflicts exist in the interaction of Western and Eastern moral systems. Since 1949 when the People's Republic of China was established, a government-supported health-care system has covered fundamental medical care for all the people. This socialist system enlarged the scope of Chinese ethics of medicine. In that period, there was a countrywide movement to promote the combination of Western medicine and traditional Chinese medicine, the so-called Integrated Chinese and Western Medicine. With the introduction of an open policy and the progress of economic reforms since the 1980s, modern medicine in China has made great progress. However, not all affordable high-tech medicine is developed and applied throughout the country. Medical ethics as a discipline is coping with many new issues today.

Modern nephrology as a discipline of medicine was developed only in the mid-1970s in China. Many physicians in China practise integrated medicine and use herbal drugs in the management of kidney disease patients. Since 1980, dialysis and transplantation have been rapidly developed in the treatment of end-stage renal disease (ESRD). However, new ethical issues have emerged and aroused many debates in the practice of nephrology in China.

The influence of traditional medicine

As early as 457 BC, there were already written records describing the symptoms and management of edema. Traditional medicine had developed its own theory and treatment in kidney diseases. As a part of the culture, it was rooted deeply in the life and thoughts of Chinese peoples and exerted enormous impact on the medical ethics of modern China (Nanjing College, 1958).

In the context of the traditional Chinese medicine, the *kidney* (*SHEN*, a counterpart of kidneys in Western medicine) is considered to be the most important among the five organ-systems (heart, liver, lung, spleen and kidney) in the body. Apart from those functions ascribed to the kidneys in Western medicine, the kidney (*SHEN*) contributes to life-essence, vigor and strength of the body, sexual competence and fertility. *SHEN* is also considered to be closely related to the other organ-systems. So Chinese people attach great importance to *SHEN* and generally take for granted that renal diseases are dangerous and terrifying because of their life-threatening and non-recoverable features. Herbs with tonic effects, widely used in the treatment of renal diseases, may cause adverse effects in patients with hypertension or a hypercatabolic state.

For the treatment of various renal diseases, there are many prescriptions in the classics of traditional medicine and in folk recipes passed on in families. Some do have therapeutic effects in nephritis, nephrosis, urinary stone diseases and uremia. The most widely known herbs, such as TW (*Tripterygium wilfordii* Hook f) in the treatment of nephrosis and rhubarb in preventing and retarding the progression of chronic renal failure, have been extensively studied with modern laboratory techniques and in clinical settings. But there are some other recipes without much scientific basis and some may even result in severe adverse reactions. For example, *Akebia quinata*, which contains aristolochic acids and is used in the treatment of urinary stone diseases and in some formulations for weight reduction, has been reported to cause acute renal failure or progressive acellular renal scarring. In some cases, the drugs are not labeled as to content and are promoted with a sense of fathomless mystery.

A large proportion of renal patients believe in herbal drugs and seek medical care first from doctors trained in traditional medicine. More patients resort to traditional medicine because they have not responded to the treatment in Western medicine, or resort to integrated medicine to enhance the efficacy of Western treatments.

The way that traditional medicine handles renal diseases has also greatly influenced the behavior of renal patients. Traditionally the diagnostic approaches need to be non-traumatic, and treatment depends mainly on oral medicine. Hence, some patients may refuse to have renal biopsies or are reluctant to undertake dialysis and transplantation even if their disease is critically severe.

There are many prohibitions regarding the treatment of kidney diseases, for example salts should be restricted with many kidney diseases, and fish or crab are usually forbidden in patients with nephritis. On the other hand, people believe that consumption of certain animal organs help to restore the function of the corresponding diseased organ in patients. Uremic patients treated with traditional remedies frequently have severe anemia, malnutrition, and disorders of electrolyte balance.

The influence of cultural—religious background and social—economic status

As in the rest of the world, medical practice in China has been influenced by its cultural and religious background. Among the theories of philosophy and religious insights that have contributed to Chinese cultural development, Confucianism and Buddhism in particular have exerted remarkable influence on the ethics of medicine. Confucianism is the most widely accepted philosophy in China not only among intellectuals, but also among the common people, and it is important because it shaped the moral system for medical practice in this country. Confucianism advocates benevolent love, righteousness, decorum, wise leadership, and sincerity. As recorded in the *Analects of Confucius*, the key principle of medicine is benevolence, and emphasizes saving lives above all other values. Life and the body have been sacred for thousands of years. The attitude toward death is also influenced by these theories. According to the doctrine of Confucianism, all parts of the body are passed on from the parents and must be protected from damage and loss; and death should be glorious with the body intact. Buddhism's belief of recycling of life also affects people's attitude toward donation of organs (or even blood, or surgical treatments). All these ideas influence profoundly the attitude of Chinese people toward the management of ESRD. The majority refuse to accept the legal principle of brain death. Living donor transplantation has been rare in the past. Renal patients, particularly in rural areas, are frequently reluctant to accept renal biopsy, hemodialysis and other operative procedures.

With the development of modern medicine and the economic/systemic reforms in China during the 1980s and 1990s, medical ethics has been developed as a coherent discipline and challenged old beliefs in clinical practice. The ethical issues in hemodialysis, organ donation, euthanasia (Shi and Yu, 1995), hospice care, bioengineering, gene therapy, and *in vitro* fertilization have now been approached systematically. Legislation and governmental regulations are being established. Medical insurance systems are starting to cover more people in urban areas, although not yet in rural regions. Ethical principles are being incorporated into medical practice, such as the primacy of the patient's interests, the needs of society, informed consent, full disclosure, competence in decision making, and equity in allocation of medical resources. People's attitudes towards organ donation and euthanasia are changing slowly but progressively.

In spite of the increasing availability of dialysis and transplantation in this country, many ESRD patients still persist with traditional treatment using herbal medicine. They may fear operative procedures and dialysis (especially hemodialysis). For some, the financial support for dialysis is not available and thus conservative treatment is the only choice. This on the one hand means that many ESRD patients are not properly treated to eliminate uremic toxins and suffer from severe anemia, malnutrition, severe bone disorders, etc. On other hand, this promotes the development of conservative treatment with Chinese herbs in the management of nephrotic syndrome and in slowing the progress of chronic renal failure.

Dialysis was introduced into China in 1960 but maintenance hemodialysis (HD) for end-stage renal disease was not initiated until 1972. It has grown rapidly since then; approximately 15000 ESRD patients are maintained on HD now. However, as compared with the total population of ESRD patients (estimated to be several hundred thousand), this is a very small percentage. China, a developing country of 1.2 billion people, has an annual gross domestic product (GDP) per capita of only 800 US dollars. Needless to say, HD is a very expensive treatment for ESRD patients in this country. The current charge for a hemodialysis treatment is 420 Chinese Yuan (50 US dollars). The average annual expense for hemodialysis per patient is 8000 US dollars, 10 times the GDP per capita. The result is that only a minority of the ESRD patients in need of replacement therapy is able to afford this expensive treatment modality. Replacement therapy for most patients is paid (entirely or partially) by government or big enterprises. To reduce the expense of HD, a widely accepted practice is to decrease the number of treatment sessions. This leads to inadequate dialysis and poor long-term outcome (Li, 1995; Li, 1996).

Hemodialysis is commonly carried out in hospital-affiliated hemodialysis centers by nephrologists and specialized nurses. Even today, there is still a shortage of hemodialysis supplies and competent staffs, relative to the needs of ESRD patients in this country. All the hemodialysis centers are located in the cities, particularly in the economically more advanced areas. Many patients start dialysis very late in the course of uremia. The criteria for the initiation of dialysis are not entirely medical, but to a large extent include the patient's financial support and the family's acceptance. Home hemodialysis is virtually non-existent in this country. Erythropoietin is only affordable for a small proportion of patients, even though erythropoietin made in China costs only half as much as the imported product. Reuse of dialyser membranes is common to cut down expense. Older patients are dialyzed if there is adequate financial support and no medical contraindication. Patients with proven viral hepatitis B infection are treated separately in most dialysis centers to prevent the spread of infection. In about 20–30% of patients, maintenance hemodialysis is discontinued for financial reasons.

Theoretically, continuous ambulatory peritoneal dialysis (CAPD) is the appropriate option for ESRD patients in rural and remote regions in China, since it should cost less and be more convenient for patients in such areas. However, imported dialysis bags are so expensive that in fact the expense of CAPD is not less than that of hemodialysis. Dialysis bags made in China do not meet quality standards, and have been associated with a high peritoneal infection rate. As a result, only a small percentage of the whole dialysis population is maintained on peritoneal dialysis. A scarcity of trained nurses in rural regions also prevents the wide application of this alternative choice of treatment for ESRD patients.

Renal transplantation in China can be traced back to the early 1960s, with the first successful clinical case in 1974. Compared with the expense of other forms of renal replacement therapy, the cost for transplantation in the long run seems to be less. In recent years, the annual number of renal transplants has increased: 1097 in 1991, 1905 in 1992, 1972 in 1993, 2382 in 1995, and 3494 in 1998 (according to the data from the China Registry of Transplantation). Virtually all the renal allografts were cadaveric, with very few living donor transplants each year. Selection criteria for transplantation are based on the first come first served principle, in addition to serological matching and tissue typing criteria.

Again, the most important factor limiting the ability of ESRD patients to receive renal transplantation is their financial support. Most of the expense of renal transplantation is for immunosuppressive drugs such as cyclosporine, mycophenolate mofetil, and monoclonal antibodies, and this expense is beyond the financial ability of 80% of the ESRD patients. However, with the availability of Chinese-made cyclosporin, which reduced the cost of renal transplantation by a third, and the improvement of short-term prognosis, more and more dialysis patients are now waitlisted for renal transplantation.

Use of organs from executed prisoners

The use of cadaveric kidneys from executed prisoners has been a common practice in this country since the 1980s. This has aroused heated debates overseas, and even condemnation and sanctions (Briggs, 1996; Cameron and Hoffenberg, 1999). Within this developing country, this practice is widely accepted by not only medical professionals and other intellectuals, but also by religious people, with very little debate. This practice has met the great demand for the treatment of the ESRD in a situation in which organs from living donors are in short supply and the definition of brain death is still not accepted. The acceptance of this practice by the public in China is due to the unique cultural background and social system of the country.

The government has imposed strict regulations on the use of cadaveric organs from executed prisoners. The principles include:

- Informed consent must be obtained from the candidate donors and their families.
- Only qualified medical centers or hospitals authorized by the government are permitted to use the organs donated by executed prisoners, and the harvested organs must be used for clinical treatment. Sales of organs or profiting from the transfer of organs is illegal and will be punished.
- The practice may not be applied in the case of minorities whose religious beliefs oppose it.

In recent years, these regulations have been strictly enforced throughout the country. Due to efforts in education and reform of prisoners, the majority of the death penalty prisoners have realized that they had harmed other people and society. Many prisoners have given explicit consent to donate, and in most cases the families have also agreed. These candidate donors, who have been convicted of murder, drug trafficking, or other serious criminal offenses believe that their donation of two kidneys is a good deed, which will save two lives and is preferable to cremation of lifesaving organs. Religious persons take consolation in the belief that their donation will be noted in the afterlife. During the process of execution, medical professionals start organ retrieval only after the coroner has confirmed the death of the donor. In all activities, including the interaction with the donor or donor's families, both officials and medical professionals are responsible for respecting wishes and feelings of the donors and their relatives.

Among the public, renal transplantation (as well as other organ transplantation) has been progressively and widely recognized as an effective and important life-saving technique. Since organ grafts from other sources are in short supply and far from meeting the need of ESRD patients, the public accept this alternative practice and acknowledge it as beneficial to society; about 3000 lives are saved each year. In Chinese minds, saving lives and relieving pain without harm to others are actions of the highest value.

Among the medical profession, 'brain death' as a practical criterion of death has been discussed for years, and this issue has been presented to a committee of the national legislature. However, this has not been approved because the resistance from the public and difficulty in application. Almost all Chinese people believe and demand that doctors should not stop their efforts to preserve life if the patient's heart is beating and the patient is breathing. Therefore, it is impossible to procure organs from victims of accidents. It is widely accepted by medical professionals that it is urgent to legislate policies for brain death and advance consent and to obtain public support. It will take more time to educate and convince the public.

Vigorous debates on medical ethical issues are helpful to optimize the practice of medicine and will benefit not only the Chinese people but also mankind throughout the world. In approaching every issue of medical ethics, not only different philosophies but also differences in cultural and history background should be taken into account. The study of ethics should be involved in extensive investigation of actual situations and offer solutions to specific problems. For medical ethical issues in China, such as the retrieval of organs for transplantation, as with other issues questioned by the Western scholars or politicians, Chinese people and medical professionals are coping with specific problems in unique ways that are appropriate for Chinese situations and practical for solving the problems for the utmost benefit of the vast majority of patients in China.

A similarity can be outlined between this practice and the issue of the family planning policy in China. The policy that one couple may have only one child or at most two once aroused heated debates and severe condemnation from those areas where people with different backgrounds hold different opinions. Now after 25 years of the application of this policy, the results show that family planning policy is pertinent to the actual situation in China. Not only China, but also the world benefits from the policy for the successful control of population and the improvement of living standards of the people in China, as well as for world population control and reduced demand for energy and materials. WHO has recently acknowledged the practice of family planning as a benefit to people of China and of the world, rather than an offense to human rights.

With the improvement of people's living standards and education, changes in values, and increased social stability, we anticipate legislative approval of brain death and acceptance of living-related organ donation. The advent of clinical xenotransplantation also holds promise for China. Chinese patients in need of renal replacement therapy are benefiting from the ever-improving medicine in this country. All Chinese nephrologists and transplant surgeons are eager to work with medical teams everywhere to meet the need of the suffering ESRD patients throughout the world.

References

Briggs, J. D. (1996). The use of organs form executed prisoners in China. *Nephrology Dialysis, Transplantation*, **11**, 38–40.
Cameron, J. S., and Hoffenberg, R. (1999). The ethics of organ transplantation reconsidered: Paid organ donation and the use of executed prisoners as donors. *Kidney International*, **55**, 724–32.
Li, Z. L. (1995). Ethical analysis and suggestion for patients with chronic renal failure and hemodialysis. *Chinese Medical Ethics*, **44**, 59–60.
Li, L. S. (1996). End-stage renal disease in China. *Kidney International*, **49**, 287–301.
Nanjing College of Traditional Chinese Medicine (ed.) (1958). *The introduction to traditional Chinese medicine*. Ren Ming Wei Shen Chu Ban She, Beijing.
Shi, D. P., and Yu, L. (1995). The situation of euthanasia in China judged from typical cases and the public opinion poll. *Chinese Medical Ethics*, **44**, 21–5.

16
India

Vivekanand Jha and Kirpal S. Chugh

Organ transplantation in India is mostly confined to transplantation of kidneys using living-related and unrelated donors and, in a small number of patients, cadaver donors. With the recent development of split transplant technique, a few liver transplants have also been performed successfully in some centers using living-related donors. The lack of infrastructure for harvesting cadaver organs has not only prevented the growth of cadaver renal donor transplant programs but also of unpaired vital organs like heart, pancreas and liver. This communication highlights the ethical aspects of kidney transplantation in developing countries in general and India in particular.

Kidney transplantation has become firmly established as the preferable modality of treatment of end-stage renal disease (ESRD) throughout the world. Advances in surgical techniques, improved immunosuppressive regimes and better management of infections have led to 1-year patient and graft survival rates in excess of 90% in most centers. In early years, living donors were the sole source of transplantable kidneys, but currently transplantation in most countries is mainly dependent on cadaver organs. Since the availability of cadaver kidneys is unpredictable, to ensure a fair and equitable distribution, organs are allotted to the most suitable recipients on the basis of certain accepted criteria. It is imperative that the potential recipients are maintained in reasonably good health until they can be transplanted. Simultaneously, refinements in dialysis techniques have enabled patients to live for many years, even decades, on maintenance hemo- and peritoneal dialysis. Quality of life is satisfactory enough so that in many instances patients choose not to enroll for transplantation and continue indefinitely on dialysis.

As the medical problems associated with kidney transplantation are on the threshold of being solved, attention is focused on getting enough organs to provide this treatment to all who need it. This has led to a search for organs from unconventional sources such as unrelated-living donors, anencephalic infants, executed criminals, and those contemplating suicide or euthanasia. Many nations have enacted 'required request' and 'presumed consent' laws directed at increasing cadaver organ retrieval. Despite all these measures, kidneys are available for transplantation only in a minority of ESRD patients (Chugh and Jha, 1995). To meet with this ever-increasing demand, procurement of organs by payment or compensation was resorted to in the past in several countries. However, because of swift condemnation by most professional societies, including the Transplantation Society and the World Health Organization, the practice was banned throughout the developed world (Chugh and Jha, 1996). In the era of instantaneous communication and easy intercontinental travel, needy patients started looking beyond the bounds of law imposed by their own countries and made India a favored destination in the 1980s. India offered a unique mix of conditions including a vast impoverished population, no laws regulating organ donation, readily available trained physicians and surgeons in the field of renal transplantation and enterprising middlemen who could bring all the interested parties together. This became the starting point of an intensely debated ethical issue in kidney transplantation, namely, commercial organ donation.

The Indian subcontinent

India is the largest and most populous country in this geographic region and is surrounded by those nations, such as Pakistan, Bangladesh, Sri Lanka, Nepal and Bhutan, which are at a more or less similar stage of socioeconomic development and have similar ethnic populations. The socioeconomic and health indicator status of the countries of the subcontinent is given in Table 16.1. One of the ways by which the economic status is judged is by estimating the number of people paying taxes. The annual income above which one must pay income tax is Rs. 60000 (US$ 1400) in India, and less than 1.5% of the population pays taxes (Mani, 1998).

The major religions practiced in the subcontinent are Hinduism (India, Nepal and Sri Lanka), Islam (India, Bangladesh and Pakistan), Buddhism (India, Sri Lanka and Bhutan) and Christianity (India and Sri Lanka). However, the level of affluence defines the social practices and lifestyles, with people of similar economic status sharing a similarity that cuts across religious boundaries.

A vast majority of population is dependent on health care provided by the government. The health expenditure covers not only medical relief, but also sanitation, water supply, immunization, infection eradication programs and family planning. Government-funded hospitals are overcrowded and understaffed, and the private for-profit hospitals are beyond the reach of over 95% of the population. There is no government-funded national or regional health insurance. Government does not permit private sector participation in insurance, including health. As a result, individuals have to fund their own medical care (Chugh and Jha, 1995).

ESRD and kidney transplantation in India

The incidence of ESRD in the Indian subcontinent has not been evaluated systematically. Estimates put the number of new patients with ESRD in India at 90–100000 per year (Chugh and Jha, 1995). Maintenance dialysis is poorly organized. The capital costs of setting up dialysis units are very high and finances are severely limited. Government hospitals have limited numbers of dialysis machines, and are in no position to provide subsidized dialysis, even to a fraction of patients. Existing units have mostly outdated machinery and poorly trained staff. This culminates in a high complication rate, and long-term survivors on maintenance hemodialysis are virtually

Table 16.1 Socioeconomic and health indicators of countries in Indian subcontinent[a]

Country	Population (millions)	Per capita GNP[b] (US$)	Purchasing power parity (US$)	Growth rate (%)	Adult literacy rate (%)	Infant mortality rate (pmp)[c]	% GDP[d] health expenditure	% of people with access to potable water
India	1000	390	1650	2.0	52	72	1.2	85
Pakistan	150	490	1590	3.1	26	74	0.8	62
Bangla Desh	125	270	1050	2.0	53	79	1.5	84
Nepal	22	210	1090	2.6	51	83	1.2	59
Sri Lanka	19	800	2460	1.3	51	18	1.4	70
Bhutan	2	400	—	2.3	54	63	2.3	—

[a] Source: *www.worldbank.org* 2000
[b] GNP: gross national product
[c] pmp: per million population
[d] GDP: gross domestic product

unknown. Moreover, these facilities are located in major cities, and it is impractical for patients living in remote rural areas to relocate themselves solely for dialysis. Unlike some Latin American countries, continuous ambulatory peritoneal dialysis (CAPD) has not become popular in India mainly because of its high cost. CAPD bags and transfer sets are not manufactured indigenously and importing them substantially raises their cost. The costs are increased further by the import duties imposed by the government. There are limited data on long-term CAPD in India, but the hot and humid climate, lack of education and compliance and poor hygienic conditions are unlikely to permit long-term complication-free survival.

The first kidney transplants were performed in India in the early 1970s. However, the results were poor and physicians and surgeons, especially in the profit-making private hospitals, were unwilling to be associated with a procedure with a low success rate. As a result, transplantation remained limited to a few major teaching hospitals in the early years. The situation changed dramatically in the 1980s with the availability of cyclosporine A, which revolutionized the outcome of transplantation and made transplants between genetically unrelated individuals a reality. More and more surgeons obtained training in the technique, and kidney transplantation increased rapidly in private hospitals located in metropolitan cities. In fact, many hospitals and nursing homes sprang up during this period with kidney transplantation as the only or the main medical activity (Chugh and Jha, 1996).

Kidney transplantation is expensive; it costs approximately US$ 1200–5000 depending on whether it is performed in a government or a private hospital. Patients must also spend US$ 3000–5000 annually on maintenance immunosuppressive therapy. Therefore, with the present system of funding, the procedure remains out of reach for most of the population, despite government subsidy.

The ethical debate on organ transplantation in developing countries like India revolves around two major issues: (1) public funding of transplantation, and (2) sale of human organs.

Public funding of organ transplantation

Should a country like India involve itself in an expensive undertaking such as organ transplantation? Can we justify the allocation of scarce public funds to transplantation when most primary health care needs are not uniformly available? Transplantation, an easily identifiable large-scale expense, has been attacked more often than other treatment modalities that are equally, if not more, expensive. According to the Indian constitution, health is a fundamental right of an individual. The worldwide experience has clearly shown that the demand for health expenditures continues to increase irrespective of the level of economic development of a country. Even in the USA, which spends more than 13% of the gross domestic product (GDP) on health services, there is never enough money to fund all health-related programs. Kidney transplantation in developing countries like India costs only a fraction of what it costs in most developed countries. The procedure itself is not technology-intensive and can be done in moderately well-equipped hospitals.

ESRD primarily afflicts the young in the Indian subcontinent. Most patients are in the 25–45 year age group, and are often the sole breadwinners of their families (Bhalla *et al.*, 1993). It is universally agreed that organ transplantation is one of the most cost-effective medical procedures compared with other modalities, which are being used to sustain organ function. Successful transplant allows the patient to return to useful productive work, which will ultimately contribute to the national wealth. Furthermore, in a socio-political system in which private sector participation in health insurance is not permitted the government is obliged to provide this facility to all its people who need it. In view of the high cost required for setting up dialysis units and the vastly superior quality of life following transplantation it would be far more profitable to focus on transplants rather than dialysis. At present, the main component of transplant costs, which makes it beyond the reach of the common citizen, is that of the immunosuppressive drugs, made more so by the duties imposed by the government. Further, there is no provision for free care of the potential cadaver donor. Whereas it might be unreasonable to expect that government subsidies would make transplant available to everyone who needs it, the least the government can do is to remove the road blocks so that the facility can become available to the general population.

It is estimated that 'rich' Indians spend over US$10 million of precious foreign exchange for medical treatment abroad every year. Though this class will always have the capacity to seek treatment abroad, a transplant program in the home country is more attractive even for rich patients, since this avoids the inconvenience of travel. India has made giant strides in the field of science and technology and has the third largest trained scientific workforce in the world. It is desirable therefore that the prevalent standard of care in the field of health, including organ transplantation, is made available even to ordinary citizens of the country. If the government does not accord the much needed priority to transplantation, it is likely to be completely taken over by the private sector healthcare industry, which would make it totally out of reach of the common citizen.

Commerce in transplantation

Living donors have always been the mainstay of kidney transplantation in India. Large families with strong interpersonal ties, combined with the knowledge that long-term dialysis was not a realistic option, frequently made related donors come forward for transplantation. Members of extended families, including cousins, uncles, aunts, nephews and nieces often volunteered to donate. Mothers are the most frequent donors, accounting for over one-third of all living donations, followed by siblings. Parents seldom accept kidneys from their children. There is a reluctance to accept a kidney from a girl of marriageable age because of the fear of reducing her chances of finding a good husband in a conservative society in which most marriages are still being arranged by parents. Absence of legislation recognizing brain death and lack of intensive care unit (ICU) facilities were considered to be the major hurdles preventing increases in cadaver transplants in the Indian subcontinent until 1994.

Transplantation using kidneys from living unrelated paid donors reared its head in metropolitan cities of India in the 1980s. The beneficiaries included recipients from within the subcontinent and from overseas, with the largest numbers coming from oil-rich Middle Eastern countries where transplant facilities were not available (Chugh and Jha, 1996). Such unregulated transplants continued for over a decade. Horror stories alleging removal of kidneys from unsuspecting individuals without their consent appeared in the lay press at regular intervals. At the same time, reports of complications in the medical literature indicated that these transplants were being performed under unacceptably low standards of medical care. Recognizing the adverse publicity of rampant commercialization in transplants, both in lay and medical press, the Indian parliament in 1995 enacted a law banning this practice. This law prohibited transplantation between anyone except immediate family members such as parents, siblings and spouses. In exceptional situations, an 'authorization committee' constituted by the government can approve organ donation outside this group, provided the committee is convinced that the donation is being made out of 'love and affection' for the recipient and no financial transaction is involved. Since health is regulated by the states under Indian constitution, the law did not become operational until ratified by the legislative assemblies of individual states. Most Indian states have done so, but five of the 31 states have still not adopted this law. Commercial transplants, therefore, continue to be legal in those states.

Recent studies have demonstrated the short- and long-term results of transplantation using kidneys from genetically unrelated donors, dubbed 'emotionally-related living donor transplants' (ERLD), to be as good as those from living-related donors, and better than the results of cadaver transplants (Chugh and Jha, 2000). Similar results from India were presented almost a decade ago using paid unrelated donors (Thiagarajan *et al.*, 1990). In the light of these observations, the potential of living-unrelated transplants to alleviate the organ shortage is being reassessed throughout the world. Though surveys carried out in North America with affluent populations and effective systems of enforcement of justice have indicated that public opinion favors non-commercial unrelated transplants (Altshuler and Evanisko, 1992), the practice of 'payment' for organs is still hotly debated. It is generally agreed that donors may be reimbursed for expenses incurred from donation, including lost wages. Whether it is ethical for kidneys to be sold for a price, like any other material possession, remains contentious. Some transplant professionals and ethicists argue that paid transplants benefit everyone involved in the act (Thiagarajan *et al.*, 1990; Radcliffe-Richards, 1991; Radcliffe-Richards *et al.*, 1998). The recipient gets a much-needed kidney, the impoverished donor gets money needed to meet vital needs and the middlemen and the health care professionals involved get incomes for their efforts. (See Chapter 7 by Hoffenberg in this volume.)

A democratic society must respect human rights and must make arrangements to safeguard medical practices from corruption and degradation. Payment for organs is not inherently unethical and it would be wrong to prohibit this contract without strong reasons. This issue involves: (1) would-be buyers (recipients), (2) would-be sellers (donors), (3) kidney-procuring agents or middlemen, (4) the medical community involved in transplantation, and (5) society at large.

Recipients

The major argument offered in favor of paid transplants is that these would allow recipients who have no other option to get transplanted, to get a new lease of life. The term 'buy or let die' was coined for this situation (Thiagarajan, 1990). Inherent in this argument is the assumption that only those who do not have a suitable related donor look for a paid donor, and that if suitable donors were available, all ESRD patients in India could undergo transplants. Reality, however, is very different. The fact is that the great majority cannot afford the costs of transplantation despite having suitable donors and are, therefore, doomed to die. Indeed, in a country with vast economic discrepancies, it would be naïve to assume that rich patients would not look into the paid donor market even if a suitable related donor were available. We are aware of several recipients who had suitable donors in the family but still preferred to buy a kidney. Broumand (1997) has recorded the case of a patient who contracted AIDS and died following a commercial kidney transplant. His sons were full of remorse at choosing an unrelated donor instead of one of them donating the kidney. The number of living-related donor transplants fell sharply in Iran after paid organ transplants were legalized, again suggesting that rich recipients preferred the market route to donation by a family member (Broumand, 1997). The assumption, therefore, that only those recipients who have no related donor and are in a situation of 'buy or let die' are forced to buy a kidney does not hold true. In our experience most recipients are desperate, care little for the donor and their interest ends the moment transplantation is performed.

Donor issues

The foremost ethical issue concerning living donors is that they should not be subjected to any harm (Shreiber, 1991). It is generally believed that donor nephrectomy carries little risk when performed by capable surgeons in appropriately equipped hospitals. However, because of the very nature of the procedure, it is likely that complications remain underreported. Deaths, although infrequent ($\approx$ 1 in 2000), do occur. Figures for major complications, such as wound infection and hemorrhage, are not available, but are likely to be higher. Thus, donor nephrectomy is not a totally risk-free procedure. Under these circumstances, what are the factors that motivate a person to donate an organ? Altruism, defined as 'doing good to others at the expense of one's own self-interest', has been considered to be the prime motivating factor for living-organ donation from the beginning (Sheil, 1995). In the context of a family or strong emotional relationship such as long-term friendship the feeling of being the one instrumental in a loved one getting 'cured of' ESRD is a source of strong emotional satisfaction for the donor. The limited risk of surgery becomes acceptable when it benefits somebody one loves and cares for. The usual preconditions for a living donation, namely that the risk to the donor must be minimal compared with the benefit to the recipient, that the donor must be extensively informed before making a choice, and that the agreement must be made willingly and under no pressure, are easily met in such situations.

The motivation of a paid donor in India is not so easy to evaluate. The population willing to donate a kidney for money is a heterogeneous mix, and can be divided into three broad groups. The first group comprises young to middle-aged illiterate males, usually landless laborers living in villages. Dissatisfied with their lot, they come to cities with the hope of finding better paying jobs. Such job seekers, however, vastly outnumber the available jobs, and most of them find themselves without any work. Having exhausted their meager savings and on the brink of starvation, they often do not have money even to go back home. At this point of time, they are approached by one of the agents, who offer them money in exchange for one of their kidneys. Desperate and without any knowledge of the actual market value of the 'reward' for their 'gift', they end up accepting whatever little is offered to them.

The second group in the 'donor market' comprises drifters and homeless people who are often addicted to alcohol and drugs and are not interested in work. Some of them are professional donors, who donate blood for money at privately run blood banks. Although the rules in India forbid donation more frequently than once in 3 months, lack of any database allows these donors to donate more frequently at different blood banks, and even at the same place under different names. Blood banks are aware of this practice, but prefer to turn a blind eye to ensure a constant supply. As a result, they are anemic, suffer from multiple nutritional deficiencies, and many are carriers of infections including hepatitis B and C and even HIV. There are numerous reports in medical literature of transmission of these infections to previously negative recipients after a commercial transplant (Chugh and Jha, 2000). In contrast to the illiterate villager, the professional donor has a better idea of the market price of his kidney, and bargains to get the most in this 'once-in-a-lifetime' opportunity. Once this finite amount has been received and squandered away, this person may even try to extract more from the recipient, the middleman or the hospital where the transplant was performed. When rebuffed, some are known to approach the press or the police with the allegation that their kidneys have been removed without their knowledge or consent. Though many such cases have been registered by the police in different parts of India, none have been proved in courts so far. There is a report from Iran, where a donor who had already sold one kidney wanted to sell the other kidney to support his drug habit. He was willing to go on maintenance dialysis, which is free there.

The third group comprises those who see kidney donation as a way to raise money to meet an immediate financial need. This could vary from paying off a debt, raising dowry for the marriage of a sister or a daughter, meeting the expenses for treatment of a family member's illness, house-building, or even buying a consumer item such as a scooter or a television. Generally, these are the people in low-paying jobs, who have no other way of raising money quickly. This kind of donation has been dubbed 'indirect altruism' because the ultimate beneficiary of the act of donation is not the kidney recipient (who is a stranger), but another person for whom the money has thus been raised.

Medical profession

Physicians play an important role in policy making and its implementation in developing countries. In general, medical professionals are ethical and concerned about patient welfare. However, idiosyncratic ethical orientations do exist amongst all professionals, including those in medicine. Illicit procurement and sale of organs could not have taken place if individual physicians and the medical community had abided by international standards and refused to perform transplantation of organs of suspicious origin. Payment to the hospital and doctors in most private hospitals depends on the number of procedures performed. In a competitive environment, professionals working in the context of a private profit-making set-up are often under overt or covert pressure by the management to maximize profits. Under these circumstances, if the program falters through donor shortage, the system of competitive covert payment (also called commission) to the middleman immediately comes into play. Such a situation often forces the 'ethical niceties' of paid donation to the background. When a service is performed solely for profit, there is often a temptation and opportunity for deception and exploitation, with faint regard for the cherished moral and ethical values of the medical profession and the society. It must be pointed out, however, that some physicians support paid organ donation not because of any bias or self-interest, but because of their commitment to the individual patient with ESRD. They feel that as physicians their main duty is to act in the best interest of the recipient, irrespective of the consequences of this act for the society.

Society

The basic principles and attitudes required for practical moral decision making by any civilized society are (1) respect for autonomy, (2) beneficence or obligation to help and care for others, (3) non-maleficence or obligation to avoid harm to others, and (4) justice or obligation to deal fairly with competing claims. The ethical attitudes attributable to the East are often compared with those of the West (Dossetor and Manickavel, 1991; Engelhardt, 1991) and a feeling is projected that because the poorer societies do not have all the amenities that are available in the West, they should not be expected to measure up to the (higher) ethical standards desirable and applicable in the advanced countries.

Western society cannot hold indirect altruism to be legitimate simply because selling a kidney is an easy way by which a perceived 'dire need' of a poor individual might be satisfied (Dossetor, 1992). Does it not burden the society with guilt? How do we define a dire need? For example, a person may consider payment of dowry for the wedding of a daughter as a dire necessity whereas the society considers it a regressive practice and tries to find ways to end it. The argument can degenerate into advocating many abhorrent practices including child labor, prostitution and even allowing individuals to sell themselves into slavery 'because there is no other way' to meet a 'dire need'. Can one justify stealing on the ground that a poor person who desperately needs something is taking it from a rich person who has an excess of it? There have been reports from East European countries of people having children who are subsequently put up for adoption by people of other countries in exchange for money. Relaxation of universally accepted ethical standards can give rise to completely unforeseen spin-offs in some societies. An Iranian militia recently started a worldwide campaign exhorting Muslims to sell one of their kidneys to offer a reward to anyone who carries out the fatwa of killing the Indian-born British author Salman Rushdie. According to one report, over 500 people including some from India, Pakistan, Iran and Lebanon have signed up to sell a kidney (news.bbc.co.uk, 1999). Organ selling is legal in Iran, and the fatwa continues to be supported by the government led by Muslim clerics.

Medical professionals have traditionally enjoyed a high degree of respect in Indian society. A feeling of disillusionment and distrust has arisen among the public because the medical profession is engaged in buying and selling human organs. Publicity about the commercial aspect of organ transplantation also has eroded the respect accorded to this noble profession. Many well-motivated persons who could have been helpful in getting public funding for ESRD treatment programs or advancing the cause of cadaver transplantation no longer wish to participate in a system in which there is corruption, exploitation and unjust distribution of organs in favor of the rich and the influential.

Strong social attitudes about the rights and obligations of men and women often influence willingness to donate or accept organs according to the gender of the donor and the recipient. Females have traditionally enjoyed lesser rights in conservative Indian society and therefore, there is a lot of pressure on wives to donate kidneys for their husbands even though there may be other suitable related donors in the family. Although donation by wives was legalized in the 1995 Indian Organ Transplantation Act, most non-commercial transplant centers accept wives only if there are no other suitable related donors in the family.

Some ethicists and medical professionals have recently argued in favor of payment for donor organs (Radcliffe-Richards, 1991; Radcliffe-Richards et al., 1998). (See also Chapter 7, by Hoffenberg in this book.) According to them, outrage at organ selling and prohibition of this practice are paternalistic, and therefore wrong. They feel that as the poor have limited choices to improve their lot, they should be allowed to make the decision to sell a kidney like any other material possession if they choose to, and prohibiting this would limit their freedom and autonomy. It has also been argued that the risk of kidney donation is less than that of a 'wretched' life in poverty, and should therefore be acceptable. It has been suggested that the act of payment itself is not wrong and should be permitted, albeit in a regulated manner. A local committee of societal peers or gatekeepers would decide whether the benefit is for the relief of a dire need that cannot be fulfilled in any other way. This committee would also help secure the benefit for which the payment is ultimately intended and protect the donor from victimization and fraud. Other suggested controls include elimination of middlemen or brokers, ban on advertising, independent psychological review of donors and recipients, independent surgical team for the donor, long-term insurance for the donor including coverage for catastrophic illness, subsidization of transplant of poor recipients by the rich, an obligation for the rich recipient to give to the community to which the donor belongs (mandated philanthropy) and no transplant of patients from other countries (Dossetor and Manickavel 1991; Sells, 1992; Radcliffe-Richards *et al.*, 1998).

At first glance, such schemes appear reasonable. However, numerous difficulties can be envisaged in their administration, both at an individual level and at a societal level. Payment to the donor would occur only after the person is found fit in all respects and actually undergoes the nephrectomy. However, a needy person is likely to express severe disappointment and dissatisfaction if doctors decide during the course of evaluation that he or she is not suitable. Instances of disgruntled rejected donors committing violence have been recorded, and in one instance, the rejected would-be donor killed a member of the prospective recipient's family (Broumand, 1997).

The question also arises as to what price society should fix for donation of a kidney. So far, it has been completely arbitrary, subject to bargaining between the donor and the middleman, dependent on the level of awareness of the donor about the value of a kidney, and the ability of the middleman to bully the donor. Should it be based on the financial status of the recipient, the donor, the urgency of recipient's need or the degree of 'matching' between the donor and recipient? Should the price be decided at an auction where the kidney would go to the highest bidder? Recently, a person put up his kidney for auction at Internet auction site E-bay, with a minimum bid of US$ 25 000 (www.ebay.com, 1999). The managers of the site, however, subsequently withdrew this advertisement. The amount requested in this instance was 20–30 times more than that paid to organ donors in India. Should organs coming from individuals belonging to different societies have different values? Inconsistency in valuation is likely to be a source of dissatisfaction for a donor who gets the lesser amount for his kidney.

Once an 'easy' way of making money becomes evident to a poor person, it becomes a temptation for him to get more through donations from other members of the family. Broumand (1997) reported a case where a paid donor after being discharged from the hospital, came back with his wife, asking that she also be accepted as a paid donor. In India, there are reports of 'communities', or 'kidney-villages' where every household has at least one member who has donated one kidney for money. In these communities, a person not willing to sell his kidney would come under increasing social pressure to follow this course of action, whatever his personal beliefs.

The advocates of regulated paid transplants assume that standards of justice and law enforcement are enforced uniformly throughout the world. It must be appreciated that proposing or making regulations is one thing, and making them work in the context of the socio-political scenario of a developing country is quite another. Transparency International, an independent watchdog body for corruption, calculates the level of fairness and transparency in public offices in different countries. In its 5th Annual Report (Cofe-Freeman and Popse 1999), India has been ranked 72nd out of 99 countries so evaluated. The committee specifically noted the lack of political will to establish an effective anti-corruption institution in the country. Therefore, placing sensitive ethical decisions like payment for organ donation in the hands of government officials and expecting them to be completely objective without being influenced by extraneous considerations is closing one's eyes to reality. A perusal of the Report shows that high standards of social justice can be found only in economically advanced countries, and paradoxically, members of such societies would not need to sell their organs for money.

We believe that the very idea of a potential recipient scouring the market for the cheapest kidney and a potential donor looking for the recipient who would pay the most fundamentally degrades human values. We also believe that no matter what the incentive, paid transplants force desperately poor people to take risks that they would not otherwise accept, and this vitiates true informed consent. Finally, the so-called freedom of an individual must be circumscribed by the needs of the society and by the greater good of social order and morality.

Finally, the process for the proposed monitoring of the donors after nephrectomy is likely to be complex and contentious. Donors come from remote rural areas that are geographically far apart and have very limited means for communication. Many programs have claimed to provide free medical care to the donor (Thiagarajan, 1990), but no data have ever been presented on such follow ups. In fact, donor follow up is practically non-existent.

Cadaver transplants

The long-term objective of ESRD treatment in countries of the Indian subcontinent, as in the rest of the world, is transplantation with cadaver donors. No objection has ever been raised by any Indian community against cadaver transplants. Altruistic organ donation is seen as an act of supreme charity by all major religions practised in the Indian subcontinent. In Hinduism, organ transplantation is as old as mythology itself. Ganesha, a major Hindu god, carries the head of an elephant. According to mythology, his father, the god Shiva, severed his head in a fit of anger but later, on repenting, transplanted an elephant's head on his body. Instances of altruistic gifting of unworldly possessions are also recorded. Yayati, a mythological character, gifted his youth to his father. Hinduism believes in the concept of 'atma' (soul) and 'sharira' (body). According to the Geeta, a holy Hindu text, the body is impermanent and perishable, and should be used towards fulfillment of one's duties and obligations. Once the soul has left the body, the latter is of no worth. The Buddhists hold similar views. None of the major Hindu religious leaders has ever expressed any opposition to organ donation. Islamic clerics in different parts of the world have endorsed the concept of brainstem death and advised the community to pledge organs after death. Certain countries with 'presumed consent' donation laws, however, exclude Muslims. India is a secular republic and cannot proscribe practices on religious grounds.

Though the Human Organ Transplant Act defined brain death and legalized cadaver transplants in India in 1995, the program still remains in infancy. There are 60000–70000 road fatalities every year in India. In theory, this should provide enough organs for transplantation of all ESRD patients. Swift transportation of the accident victims to intensive care units with life support systems, quick ascertainment of brain death and identification of a suitable recipient are essential for the success of a cadaver program. However, the government lacks the resources and the will to support complex medical technology and implement the monitoring procedures needed to make this program work. In the limited number of cadaver transplants performed in India, the donor organs have gone to recipients from the same hospital, or in rare cases, to another hospital in the same city.

The role of ICU staff in identifying and caring for potential donors is vital to the success of cadaver transplants (Quah, 1992). However, the staff often feel that their primary responsibilities do not lie in this direction, and that they get no direct benefit from this process. Moreover, very few hospitals have ICUs with ventilators, and there are always very sick patients waiting to get a scarce ventilator. It would be unethical to deny entry to a patient whose life could be saved by a ventilator in order to take care of a brain-dead cadaver donor. It is essential that ICU staff be sensitized to the fact that cadaver organs would go towards saving the lives of more than one person. They should be made to feel that they are an important link in the chain of transplantation, and should be brought into the mainstream by highlighting their role in the publicity that is normally cornered by the transplant surgeons and nephrologists.

Mobilizing public opinion is fundamental to the success of a national cadaver transplant program. The attitudes, values and behavior of the public are influenced by many factors. A low literacy level impedes understanding of information about the success, implications and need for organ donation. Heterogeneity in language and the dispersion of population over vast rural hinterlands make educational campaigns and transmission of accurate information on transplantation extremely difficult.

It needs to be emphasized that even though India has gained notoriety as the cradle of paid transplants, commercialization in transplantation is not solely an Indian phenomenon. Reports indicate that at various times it has been practiced in South America, the Philippines, Egypt, Iran, Iraq and Turkey, with active involvement of professionals from affluent European, Middle Eastern and other Asian countries (Abouna *et al.*, 1991; Daar, 1992; Chugh and Jha, 1996, 2000; news.yahoo.com 1999).

The debate on the place of payment in transplantation will certainly go on until poverty, the cause that gives rise to such a situation, is eradicated. The balance of access and distribution puts the rich always at the receiving end and the poor at the giving one. This can be considered analogous to the rich being able to buy their way out of a national duty, or to get a job for a consideration, to the detriment of an equally deserving person from a socially disadvantaged group. It is our argument that there should be only one set of ethical principles throughout the world. Relaxation of moral standards in any country opens the door to the slippery slope of corruption, exploitation and degradation.

References

Abouna, G. M., Sabawi, M. M., Kumar, M. S. A., and Samham, M. (1991). The negative impact of paid organ donation. In (eds Land, W., and Dossetor, J. B.) *Organ replacement therapy: Ethics, justice, commerce*, pp. 164–72. Springer-Verlag, Berlin.

Altshuler, J. S., and Evanisko, M. J. (1992). Financial incentives for organ donation: the perspectives of health care professionals. *Journal of the American Medical Association*, **267**, 2037–8.

Bhalla, V. P., Gupta, S., and Nundy, S. (1993). Public funding of organ transplantation: Is it justifiable? In (eds Kapoor, V. K., Ghosh, P. K., Bhandari, M., and Agarwal, S. S.) *Perspectives on organ transplantation*, pp. 53–7. Churchill Livingstone, New Delhi.

Broumand, B. (1997). Living donors: The Iran experience. *Nephrology, Dialysis, Transplantation*, 1830–1.

Chugh, K. S., and Jha, V. (1995). Differences in the care of ESRD patients worldwide: Required resources and future outlook. *Kidney International*, **48** (suppl 50), S7–S13.

Chugh, K. S., and Jha, V. (1996). Commerce in transplantation in third world countries. *Kidney International*, **49**, 1181–6.

Chugh, K. S., and Jha, V. (2000). Problems and outcomes of living unrelated donor transplants in the developing countries. *Kidney International* **57** (suppl 74), 131–5.

Cote-Freeman, S. and Pope, J. (Eds.) The coalition against corruption, Fifth annual report. Transparency International, Berlin, 1999.

Daar, A. S. (1992). Nonrelated donors and commercialism: A historical perspective. *Transplantation Proceedings*, **24**, 2087–9.

Dossetor, J. B. (1992). Rewarded gifting: Is it ever ethically acceptable? *Transplantation Proceedings*, **24**, 2092–4.

Dossetor, J. B., and Manickavel, V. (1991). Ethics in organ donation: Contrast in two cultures. *Transplantation Proceedings*, **23**, 2508–11.

Engelhardt, H. T. Jr. (1991). Is there a universal system of ethics or are the ethics culture-specific? In (eds Land. W., and Dossetor, J. B.) *Organ replacement therapy: Ethics, justice, commerce*, pp. 147–53. Springer-Verlag, Berlin.

http://www.ebay.com: Kidney–Fully functional kidney for sale (Item#153213006). 26 August 1999.

http://news.bbc.co.uk/hi/english/world/middle_east/newsid_581000/581258.stm: Iranians offer kidneys for Rushdie's head. 1999.

http://news.yahoo.com. Philippines to stop commercial sale of kidneys. 3 September 1999.

Mani, M. K. (1998). The management of end-stage renal disease in India. *Artificial Organs*, **22**, 182–6.

Quah, S. R. (1992). Social and ethical aspects of organ transplantation. *Transplantation Proceedings*, **24**, 2097–8.

Radcliffe-Richards, J. (1991). From him that hath not. In (eds Land, W., and Dossetor, J. B.) *Organ replacement therapy: Ethics, justice, commerce*, pp. 191–6. Springer-Verlag, Berlin.

Radcliffe-Richards, J., Daar, A. S., Guttmann, R. D., Hoffenberg, R., Kennedy, I., Lock, M., Sells, R. A., and Tilney, N., for the International Forum for Transplant Ethics (1998). The case for allowing kidney sales. *Lancet*, **351**, 1950–2

Sells, R. A. (1992). Toward an affordable ethic. *Transplantation Proceedings*, **24**, 2095–6

Sheil, A. G. R. (1995). Ethics in organ transplantation. *Transplantation Proceedings*, **27**, 87–9.

Shreiber, H-L. (1991). Legal implications of the principle *Primum nihil nocere* as it applies to live donors. In (eds Land, W., and Dossetor, J. B.) *Organ replacement therapy: Ethics, justice, commerce*, pp. 13–17. Springer-Verlag, Berlin.

Thiagarajan, C. M., Reddy, K. C., Shunmugasundaram, D., Jayachandran, R., Nayar, P., Thomas, S., and Ramachandran, V. (1990). The practice of unconventional renal transplantation (UCRT) at a single center in India. *Transplantation Proceedings*, **22**, 912–4.

17
Africa
Sarala Naicker

Africa is a vast and diverse continent comprising 53 countries and approximately 760 million people. It extends over 30 million km^2 and is home to people of different ethnic origins, religions and languages. Continuing global population growth and rapid urbanization has forced many millions of city dwellers to live in overcrowded and unhygienic conditions, where lack of clean water and inadequate sanitation foster breeding grounds for infectious diseases. Migration and the mass movement of millions of refugees or displaced persons from one country to another, as a result of wars and civil turmoil, have added to the problems of overcrowding and poverty.

Relationship between wealth and healthcare

Countries are classified into low, middle and high income groups according to World Bank criteria (World Development Report, 1993); the main criterion being gross national product (GNP) per capita per year in US dollars. Low income is $635 or less, high income $7911 or more. The richest 20% enjoys 82.7% of world income, with the poorest 60% of the world's population earning 5.6% of world income (Abbasi, 1999).

Ever-increasing debt is the main explanation for the widening gap between the wealthiest and poorest countries; the 40 heavily indebted poor countries owe more than twice what they earn in a year from exports. Africa spends twice as much repaying debt as it does on health care. There is an inverse correlation between a country's GNP and its infant mortality rate, being 8.5 per 1000 live births in the industrialized world, 90.6 in the developing world and 155.5 in the least developed nations. Life expectancy correlated with GNP, with the average life expectancy of 52 years in sub-Saharan Africa and 76 years in established market economies (Europe and USA).

Per capita expenditure per year on health care ranges from 9 US dollars (Nigeria), 29 US dollars (Senegal), and 100 US dollars (North Africa) to 158 US dollars (South Africa); health care expenditure in Europe is approximately 2000 US dollars. Population per doctor ranges between 5000 and 15000, with one doctor per 60000 people in Ethiopia and Equatorial Guinea.

Health problems in the developing world

The World Health Report (1997a) outlines the causes of death in the developing and developed world. Infectious diseases are the world's leading cause of death (43% of all deaths in the developing world compared with 1.2% in the developed world), with 4.4 million deaths due to acute respiratory infections, 3.1 million due to diarrhoeal disease, 3.1 million due to tuberculosis and 2.1 million due to malaria. HIV/AIDS-related deaths are in excess of 1 million. About half the world's population is at risk of many endemic diseases. Diseases that had seemed to be controlled such as tuberculosis and malaria have become a major health problem, with problems of resistance to therapy. New diseases, such as AIDS, have reached epidemic proportions especially in sub-Saharan Africa. The outlook for many individuals in the developing world is that if they manage to survive the killer infections of infancy, childhood and maturity, they will become exposed in later life to non-communicable diseases.

Increasingly, health is influenced by social and economic circumstances. Any improvements in health thus demand integrated, comprehensive action against all the determinants of ill-health.

Major health problems in Africa

A questionnaire sent by the author to colleagues in the various regions of Africa revealed that the major health problems in Africa are AIDS, tuberculosis, malaria, gastroenteritis and hypertension. This emphasizes again the problem of infections in Africa. Hypertension affects about 20% of the adult population, an estimated 691 million people worldwide. It is one of the major risk factors for heart disease, stroke and kidney failure. Strokes and other cerebrovascular diseases are the second most common worldwide cause of death, accounting for 4.6 million deaths worldwide (of which two-thirds are in developing countries).

Diabetes mellitus may present one of the most daunting challenges in the future. The number of persons with diabetes in Africa is currently estimated to be about 135 million; this number is expected to rise to about 300 million by the year 2025. While the increase in cases will exceed 40% in developed countries, it is anticipated to be in the order of 170% in developing countries (World Health Report, 1997b).

Patterns of renal disease

There is a wide variation in the patterns of renal disease in different geographical areas. Accurate and comprehensive statistics are lacking. Glomerulonephritis in South Africa is characterized by a high frequency in blacks, a lesser frequency in Indians and a lower frequency in whites. There is a greater frequency of nephrotic syndrome, when compared with the temperate regions of the world: in Zimbabwe accounting for 0.5% of all hospital admissions; in Kwa Zulu Natal, South Africa 0.2%; 2% in Uganda and 2.4% in Nigeria (Seedat, 1996). It appears that the milieu of chronic parasitic, bacterial and viral infections predisposes to an increased prevalence of glomerulonephritis.

North Africa

The principal causes of renal disease in North Africa (comprising Morocco, Algeria, Tunisia, Libya and Egypt) are glomerulonephritis (18–24%), interstitial nephritis

(14–32%), diabetes mellitus (5–20%) and nephrosclerosis (5–18%) (Barsoum, 1998). Proliferative glomerulonephritis is the most prominent of these diseases, probably reflecting the environment of bacterial and parasitic infections. IgA nephropathy is rare, constituting 0.2–3.8% of renal biopsies. Childhood nephrotic syndrome is characterized by a high frequency of steroid resistance and histologically by focal and segmental glomerulosclerosis (23–34%) and proliferative glomerulonephritis (10–32%) (Barsoum, 1998).

Schistosomiasis

This parasitic disease is prevalent in Africa and is responsible for considerable morbidity in the northwest, where both *S. haematobium* and *S. mansoni* species may cause renal disease. *S. haematobium* infections are responsible for about 20% of renal failure in the Egyptian dialysis population. This differs from the situation in southern Africa where *S. haematobium* is endemic in the east but is an infrequent cause of renal failure. *S. mansoni*-associated glomerulopathy is responsible for about 10% of renal failure in the Egyptian dialysis population (Barsoum, 1998).

Amyloidosis

The prevalence of amyloidosis varies between 4 and 9% among patients attending renal clinics in North Africa. The aetiology is tuberculosis (10% in Egypt; 40% in Algeria and Tunisia), familial Mediterranean fever (11.6–30%), schistosomiasis (15% in Egypt) and hydatid disease (3% of cases in Tunisia). Chronic suppuration is the major cause of renal amyloidosis (Barsoum, 1998).

Sickle cell anaemia

Sickle cell anaemia is endemic in Africa with a prevalence of 8–10% in the northern regions. Sickle anaemia has been reported to be responsible for up to 20% of mesangiocapillary glomerulonephritis in Tunisia.

Post-infectious glomerulonephritis

Streptococcal pharyngitis and skin infections still frequently cause post-infectious glomerulonephritis. Chronic salmonellosis (complicating schistosomiasis) is associated with glomerular and interstitial lesions. Hepatitis B viral infections present with membranous nephrotic syndrome in children in southern and western Africa (Seggie *et al.*, 1984) while in adults it tends to be a more proliferative lesion. Hepatitis C virus infection may be implicated in the pathogenesis of type 1 mesangiocapillary glomerulonephritis in Egypt.

South Africa

The pattern of renal disease in South Africa has been reviewed recently (Naicker, 1998). Several authors have described the pattern of glomerulonephritis. In a 6-year study of 252 blacks and 75 Indians with primary glomerulonephritis in Durban, 35.7% of black adults had mesangiocapillary glomerulonephritis, 21.4% had membranous nephritis and 10.7% had minimal change disease. The histology in Indians was that of mesangiocapillary glomerulonephritis in 13.3%, membranous in 21.3% and minimal change disease in 21.3% (Seedat et al., 1988). This study revealed a 0.8% prevalence of IgA nephropathy in blacks compared with 13.3% in Indians. This low prevalence of IgA nephropathy in blacks was confirmed in the Western Cape in a 7-year study of 872 renal biopsies where IgA nephropathy occurred in 34 (3.8%) of all biopsies: 15 (44.1%) were white, 18 (52.9%) in mixed race groups, 1 (2.9%) Indian, and none were black (Swanepoel et al., 1989). The low prevalence of minimal change disease in blacks was confirmed in a study of 74 black and 56 Indian children with nephrotic syndrome (Coovadia et al., 1979): minimal change disease occurred in 13.5% of black children and 75% of Indian children; membranous nephropathy occurred in 29.8% of black and 3.6% of Indian children. In another study, membranous nephropathy occurred in 16.2% of 388 children (Wiggelinkhuizen and Sinclair-Smith, 1987), of whom 51.9% were black and 20.9% were mixed race, and hepatitis B virus was identified in 73% of these patients, in a population group where the hepatitis B carrier rate is 10%.

Prevalence data for HIV-associated nephropathy are not available for South Africa or Africa in general. In a renal biopsy study of 21 black HIV-positive patients at Baragwanath hospital in Johannesburg, HIV-associated nephropathy was present in 62% (Pantanowitz et al., 1999). HIV surveillance studies at King Edward VIII hospital in Durban for 1 day in February 1995 showed that 19% of all admissions were HIV related; 30.8% of deaths were HIV related; in 1999, 30% of women attending the antenatal clinic were HIV positive.

East Africa

It is estimated that 2–3% of medical admissions in tropical countries are due to renal-related complaints, the majority being the glomerulonephritides which, in East and Central Africa, are characterized by poor response to treatment and progression to renal failure. Renal disease, especially glomerular disease, is more prevalent in Africa and seems to be of a more severe form than that found in Western countries (Kibukamusoke, 1968; Nseka and Tshiani, 1989). The commonest mode of presentation is the nephrotic syndrome, with the age of onset at 5–8 years. Various infective agents are implicated in the aetiology, including *Plasmodium malariae*, schistosomiasis, hepatitis B virus, streptococcal infections, syphilis, leprosy, filariasis and hydatid disease (McLigeyo, 1990). Genitourinary tuberculosis has been reported to represent 0.43% of all urological admissions in Nairobi (Otieno, 1983).

Acute renal failure

Major causes of acute renal failure are malaria, gastroenteritis, AIDS, infections and traditional medicines in large parts of Africa. The unavailability of medical help in many areas, the vast distances involved and lack of transport may cause delays in receiving treatment. Training in the basic principles of prevention, diagnosis and initial therapy needs to be implemented. Acute renal failure constituted 5% of central hospital admissions in Zimbabwe in 1996 (Ndhlovu, personal communication). Herbal remedies accounted for 10.9% of all cases of acute renal failure in East Africa (Adu and Kibukamusoke, 1984; Otieno *et al.*, 1991). Local beliefs, especially in rural areas, attribute symptoms of disease to evil spirits. This results in a tendency to avoid seeking medical aid and to resort to traditional healers and witch-doctors at the outset.

Chronic renal failure

Several studies have demonstrated the high incidence of chronic renal disease among black Americans (Easterling, 1977; Mausner *et al.*, 1978; Rostand *et al.*, 1982). Unfortunately, there are no reliable statistics in all African countries. However, there is a general impression that it is at least 3–4 times more frequent than in more developed countries; this is substantiated by analysis of the causes of death, reporting that uraemia accounts for 1–1.5% of total annual deaths among Egyptians, both in the predialysis era and for two decades thereafter (Barsoum *et al.*, 1974). These figures are comparable with those of other countries in the region with similar socio-economic standards (Abdulla, 1979; Abdullah, 1981). Therefore, calculations suggest that death from renal disease must be in the range of 200 per million of the general population (Barsoum, 1992). The reported annual new patient load ranges between 34 and 200 per million population for North Africa (Barsoum, 1998).

Statistics of the South African Dialysis and Transplant Registry (SADTR) reflect the patients selected for renal replacement therapy and do not accurately reflect the aetiology of chronic renal failure, as few patients with diabetic end-stage renal disease are offered dialysis or transplantation because of associated co-morbid conditions. In 1994, glomerulonephritis was recorded as the cause of ESRD in 1771 (52.1%) of patients and hypertension in 1549 (45.6%) of patients by the SADTR (du Toit *et al.*, 1994). In a study of 394 patients from 1974 to 1981 in Natal, hypertension was reported as the cause of ESRD in 32% of blacks, 24% of Indians and 29% of mixed race patients; glomerulonephritis in 25% blacks, white and Indians and 33% of mixed race patients; analgesic nephropathy occurred predominantly in whites, causing ESRD in 33% (Seedat *et al.*, 1984). In contrast, a study of ESRD in Johannesburg showed that glomerulonephritis occurred in 32%, analgesic nephropathy in 21% and hypertension in 2% (Meyers *et al.*, 1983). In a 6-year study of 3632 patients with ESRD, based on SADTR statistics, hypertension was reported to be the cause of ESRD in 4.3% of whites, 34.6% of blacks, 20.9% mixed race group and 13.8% of Indians, with 15.9% of essential hypertensives resulting in ESRD and 57% of these undergoing malignant change (Veriawa *et al.*, 1990).

Hypertension is common in the urban black population in Africa (Mabayoje *et al.*, 1992). Prevalence studies in the adult population of Natal showed that hypertension was present in 25% of urban Zulus, 17.2% of whites and 14% of Indians (Seedat, 1983). Malignant hypertension is an important cause of morbidity and mortality among urban black South Africans, with hypertension accounting for 16% of all hospital admissions.

In a 10-year study of 368 patients with chronic renal failure in Nigeria, the aetiology of renal failure was undetermined in 62%. Of the remaining patients whose aetiology was ascertained, hypertension accounted for 61%, diabetes mellitus for 11% and chronic glomerulonephritis for 5.9% (Mabayoje et al., 1992). Patients with chronic renal failure constituted 10% of all medical admissions in this centre. Chronic glomerulonephritis and hypertension are principal causes of chronic renal failure in tropical Africa (Nseka and Tshiani, 1989) and East Africa (together with diabetes mellitus and obstructive uropathy) (McLigeyo and Kayima, 1993).

Renal replacement therapy in Africa

The availability of dialysis and transplantation is very variable in Africa. Table 17.1 shows treatment rates of 30–186.5 per million population (pmp) in countries with more established programmes. Services are still predominantly urban and therefore generally inaccessible to the poorer, less-educated rural patient.

South Africa

Situated on the southern tip of Africa, with a surface area of approximately 1.2 million km^2, South Africa's population is 76.2% black, 13.3% white, 8.6% 'mixed' and 2.6% Asian origin. Most urban black localities have a poor infrastructure of services and, with rapid urban migration, there has been a proliferation of shanty towns and squatter camps. The rural black population has poor access to public services.

Since 1994, major constitutional changes have occurred; inequalities in the health structure are being addressed with an emphasis on primary health care and free treatment for children under 6 years and pregnant women.

The South African Dialysis and Transplant Registry report of 1994 showed that 3399 patients (99 pmp) were alive on treatment for end-stage renal failure, with 754 new patients having commenced therapy in 1994, hospital haemodialysis in 1051 patients (30%), home haemodialysis in 26 patients, continuous ambulatory peritoneal dialysis in 448 patients, and intermittent peritoneal dialysis in 13 patients. Two hundred and ninety-nine transplants were performed in 1994, 253 from cadaver donors, 35 from living-related donors and 11 from unrelated donors, with a total of 1578 functioning grafts at year end; the transplant rate was 8.7 pmp. The bulk of cadaver donors are from the white and mixed race groups (21.9% of the population); following

Table 17.1 Renal replacement therapy in Africa (1993–1996)

Country	Population (millions)	GNP per capita[a] (US dollars)	Dialysis (pmp)[b]
Algeria	28.0	2170	78.5
Egypt	60.0	1000	129.3
Libya	5.1	1800	30.0
Morocco	27.0	1010	55.6
Tunisia	8.7	1260	186.5
South Africa	34.4	2560	99.0

[a] GNP: gross national product
[b] pmp: per million population

intensive public and media campaigns cadaver donors are very slowly being retrieved from the black and Indian groups. The Indian group in South Africa, which is divided into Moslems, Hindus and Christians, has been reluctant to donate cadaver organs because of religious and cultural reasons. The black group has had many problems with organ donation: many potential donors were unidentified because of the previous migrant labour system; the elders in the family (who are in distant rural areas) had to be consulted before consent could be given. A survey conducted between 1987 and 1990 showed that over 70% of blacks and whites would be prepared to donate their own organs or those of a close relative (Pike et al., 1992).

The 28 renal facilities are situated in the larger towns and cities, with eight units offering both dialysis and transplantation. The majority of renal units are in the public sector and are funded by government; the private dialysis units are re-imbursed by medical insurance or patients' private funds. Because of financial constraints, the National Health Department, in consultation with nephrologists, has formalized a protocol for the management of ESRD: state facilities will offer renal replacement therapy only to patients who are eligible for a transplant. There are no constraints of sex, race or social status; dialysis is offered to transplantable patients who are able to attend for treatment. This process was tested in the Supreme and the Constitutional Courts by a patient with diabetic ESRD with ischaemic heart disease and cerebrovascular disease (*Soobramoney* v *Minister of Health KwaZulu Natal*, Constitutional Court, 1997). The legal view was that, in the context of budgetary constraints and many competing priorities, the state was justified in limiting treatment to those who are likely to derive the most benefit over the long term. Respect for human rights calls for the provision of essential health services to all (within the limits of available resources).

With the low transplant rate in South Africa, haemodialysis units are saturated and it is becoming difficult to accommodate new patients unless they have a related donor or are able to undertake continuous ambulatory peritoneal dialysis; peritonitis and the high costs of peritoneal dialysis fluids also limit this option.

North Africa

Table 17.1 shows the number of patients per million on dialysis in North Africa ranging from 30 pmp (Libya) to 186.5 pmp (Tunisia). The majority of patients are treated by hospital haemodialysis; continuous ambulatory peritoneal dialysis is gradually being implemented in Tunisia. The majority of the patients in Egypt are dialyzed in state-owned units funded by government; about a third of patients are treated in private dialysis clinics, which are partly funded by government. The bulk of the cost of dialysis is met by these patients themselves (either from income, medical insurance or funds raised by non-governmental organizations). Renal transplantation is limited by the lack of cadaver transplants, hence the large number of living-unrelated transplants in Egypt, with over 3000 unrelated transplants over the decade from 1980 to 1990. Living-unrelated transplants have been banned in Egypt since 1992 (Barsoum, 1998). In Tunisia, 73% of renal transplants are from related donors and 26% from cadaver donors, with a transplant rate of 4.3 pmp (Ben Abdallah, 1999, unpublished data).

Rest of Africa

Dialysis and transplant programmes in the rest of Africa are dependent on the availability of funding and donors.

- Namibia: currently, there are two patients on haemodialysis, five on CAPD and 20 transplant recipients, who are funded privately (Oosthuizen, personal communication).
- Zimbabwe: there are 59 patients on haemodialysis, 38 CAPD patients and four transplant recipients. Funding is primarily from private sources or medical insurance (Ndhlovu, personal communication).
- Botswana: has four patients on CAPD and three transplant recipients, all funded privately (Assounga, personal communication).
- Sudan: has 180–200 patients on haemodialysis, 150 patients on intermittent peritoneal dialysis and 300 transplant recipients. Funding is mainly governmental, with some funds from donations from national societies and individuals abroad (Suleiman, personal communication).
- Congo-Brazzaville: has 30 patients on CAPD, two patients on haemodialysis and six transplant recipients (Assounga, personal communication).
- Kenya: haemodialysis and CAPD are practised in Kenya in both governmental and private facilities; there are 80 patients on haemodialysis, 20 on CAPD and a variable number on intermittent peritoneal dialysis. Living-related donors are the main source of transplants and approximately two transplants are undertaken weekly (Were, personal communication).
- Tanzania: has intermittent haemodialysis for patients with acute renal failure or chronic patients being prepared for kidney transplants abroad. There is no peritoneal dialysis in Tanzania.
- Nigeria: offers haemodialysis, CAPD and intermittent peritoneal dialysis depending on availability of funds. Patients were previously referred to Europe for renal transplantation, which is currently being established in Nigeria.
- Cameroon: offers all modalities of dialytic support to limited numbers of patients, depending on funding.
- Cote d'Ivoire: has a few haemodialysis and renal transplant patients, with the patients being transplanted in other countries.
- Ethiopia: has haemodialysis and peritoneal dialysis facilities for acute renal failure.

The dilemma of renal replacement therapy in Africa

Poverty and the high cost of dialysis and organ transplantation raise many ethical issues: in spite of legal measures and a strict code of conduct for the medical profession, attempts to be equitable have been unsuccessful in many countries. The chances of rich or influential patients obtaining dialysis and a transplant are much better than those of the poor, hence the proliferation of living unrelated transplants on a commercial basis in some countries. Presently, the trade in organs is forbidden by law in most countries in Africa but rich patients then go to a country abroad that does not have such restrictions and have the transplant there. While this may not be equitable, there is debate regarding the ethical aspects: is it ethical to prevent a person who is able to pay for treatment from receiving it? Is it ethical to prohibit a destitute person from selling a kidney, when the sale of this organ may rescue his family from starvation and illness (Cameron and Hoffenberg, 1999)?

Much controversy occurs over the issue of whether dialysis and transplantation should be available in developing countries. These facilities, together with other 'expensive' treatments such as *in vitro* fertilization and cancer chemotherapy, are available in many countries in Africa. In countries where these therapies are not available, the rich obtain such treatment outside their country of residence. Should health ministries in developing countries continue to defray the exorbitant costs of overseas treatment for a select privileged few while the majority are deprived of basic amenities?

It would be unethical to stop chronic dialysis and transplantation in countries where these programmes are entrenched; it would be justifiable to facilitate equitable access to treatment by formulating guidelines as to who is to receive such treatment. In 'low income' countries, it would be difficult to justify expensive high-technology programmes, when basic requirements such as clean water, housing, education, employment and primary health care should take priority. Middle income countries, having formulated health care priorities, should be able to meet these needs as well as provide chronic dialysis and transplantation. Because health care must be rationed, it should be done fairly within, rather than between types of treatment (Klein, 1995). Reduction in resources should be spread in equal proportions over all categories of high-technology treatment.

It is unlikely that chronic dialysis would be offered to all patients and a selection process would be necessary, resulting in an ethical dilemma as to how to allocate treatment; such a selection process would be justifiable if criteria for treatment are carefully formulated by nephrologists, health administrators, ethicists and community and patient representatives and affords equitable access to treatment (without any bias regarding race, gender or socio-economic status). The goal should be to have a circumscribed chronic dialysis programme, with as short a time on dialysis as possible, and to increase the availability of transplantation (both living related and cadaver). This is my view, as well as that of many South African and African nephrologists. Some nephrologists may feel that it is their duty to defend the rights of all uraemic patients to be dialysed irrespective of available funds or limitations in resources.

Medical education in developing countries should include resource management in the curriculum.

Strategy for treatment of renal failure in Africa

Ideally, every end-stage chronic renal failure patient should have access to dialysis. The reality is that there is not enough money for health care in the developing world, particularly for expensive and chronic treatment such as renal replacement therapy. When dealing with competing priorities, ESRD treatment may be deemed socially unfair by health administrators and other health-care personnel as it consumes a sizable portion of the health budget but benefits only a few hundred patients per million population. Clear criteria are required as to the just and equitable allocation of scarce resources. There is an ethical dilemma when considering how these resources should be allocated; dialysis committees may be needed (as was the case previously in Europe and the USA) to facilitate this process. The Department of National Health in South Africa, in consultation with nephrologists and health administrators, has proposed that patients with end-stage chronic renal failure should only be offered dialysis in a state facility if they are eligible for a kidney transplant, thus excluding patients with serious co-morbid conditions. It has been recommended that potential chronic dialysis patients should be discussed by a dialysis review committee; there should be no bias regarding race, gender, religion, social or financial status. There is consensus in South Africa that dialysis needs to be 'rationed' because of financial constraints, while transplantation would be supported and promoted. Living unrelated transplants may only occur after review by an ethics committee and consent from the Minister of Health. Sale of organs is prohibited by law. The structure of review committees should be such as to include a variety of health-care personnel (nephrology physicians and nurses), social workers, psychologists, medical administrators, patient/community members; access to a hospital or university ethics committee would also assist especially in the event of difficult decisions when excluding patients from dialysis. This should minimize bias and promote equity of access to treatment. This scenario works well in areas of South Africa with an active cadaver transplant programme; in areas where cadaver transplants are few in numbers, dialysis programmes are becoming saturated and the situation may arise soon, where no dialysis may be offered once all available dialysis slots are occupied and the budget for CAPD fully utilized, thus promoting a first-come, first-treated situation for those who qualify for treatment. The wealthy would not be restricted and would be able to receive treatment in the private sector, irrespective of their physical status and co-morbid illnesses.

Proposals to cancel third-world debt repayments should be acted on and these funds rechanneled to social benefits: housing, provision of clean water, education and health. Efforts should be made to optimize therapy of renal disease and renal failure globally and particularly in developing countries. Strategies should be developed to manage conditions such as hypertension and diabetes mellitus at the primary health-care level in an effort to decrease the incidence of chronic renal failure. In areas where there are insufficient numbers of physicians, nurses and other allied health workers could be trained to manage these conditions at a local level, with clearly defined criteria for referral of patients. Patients with renal disease should be referred to a nephrologist at an early stage so as to institute measures to retard progression and plan timely transplantation and/or dialysis; this is particularly important where related donors may be available, as a cost-effective strategy.

All or most countries should be able to offer dialytic support for acute renal failure. Where economically feasible, the next stage would be to develop a transplant programme (utilizing living-related and cadaver donors); this may not be possible in the 'low income' countries. It requires government support, legislation, extensive campaigns to educate the public and medical profession, development of trauma and intensive care units, efficient organ donor retrieval and transplant teams and funding; following this, legislation for presumed consent with a facility for opting out should be implemented. The major religions in Africa are Christianity and Islam, which are supportive of organ donation. The Muslim clergy accepted the concept of brainstem death at conferences in Kuwait in 1985 and Jordan in 1986 but this was later disputed by medical and political groups. The Islamic Organization of Medical Sciences in 1996 approved the recovery of organs from brainstem dead persons (Gabr, 1998). All religions express concern for the welfare of mankind and most religious leaders accept organ transplantation as a means of saving life. Intensive public awareness campaigns are necessary to improve the rate of cadaver transplantation in Africa. Legislation on organ transplantation in developing countries needs to be clear on the criteria for brainstem death, requirements for consent for living and cadaver donors, regulations for institutions and health professionals regarding cadaver and living donation of organs and a registry of potential recipients and donors.

Negotiations should take place between governments and pharmaceutical and dialysis companies to look at the cost-structure of immunosuppressives and dialysis fluids and dialysis membranes so as to make treatment more affordable. Measures to decrease usage of Cyclosporine A by concomitant use of Ketoconazole or withdrawing Cyclosporine use after 6–12 months may be implemented. Chronic dialysis (both haemodialyis and CAPD) should only be available in developing countries if there is an active transplant programme, so that the numbers on dialysis will not rapidly mushroom out of control. National non-governmental organizations may be able to support part of the costs; the National Kidney Foundation of Singapore is an excellent model. Dialysis facilities should be planned regionally and be easily accessible to patients, so that they do not have to travel long distances. CAPD is currently an expensive treatment modality in Africa. Efforts should be made to have the cost of CAPD fluids reduced, so that this treatment could be freely available in Africa. After initial training on CAPD, the patient is not dependent on frequent visits to a dialysis centre. The use of CAPD in conjunction with an active transplant programme is an appealing strategy for Africa.

References

Abbasi, K. (1999). The World Bank and world health. Healthcare strategy. *British Medical Journal, South African Edition*, 7, 376–9.

Abdulla, K. (1979). Chronic renal failure in Northern Iraq. *Iraqi Medical Journal*, 27, 43–6.

Abdullah, M. S. (1981). Development of renal services in Kenya. *East African Medical Journal*, 30, 9–10.

Adu, J., Kibukamusoke, J. W. (1984). Acute renal failure in the tropics. In *Tropical Nephrology*, pp. 199–215. (ed. Kibukamusoke, J. W.) Citforge, Canberra, Australia.

Barsoum, R. S. (1992). Ethical problems in dialysis and transplantation: Africa. In *Ethical problems in dialysis and transplantation*, pp. 169–82. (eds Kjellstrand, C. M., and Dosseter, J. B.), Kluwer Academic, Dordrecht.

Barsoum, R. S. (1998). Renal disease in indigenous populations: North Africa. *Nephrology*, 4, S29–S32.

Barsoum, R. S., Rihan, Z. E., Ibrahim, A. S., and Lebstein, A. (1974). Long term intermittent haemodialysis in Egypt. *Bulletin of World Health Organization*, 51, 647–54.

Cameron, J. S., and Hoffenberg, R. (1999). The ethics of organ transplantation reconsidered:

Paid organ donation and the use of executed prisoners as donors. *Kidney International*, **55**, 724–32.

Combined report on maintenance dialysis and transplantation in the Republic of South Africa (1994). In *South African Dialysis and Transplantation Registry Report.* (eds du Toit, E. D., Pascoe, M., MacGregor, K., and Thomson, P. D.) Cape Town, South Africa.

Coovadia, H. M., Adhikari, M., and Morel-Maroger, L. (1979). Clinico-pathological features of the nephrotic syndrome in South African children. *Quarterly Journal of Medicine*, **48**, 77–91.

Easterling, R. E., (1977). Racial factors in the evidence and causation of end stage renal disease. *Transactions of the American Society Artificial Internal Organs*, **23**, 28–33.

Gabr, M. (1998). Organ transplantation in developing countries. *World Health Forum*, **19**, 120–3.

Kibukamusoke, J. W. (1968). Kidney disease in the tropics. *East African Medical Journal*, **45**, 632–7.

Klein, R. (1995). Priorities and rationing: pragmatism or principles? *British Medical Journal*, **311**, 761–2.

Mabayoje, M. O., Bamgboye, E. L., Odutola, T. A., and Mabadeje, A. F. B. (1992). Chronic renal failure at the Lagos University Teaching Hospital: a 10 year review. *Transplantation Proceedings*, **24**, 1851–2.

Mausner, J. S., Clark, J. K., Coles, B. I., and Menduke, H. (1978). An areawide survey of treated end stage renal disease. *American Journal of Public Health*, **68**, 166–9.

McLigeyo, S. O. (1990). Nephrotic syndrome in the tropics (editorial). *East African Medical Journal*, **67**, 377–80

McLigeyo, S. O., and Kayima, J. K. (1993). Evolution of nephrology in East Africa in the last seventy years–studies and practice. *East African Medical Journal*, **70**, 362–8.

Meyers, A. M., Furman, K. I., Botha, J. R., Milne, F. J., Thomson, P. D., Louridas, G., *et al.* (1983). The treatment of end stage renal disease at the Johannesburg Hospital: a 17 year experience. Part 1. The role of dialysis. *South African Medical Journal*, **64**, 515–21.

Naicker, S. (1998). Patterns of renal disease in South Africa. *Nephrology*, **4**, S21–S24.

Nseka, M., and Tshiani, K. A. (1989). Chronic renal failure in tropical Africa. *East African Medical Journal*, **66**, 109–14.

Otieno, L. S. (1983). Genitourinary tuberculosis at Kenyatta National Hospital (1973–1980). *East African Medical Journal*, **60**, 232–7.

Otieno, L. S., McLigeyo, S. O., and Luta, M. (1991). Acute renal failure following use of herbal remedies. *East African Medical Journal*, **68**, 993–8.

Pantanowitz, L., Goetach, S., Butler, O., Katz, I. J. (1999). Renal biopsies of HIV positive patients at Baragwanath hospital 1989–1997. Abstracts of African Congress of Nephrology, Durban. *Kidney International*, **55**, 2130.

Pike, R. E., Odell, J. A., and Kahn, D. (1992). Public attitudes to organ donation in South Africa. *Transplantation Proceedings*, **24**, 2102.

Rostand, S. G., Kirk, K. A., Rutsky, E., and Pate, B. A. (1982). Racial differences in the incidence and treatment of end stage renal disease. *New England Journal of Medicine*, **306**, 1276–9.

Seedat, Y. K. (1983). Race, environment and blood pressure: the South African experience. *Journal of Hypertension*, **1**, 7–12.

Seedat, Y. K., Naicker, S., Rawat, R., and Parsoo, I. (1984). Racial differences in the causes of end stage renal failure in Natal. *South African Medical Journal*, **65**, 956–8.

Seedat, Y. K., Nathoo, B. C., Parag, K. B., Naiker, I. P., and Ramsaroop, R. (1988). IgA nephropathy in Blacks and Indians of Natal. *Nephron*, **50**, 137–41.

Seedat, Y. K. (1996). Ethnicity, hypertension, coronary heart disease and renal diseases in South Africa. *Ethnicity & Health*, **1**: 349–57.

Seggie, J., Nathoo, K., and Davies, P. G. (1984). Association of hepatitis B (HB_S) antigenaemia and membranous glomerulonephritis in Zimbabwean children. *Nephron*, **38**, 115–9.

Swanepoel, C. R., Madaus, S., Cassidy, M. J. D., Temple-Camp, C., Van Diggelen, N. T., Pascoe, M. D., *et al.* (1989). IgA nephropathy: Groote Schuur Hospital experience. *Nephron*, **53**, 61–4.

Veriawa, Y., du Toit, E., Lawley, C. G., Milne, F. J., and Reinach, S. G. (1990). Hypertension as a cause of end stage renal failure in South Africa. *Journal of Hypertension*, **4**, 379–83.

Wiggelinkhuizen, J., and Sinclair-Smith, C. (1987). Membranous glomerulonephropathy in childhood. *South African Medical Journal*, **72**, 184–7.

World Development Report (1993). *Investing in Health. World Development Indicators*. World Bank, New York, University Press.

The World Health Report (1997a). Fighting disease, fostering development. *World Health Forum*, **18**, 1–8.

The World Health Report (1997b). Conquering suffering, enriching humanity. *World Health Forum*, **18**, 248–60.

INDEX

abortion 65
Abram, H. 11
absolutism 35–6
abusive patients 91, 94, 104, 106
academic medicine 218–19
access to health care 214–15
action guides 32
adolescents, compliance issues 189
advance care planning 117–19
advance directives 49–50, 117–19, 226, 228–9
affirmative defense 40
Africa 255–67
   diabetes 256
   hypertension 256, 259
   religion 265
   renal disease 256–8
   renal failure 258–60
   renal replacement therapy 260–5
aged patients 88–9, 99–100, 203, 205–6
   overtreatment 224
Aid to Capacity Evaluation 116
AIDS 101
Akebia quinata 235
Alexander, S. 6, 26
allocation
   defined 85
   macro-/micro-allocation 13–14
   organs 73–5, 150–1, 154–63
   resources 13–14, 20, 21, 151, 201–11, 264
Alport syndrome 168, 169, 170, 193
altruism 132
American Society of Nephrology 7–8
amyloidosis 257
anencephaly 139, 191
animal rights 151–2
authority rules 32
autonomy 31, 123

Bard, S. 25
Bartter's syndrome 169
Belmont Report 27, 31
beneficence 31
bioethics 27, 31–2
Bland, A. 70
Botswana 262
brain death 40, 225, 239, 265
Brody, B. 36
Buddhism 224, 236

Cabot, R. 25
cadaveric organs 12, 70–2, 77–8, 140–2, 238, 252–3, 260–1

Cameroon 262
capacity 45–9, 50, 66, 116–17
cardiovascular complications 159–60
case example 37–9
casuistry 33–4, 36
children 183–97
   compliance issues 188–90
   dialysis/transplantation choice 184–6
   infants 186–7
   informed consent 50, 65, 183–4
   living-related donors for 190–1
   as organ donors 190
   prioritizing 191–2
   screening 187–8
   see also genetic disease
China 234–40
   culture 236
   dialysis 236–7
   executed prisoners, organs from 140–2, 238
   family planning 239
   nephrology 234
   religion 236
   socioeconomics 237–8
   traditional medicine 234, 235
   transplantation 237–8
clinical ethics, defined 25
clinical guidelines 18–19, 55–6, 217
cloning 78
codes of conduct 36
coercion 116
commercial interests 215–18, *see also* selling organs
common sense 36
communitarian perspective 35
comorbidity 100–2
compassion 54, 105
compliance 91–5, 104–6, 188–90
Confucianism 224, 236
Congo–Brazzaville 262
consequentialist theory 29
continuous ambulatory peritoneal dialysis 237, 244, 265
contracting in/contracting out 71–2, 135, 161–2, 163–4
coronary artery disease 159–60
cost control 203–8
Cote d'Ivoire 262
counseling 172–3, 177
Cruzan, N. 27
cultural issues 35–6, 123–4, 236
cystinuria 169
cytomegalovirus 160

death
  assisted 43, 68, 226
  brain death 40, 225, 239, 265
  letting die–killing distinction 43
  passive euthanasia 41
decisional capacity 45–9, 50, 66, 116–17
dementia 103–4
deontological theory 29–30
developing countries
  health problems 255–6
  renal replacement therapy controversy 263
diabetes
  in Africa 256
  dialysis 86–7, 101
  transplantation 160
  X-linked nephrogenic diabetes insipidus 169
dialysis
  continuous ambulatory peritoneal 237, 244, 265
  at home 6, 7
  legal issues 65–70
  payment policy 16
  refusal 67–8, 229–30
  units, medical directors 216–17
  withdrawing/withholding 17–18, 19, 69–70, 110, 227–8
disability-adjusted life years (DALYs) 202, 204
disclosure 67, 115
discrimination 13
disease management 56
do-not-resuscitate orders 49, 119–21
donation, *see* organ donation
double agency 40
double effect 40–1
Down s syndrome 89
Dukeminier, J. 11–12

East Africa, renal disease 258
economic approach 36–7
economic issues 36–7, 85–6, 212–20, 244–5, *see also* resource allocation
education 218–19
Egypt 261
elderly 88–9, 99–100, 203, 205–6
  overtreatment 224
embryo wastage 64–5
emergencies 66, 159
end-of-life care 110–29
  conflicts 121–3
  cultural issues 123–4
  family feedback 114
  pain management 114–15
  quality 111–13, 124–5
Epstein Barr virus 161
ethic of care 35
ethical dilemmas 28, 212–20
ethical issues, defined 28
ethical problems
  approaches to 32–9

  defined 28
  resources 55–7
  reviewing 44
ethical theory and principles 24–62
  defined 28, 29
  historical aspects 25–8
  terminology 28
ethics, defined 28
ethics committees 27, 56, 95–6
Ethiopia 262
Eurotransplant Kidney Allocation System 156–7
euthanasia 41, 226
executed prisoners, organs from 140–2, 238
experiment–therapy debate 7–9
extraordinary–ordinary distinction 42

Fabry s disease 169
family planning 175–8
Fanconi syndrome 169
feminine perspective 35
fixed budgets 206
Fletcher, J. 25
Food and Drugs Administration 4
Freund, P. 10–11
futility 53–4, 69, 90–1, 102–3, 122, 213–14

general physicians 213–14
genetic disease 167–82, 192–4
  counseling 172–3, 177
  family planning 175–8
  family responsibility 178–9
  individual s knowledge of 170–2
  modifying 174–5
  preimplantation diagnosis 176–7
  prenatal diagnosis 64–5, 175–6
  screening 192–3
geographical variability in treatment 85–6
George W. Gay Lecture 10
glomerulonephritis 257–8
God Committee 6, 26
Gottschalk Report 8–9
guidelines 18–19, 55–6, 217

herbal medicine 235
hereditary disease, *see* genetic disease
Hinduism 252
Hippocrates 25, 212
historical perspectives 3–23, 25–8
HIV 258
HLA-matching 155–6
home dialysis 6, 7
hypertension 256, 259

IgA nephropathy 258
India 241–54
  cadaver transplantation 252–3
  dialysis 242, 244
  paid donors 246–7, 248, 250, 253
  related live donors 245

religion 242, 252
  socioeconomics 242, 243
  transplantation 241, 244–53
industrialization 215–18
infants 186–7
infection risks 145–8, 160–1
informed consent 31, 45–6, 67, 115–17, 225–6, 229–30
  pediatrics 50, 65, 183–4
  xenotransplantation 149–50
Institute of Medicine 17–18, 144–53
institutional approach 36
interactive counseling 172–3, 177
Internet resources 57, 171, 177
interpretive ethics 173
intuition 36
Islam 265

Jackson, H.M. 7
Japan 223–33
  advance directives 226, 228–9
  dialysis 226–30
  ethical issues 225–30
  euthanasia 226
  health care system 223–4
  informed consent 225–6, 229–30
  overtreatment of elderly 224
  religion 224
  transplantation 227, 230
Johnson, L.B. 4
justice 31, 161

Kantian deontology 29–30
Kenya 262
Kidney Disease Control Program 9–10
kidneys, *see* organ donation; organs
Kolff, W. 25

Leake, C. 25
legal issues 37, 63–81
Levinsky, N. 7
life expectancy 101
limiting treatment 52–3
live donors
  legal issues 75–7
  related 155, 163, 190–1, 245
  risks 247
  unrelated 136–7, 155, 163, 246, 261

Maimonides 212
manipulation 116
means testing 207–8
media interest 6, 26
mediation 122–3
Medicaid 4
medical directors 216–17
Medicare 3–4, 14–17
mental deficiency 89–90, 104, 230
moral rules 32

moral theories and traditions 28–30
morality 28
morals 28

Namibia 262
National Institutes of Health 5
National Kidney Foundation
  experiment–therapy debate 7
  Honolulu Conference (1976) 16–17
Nigeria 262
non-compliance 91–5, 104–6, 188–90
non-heart beating donors 163
non-maleficence 31
North Africa
  renal disease 256–7
  renal replacement therapy 261
Nuremberg Code 25

opting in/opting out 71–2, 135, 161–2, 163–4
organ donation
  altruistic motive 132
  anencephalic sources 139, 191
  cadaveric 12, 70–2, 77–8, 140–2, 238, 252–3, 260–1
  by children 190
  by executed prisoners 140–2, 238
  family conflicts 12
  live donors
    legal issues 75–7
    related 155, 163, 190–1, 245
    risks 247
    unrelated 136–7, 155, 163, 246, 261
  non-heart beating donors 163
  opting in/opting out 71–2, 135, 161–2, 163–4
  paired kidney exchange 134
  payment for 12, 131–4, 246–7, 248, 249, 250–2, 253
  from persistent vegetative state patients 137–9
Organ Procurement and Transplantation Network 157–8
organs
  allocating 73–5, 150–1, 154–63
  compatibility 155–6
  exchange programmes 156–9
  increasing supply 163–5
  selling 12, 131–4, 246–7, 248, 249, 250–2, 253
Osler, W. 25
overtreatment 86, 224

Page, I. 7
pain management 114–15
paired kidney exchange 134
pancreas–kidney transplantation 160
passive–active distinction 42
paternalism 41, 187
patient selection 6, 8, 11–13, 17–18, 21, 87–8, 99–109
  age 88–9, 99–100, 191–2, 205–6

patient selection (*cont.*):
  committees 6, 26, 264
  comorbidity 100–2
  medical criteria 204–5
  mental status 89–90, 102–4
  signed-up donors 161–2
pediatrics, *see* children
Percival, T. 25
persistent vegetative state
  organs from 137–9
  withdrawing treatment 27, 70, 102–3
philosophical distinctions 42–3
physician
  general/specialist 213–14
  judgment 206–7
pluralistic casuistry 36
polycystic kidney disease 168, 169, 194
Polycystic Research Foundation 171
preimplantation diagnosis 176–7
prenatal diagnosis 64–5, 175–6
press interest 6, 26
prima facie duties 30
principlism 32–3
priority-setting 210
prisoners
  executed, organs from 140–2, 238
  research on 139–40
procedural rules 32
professional codes 36
proportionality 31
prudential reasoning 36
psychosis 89–90
Public Health Service Act 15
Public Law 92–603 (Section 299I) 4, 15

quality-adjusted life years (QALYs) 202, 204
Quinlan, K.A. 27

race 184, 190
rapid cycle change 113
rationing 6–7, 9–11, 19–20, 21, 86–7, 206
  implicit/explicit 214
reflective equilibrium 34
refusing treatment 27–8, 51–2, 53, 66, 67–8,
  229–30
Regional Medical Programs 10
relational approach 35
relativism 35–6
religion 68, 224, 236, 242, 252, 265
renal tubular acidosis (RTA) 169, 170
report cards 113
research
  on animals 151–2
  industrial sponsorship 218
  subjects 27, 139–40
resource allocation 13–14, 20, 21, 151, 201–11,
  264
RPA–ASN guideline 18–19
Rush, B. 25

Sanders, D. 11–12
scarcity 5–7, 10, 20
schistosomiasis 257
Scribner, B. 5, 6–7
Seattle Artificial Kidney Center 6
secondary gain 93
self-determination 31, 123
selling organs 12, 131–4, 246–7, 248, 249, 250–2,
  253
Shintoism 224
sickle cell anaemia 257
Siemsen, A. 16
social attitudes 148–9, 249–52
socioeconomics 237–8, 242, 243, 255
solidarity model 161–2
South Africa
  renal disease 257–8
  renal replacement therapy 260–1, 264
specialist physicians 213–14
substantive rules 32
Sudan 262
suicide 43, 68
SUPPORT 101
surrogate (substitute) decisions 50–1, 116–17, 229
symptom management 114–15

Tanzania 262
teleological theory 29
terminal illness 100–2
therapeutic exception/privilege 41
Tower J. 15
transplantation
  cardiovascular complications 159–60
  children, priority to 191–2
  Coordinators 164
  cost factors 244–5
  diabetes 160
  experiment–therapy debate 8
  infection risks 160–1
  see also organ donation; organs; xenotransplan-
    tation
treatment
  limiting 52–3
  refusing 27–8, 51–2, 53, 66, 67–8, 229–30
  withdrawing/withholding 17–18, 19, 41, 42–3,
    52, 69–70, 110, 227–8
Tripterygium wilfordii 235

Ulysses contract 41–2
undertreatment 86–7
United Kingdom
  rationing 19–20
  resource allocation 20
  Transplant Support Service Authority 158–9
United Network for Organ Sharing 157–8
United States of America, health care
  Medicaid 4
  Medicare 3–4, 14–17
  pre-Medicare 3, 5–14

utility 29, 31

values history 47–9
Veterans Administration 6
virtues approach 34–5
voluntariness 115–16

Wadlington, W. 11
withdrawing/withholding treatment 17–18, 19, 41, 42–3, 52, 69–70, 110, 227–8

xenotransplantation 144–53
  animal rights issues 151–2
  funding 151
  infection risks 145–8
  informed consent 149–50
  organ allocation 150–1
  social issues 148–9

Zimbabwe 262
Zwick, C. 10